Yi-Ping Phoebe Chen (Ed.)

Bioinformatics Technologies

Yi-Ping Phoebe Chen (Ed.)

Bioinformatics Technologies

With 129 Figures and 50 Tables

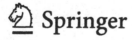 Springer

Yi-Ping Phoebe Chen (Ed.)
School of Information Technology,
Faculty of Science and Technology,
Deakin University, Australia
Email: phoebe@deakin.edu.au

ACM Computing Classification (1998): J.3, I.5, H.3

ISBN 3-642-42202-0 Springer Berlin Heidelberg New York

Springer is a part of Springer Science+Business Media

springeronline.com

© Springer-Verlag Berlin Heidelberg 2005
Softcover re-print of the Hardcover 1st edition 2005

Typesetting: By the author
Cover design: KünkelLopka, Heidelberg
Production: LE-TeX Jelonek, Schmidt & Vöckler GbR, Leipzig
Printed on acid-free paper   45/3142/YL - 5 4 3 2 1 0

Preface

This book arose primarily out of a compelling need for a comprehensive reference in bioinformatics that will cater to students, research, and industry. We strongly believe that this new field evolved from the active interaction of two fast-developing disciplines: biology and information technology. Solving modern biological problems requires advanced computational methods. Key techniques include database management, data modeling, pattern recognition, data mining, query processing, and visualization of biological data. Until very recently, virtually all public databases were based on large flat files stored in simple formats. Navigation among databases required expert knowledge and considerable patience. The huge quantities of biological data and escalating demands of modern biological research increasingly require the sophistication and computing power of information technology (IT) tools. More specifically, optimal use of these tools requires proximal information – knowing which data points are in the surrounding area of others. In this book, we will present methodologies and data structures for arriving at high quality biological information, which can then be used as foundation to develop practical tools for clustering and visualization in biological data mining and database management.

Throughout the book, we will demonstrate the application of well established concepts and techniques of information technology to the management and analysis of biological data. Biological analysis requires the integration of software tools used in data mining, such as clustering, classification, decision trees and decision tables, and sequence and structural modeling such as data modeling. A distinctive feature of our book is the integration of advanced database technologies with visualization techniques such as query-interactive user interfaces, visual descriptions, and advanced 3-D visual modeling.

Biological data continue to grow exponentially in size and complexity. As a result, they introduce new data types not previously seen even in molecular biology. It is vital and urgent that advanced information technologies, in particular, database technologies and visual analysis, be applied to support biological research and innovation based on biological data. Specific IT-motivated activities are taking root in some parts of the biological research community, and we foresee that they will benefit information technology.

"Bioinformatics technologies" is a comprehensive book that covers these two important areas, viz., IT and biology, which have become interwoven in recent years. Many international experts have made contributions to this book. Each article is written in a way that a practitioner of bioinformatics can easily understand and then apply the knowledge gained to extract useful information from biological data. Each article covers one topic, and can be read independently of each other. The book provides both a general survey of the topic and an in-depth exposition of the state-of-the-art. Practitioners will certainly find this book very resourceful and handy when looking for solutions to practical problems in bioinformatics. Researchers can use this book as a source for obtaining background information, current trends and developments; this provides them also with the most important references on these topics.

The book covers the basic principles and applications of bioinformatics technologies. It also contains many articles that specifically address bioinformatics databases and emerging topics in bioinformatics technologies such as patterns discovery, data mining, simulation and visualization. The central issue in bioinformatics is how to transform biological data into meaningful and valuable information. It implies that the biological knowledge related to the problem domain is incorporated into the requirements analysis phase of the bioinformatics.

However, it has been recently recognized that in the twenty-first century bioinformatics will play an increasingly important role. For this reason, the international conference series on Asia-Pacific Bioinformatics (first bioinformatics conference in the IT domain) was founded in 2002. The underlying goal behind this conference series is to recognize the interdisciplinary nature of bioinformatics in the interplay between biology and IT and how information technology can be applied to biology.

Even though a great deal of attention is paid to this area in terms of research and investment, the theoretical understanding needs further refinement to bring the outcome of the biological analysis effectively to the service of mankind. In editing this book, this viewpoint has been carefully taken into consideration to conceptually organize the recent progress in bioinformatics.

The book is organized into twelve chapters that cover twelve important technologies in bioinformatics.

Chapter1, Introduction to Bioinformatics, provides an overview of bioinformatics technology, and different techniques within bioinformatics. Further, it introduces the relationships between the other chapters.

Chapter 2, Overview of Structural Bioinformatics, presents an overview of structural bioinformatics. The chapter describes organization of structural bioinformatics, the Protein Data Bank, secondary resources and applications, and using structural bioinformatics approaches in drug design. It also includes structural classification, structure prediction, functional assignments in structural genomics, protein-protein interactions and protein-ligand interactions. The role of structural bioinformatics in systems biology is also briefly discussed.

Chapter 3, Database Warehousing in Bioinformatics, deals with the basics in database warehousing, transforming biological data into knowledge, data warehouse architectures and data quality in bioinformatics.

Chapter 4, Data Mining for Bioinformatics, discusses the basics of data mining applicable to bioinformatics. The main types of data analysis, namely, biomedical data analysis, DNA data analysis, protein data analysis and microarray data analysis, are elaborated upon. Biomedical data analysis includes a major nucleotide sequence database, a protein sequence database, a gene expression database, and software tools for bioinformatics research. DNA data analysis covers DNA sequence and DNA data analysis. Protein data analysis encompasses protein and amino acid sequence and protein data analysis.

Chapter 5, Machine Learning in Bioinformatics, dwells on the theory behind machine learning applied to bioinformatics. It includes neural network architectures and applications. We also describe other machine learning techniques, such as genetic algorithms and fuzzy systems.

Chapter 6, Systems Biotechnology: a New Paradigm in Biotechnology Development, describes a new paradigm in biotechnology development called system biotechnology. It covers integrative approaches and *in silico* modeling and simulation of cellular processes.

Chapter 7, Computational Modeling of Biological Processes with Petri Net-Based Architecture, describes computational modeling of biological processes with a Petri net-based architecture, a hybrid Petri net and a hybrid dynamic net, and a hybrid functional Petri net. The chapter also covers the implementation of a HFPNe in a genomic object net and the modeling of biological processes with a HFPNe and a genomic object net and its visualizer.

Chapter 8, Biological Sequence Assembly and Alignment, illustrates biological sequence assembly and alignment. It covers large-scale sequence assembly, Euler sequence assembly, PESA sequence assembly, large-scale pairwise sequence alignment, large-scale multiple sequence, alignment, and load balancing and communication overheads.

Chapter 9, Modeling for Bioinformatics, covers the basics of modeling techniques related to bioinformatics. It includes the major modeling techniques, namely, hidden Markov modeling for biological data analysis, comparative modeling and molecular modeling. An elaborate discussion is made to apply hidden Markov modeling on biological data to have sequence identification, sequence classification, and multiple alignment generation. Comparative modeling comprises protein comparative modeling, comparative genomic modeling, and probabilistic modeling. The probabilistic modeling encompasses Bayesian networks, stochastic context-free grammars, and probabilistic Boolean networks. Finally, we describe molecular modeling, which deals with molecular and related visualization applications, molecular mechanics, and modern computer programs used in molecular modeling.

Chapter 10, Pattern Matching for Motifs, addresses the issues in pattern matching for discovering motifs. Topics include gene regulation and promoter organization. We include motif recognition and motif detection strategies. The chapter also includes two different approaches, namely, the single gene multi-species approach and the multi-gene multi-species approach.

Chapter 11, Visualization and Fractal Analysis of Biological Sequences, deals with visualization and fractal analysis of biological sequences. It elaborates on the fractal analysis, the recurrent iterated function system model, the moment method to estimate the parameters of the IFS (RIFS) model, multifractal analysis, the DNA walk model, and chaos game representation of biological sequences. Two-dimensional portrait representation of DNA sequences and one-dimensional measure representations of biological sequences are also introduced.

Chapter 12, Microarray Data Analysis, discusses the techniques used to analyze microarray data and microarray technology used for genome expression study, image analysis for data extraction, and data analysis for pattern discovery.

In a rapidly expanding area such as bioinformatics, no book can claim to cover the topics that suit the interests of everyone. However, it is hoped that this book is comprehensive enough to serve as a useful and handy guide for both practitioners and researchers. This book will help both IT professionals and biologists to understand the bioinformatics world.

We would like to thank all authors who contributed the chapters in this book, without whom the mission would have been impossible. Special thanks to the reviewers for their professional inputs. We thank Ricky Chen and Chinnu Subramaniam for helping us check parts of the manuscript at short notice. We have taken care to cite referenced work. If we have missed any citation, we apologize for the lapse. We thank all researchers for their permission to use their figures in this book. We also wish to thank the Springer publisher Ralf Gerstner for his final step of checking and timely help before publication. Finally, we wish to thank our families and friends for their support.

We are sure that some errors may stay behind in the book. Your input for improvement will be helpful for future reprints and editions. Comments, corrections, and constructive suggestions should be sent to Springer or by electronic mail to phoebe@deakin.edu.au

January 2005   Yi-Ping Phoebe Chen

Contents

1 Introduction to Bioinformatics

Yi-Ping Phoebe Chen [1, 2]

[1] School of Information Technology
Faculty of Science and Technology
Deakin University, 221 Burwood Highway, VIC3125, Australia
[2] Australian Research Council (ARC) Centre in Bioinformatics

1.1 Introduction

This book is an introduction to what has come to be known as Bioinformatics and Bioinformatics Technologies. The material in this book is presented from a non-biologist's perspective, where emphasis is placed on basic concepts of Bioinformatics and technologies used to discover interesting biological data patterns unknown in large datasets. For a biologist, this book will present useful information on technologies that can be applied. Various methods that focus on the development of scalable and efficient bioinformatics technologies tools are discussed. In this chapter, you will learn how Bioinformatics is a part of the natural evolution of database technologies, why data mining, data modeling, machine learning, pattern matching, and visualization are important, and how they are defined. You will also learn about the general architecture of bioinformatics technologies and its applications. Why is it so important to understand biological problems? How can one understand a biological problem? How can one understand biological worlds from the points of view of information technology, computer science, mathematics, and commerce? These questions are briefly answered. Furthermore, various types of biological data are discussed. This book explains the technologies that can be used for analysis, the nature of biological knowledge that can be found, and the bioinformatics tools that can be applied. Finally, challenging research issues for building bioinformatics technologies, tools, and applications of the future are also discussed.

1.2 Needs of Bioinformatics Technologies

What is bioinformatics? Why is bioinformatics important? Bioinformatics has attracted a great deal of attention from various disciplines, such as information technology, mathematics, and non-traditional biological sciences in recent years. This is due to the availability of enormous amounts of public and private biological data and the compelling need to transform biological data into useful information and knowledge. Understanding the correlations, structures, and patterns in biological data are the most important tasks in bioinformatics. The information and knowledge from these disciplines can then be wisely used for applications that cover drug discovery, genome analysis and biological control.

Bioinformatics can therefore be considered to be the combination of several scientific disciplines that include biology, biochemistry, mathematics, and computer science. It involves the use of computer technologies and statistical methods to manage and analyze a huge volume of biological data about DNA, RNA, and protein sequences, protein structures, gene expression profiles, and protein interactions.

Specifically, bioinformatics encompasses the development of databases to store and retrieve biological data, of algorithms and statistics to analyze and determine relationships in biological data, and of statistical tools to identify, interpret, and mine datasets. Figure 1.1 illustrates the underlying definition of bioinformatics (Baxevanis and Ouellette, 2001; Kuonen, 2003; Baldi and Brunak, 2001; and Westhead et al., 2002).

The field of bioinformatics plays an increasing role in the study of fundamental biological problems owing to the exponential explosion of sequence and structural information with time (Ohno-Machado et al., 2002). Figure 1.2 shows the exponential growth of GenBank.

As an example, the number of entries in a database of gene sequences in GenBank has increased from 1,765,847 to 22,318,883 in the last five years. These entries tend to double every 15 months (Benson et al., 2002).

There are two major challenging areas in bioinformatics: (1) data management and (2) knowledge discovery.

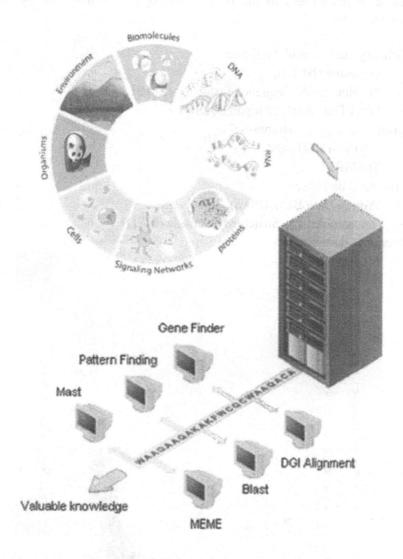

Fig. 1.1. A illustration of a bioinformatics paradigm (adapted from
http://www.bioteach.ubc.ca/Bioinformatics/whatisbioinform/)

With the emergence of high-throughput technologies such as whole genome sequencing and DNA microarrays, large volumes of data are generated. The efficient management of this biological data is desirable.

A challenge to data management involves managing and integrating
the existing biological databases. There are several types of databases

available to researchers in the field of biology. The most widely used among them are

- primary nucleic acid databases
  - GenBank (NCBI),
  - the Nucleotide Sequence Database (EMBL), and
  - DNA Data Bank of Japan (DDBJ)
- protein sequences databases
  - SWISS-PROT, and
  - TrEMBL
- structural databases
  - Protein Data Bank (PDB), and
  - Macromolecular Structure Database (MSD)
- literature databases
  - Medline

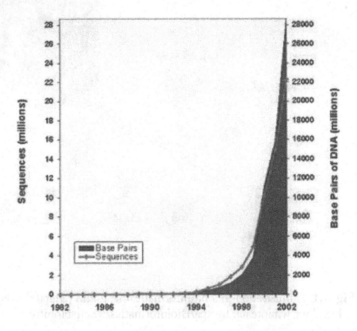

Fig. 1.2. The growth of data in GenBank (source:
http://www.ncbi.nih.gov/Genbank/genbankstats.html)

However, in some situations, a single database cannot provide answers to the complex problems of biologists. Integrating or assembling information from several databases to solve problems and discover new knowledge are other major challenges in bioinformatics (Kuonen, 2003; Ng and Wong, 2004; Wong, 2000; and Wong, 2002).

The transformation of voluminous biological data into useful information and valuable knowledge is the challenge of knowledge discovery. Identification and interpretation of interesting patterns hidden in trillions of genetic and other biological data is a critical goal of bioinformatics. This goal covers identification of useful gene structures from biological sequences, derivation of diagnostic knowledge from experimental data, and extraction of scientific information from the literature (Han and Kamber, 2001; Jagota, 2000; Narayanan et al., 2002; and Ng and Wong, 2004).

1.3 An Overview of Bioinformatics Technologies

The term "bioinformatics" has been used with different meanings by different groups of scientists and researchers (Perry, 2000). According to these researchers, it means all bioinformatics activities related to genomics that focus on chromosome mapping and sequencing, and on exploring the functions of genes, functional genomics, and structural genomics. Besides supporting genomics, information technology supports a wide range of biosciences, such as human brain science and plant architecture, and computational biology. The data are characterized by variety and heterogeneity: they are related to different organic structures, environments, and spatial scales, and derive from multiple sources. Database management, artificial intelligence, data mining, and knowledge representation can provide key solutions to the challenges posed by biological data. However, these approaches require powerful and sophisticated computational tools to provide efficient solutions to very complex problems. Exciting opportunities are emerging by integrating molecular biology components of bioinformatics with computational, physiological, morphological, taxonomic, and ecological components. Addressing these challenging issues will help the life sciences to access, retrieve, analyze, and visualize data and relationships in a collaborative work environment. Even biomedical and health informatics can benefit from bioinformatics technologies.

Bioinformatics can be viewed as naturally evolving from computer and biological sciences. This evolution has been investigated in the development of the following functionalities:

- biological data collection such as NCBI (http://www. ncbi.nih.gov/), GeneBank, DDBJ and PDB,

- biological data creation such as the human genome project, gene discovery and gene expression,
- biological databases such as EMBL, EMBI and SWISS-PROT,
- biological data management such as bioinformatics data warehousing and Sequence Retrieval Systems (SRS),
- biological data structures such as structural bioinformatics,
- biological modeling such as HMM, comparative modeling, probabilistic modeling and molecular modeling,
- biological data analysis and exploration such as bioinformatics data mining, and biological understanding such as machine learning and pattern matching and visualization of biological sequences,
- sequence analysis: sequence assembly and alignment, and
- biological processes.

Bioinformatics technology is an interdisciplinary field, a confluence of a set of technologies, as shown in Fig. 1.3. It includes database technologies, data mining, structures, process, modeling, visualization, machine learning, pattern matching, networks, and tools.

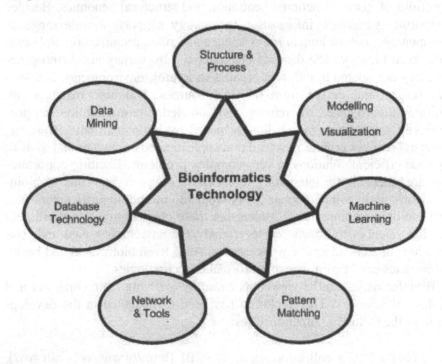

Fig. 1.3. Technologies within Bioinformatics

The existing research in bioinformatics is related to knowledge discovery, sequence analysis, structure analysis, and expression analysis. Sequence analysis is the discovery of functional and structural similarities and differences between multiple biological sequences. This can be done by comparing the new (unknown) sequence with well-studied and annotated (known) sequences. Scientists have found that two similar sequences possess the same functional role, regulatory or biochemical pathway, and protein structure. If two similar sequences are from different organisms, they are said to be homologous sequences. Finding homologous sequences is important in predicting the nature of a protein. This helps greatly in the development of new drugs, and in the performance of phylogenetic analysis. One proposed method for sequence comparison is sequence alignment. It is a procedure for base-by-base comparison of two (pairwise) or more (multiple) sequences by searching for a series of individual characters or character patterns that are in the same order in the sequences. To search for an identical character or character patterns, the string matching technique is widely used. Another active research area in the field of sequence analysis is gene prediction. Gene prediction is the process of detecting meaningful signals in uncharacterized DNA sequences. Gene prediction uses homology search to acquire knowledge of the interesting information in DNA. Figure 1.4 illustrates the existing works in knowledge discovery in bioinformatics.

Structure analysis is the study of proteins and their interactions. Proteins are complex biological molecules composed of a chain of units, called amino acids, in a specific order. They are large molecules required for the structure, function, and regulation of the body's cells, tissues, and organs. Each protein has unique functions. The structures of proteins are hierarchical and consist of primary, secondary, and tertiary structures. In other words, at the molecular level, proteins can be viewed as 3D structures. The understanding of protein structures and their functions leads to new approaches for diagnosis and treatment of diseases, and the discovery of new drugs. Current research on protein structural analysis involves comparison and prediction of protein structures.

Expression analysis includes gene expression analysis and gene clustering. Basically, gene expression analysis is a study that determines the similarities or differences of genes expressed in a particular cell type or tissue. Gene expression, represented by a matrix, can be determined in two ways. First, comparing the expression profiles of genes: if the expression profiles are similar, the genes are co-regulated and functionally related. Second, by comparing the expression profiles of samples, one can consider whether genes are expressed differently. Gene clustering aims to group together genes having similar expression profiles. Genes in a specific group are co-regulated and functionally related to each other rather than to genes in different groups. Due to the complexity and gigantic volume of biological data, the traditional computer science techniques and algorithms fail to solve the complex biological problems in the real world.

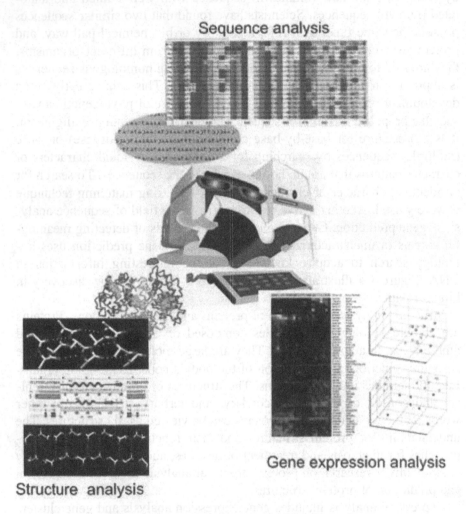

Sequence analysis

Gene expression analysis

Structure analysis

Fig. 1.4. Knowledge discovery in Bioinformatics

1.4 A Brief Discussion on the Chapters

This book covers information technology as applicable to Bioinformatics. Chapter 1 provides an overview of bioinformatics and briefly discusses the interrelationships between the different disciplines such as biology and computer science. Furthermore, it lists in a nutshell the technologies and tools used in bioinformatics.

Chapter 2 provides an overview of structural bioinformatics. The resources of protein structures such as the Protein Data Bank (PDB), and tools and their applications are also discussed. It also covers structural classification, structure prediction, and functional assignments in structural genomics. Further, protein-protein interactions and protein-ligand interactions are clearly explained. The future of structural bioinformatics is also explored in this chapter. Chapter 2 offers a clear and concise overview that forms the foundation for Chap. 3 and part of Chap. 4.

Chapter 3 deals with the basics of database warehousing related to Bioinformatics. It dwells on the organization of bioinformatics data, and the techniques used to transform the data into meaningful information and knowledge. Data is stored in different databases located in different parts of the world, in different formats. This creates insurmountable problems for the bioinformatics community in the extraction of meaningful and reliable information. A detailed discussion is presented on data warehouse architectures and data quality to address these problems. This becomes the basis for data mining, discussed in the subsequent chapter.

Chapter 4 discusses techniques used in data mining for bioinformatics, such as biomedical data analysis, DNA data analysis, and protein data analysis. In order to discover knowledge from the vast genomic and proteomic data, we need tools to deal with the data. Pattern discovery tools and visualization tools are discussed in this chapter. A brief discussion is presented on the theory underlying DNA and protein sequences. The analytical techniques for DNA sequence comparison, gene prediction, and phylogenic analysis are subsequently explained. In the case of protein data analysis, the popular techniques, such as neural networks and HMM, and tools such as DALI and VAST, are elaborated to throw light on the secondary and tertiary protein structures. In order to mine reliable knowledge from biological data, efficient machine learning techniques are needed. These can be found in Chap. 5.

As the growth of biological data has been enormous in the last decade alone, we need to have less-time-consuming and more-reliable techniques to deal with this situation. This can be done effectively only when artificial intelligence (AI) is introduced into the processing, as exemplified in the mature engineering fields. This opens new avenues for introducing the proven AI techniques for analyzing genome and proteome. Chapter 5 deals with the major machine learning techniques, namely, artificial neural networks, genetic algorithms, and fuzzy systems. The newly evolving support vector machine is also covered in brief. Further, this chapter explains the underlying issues of these machine learning techniques when applied to complex biological data.

Chapter 6 introduces an integrated approach, called systems biotechnology, to understand the underlying biological processes and solve the complex biological problems. The knowledge gained so far will help us to look at problems in an interrelated way. In systems biotechnology, various components, namely, experimental finding, modeling and simulation, and knowledge discovery are combined as a single system to gain insight into any biological organism. An interesting discussion can be found on the analysis of the *E. coli* genome using this approach. The chapter also discusses how a biotechnology process can be developed in a rational and systematic way. The tools necessary to implement this approach are also described in this chapter. One of the crucial components of this approach is the modeling of biological processes and data. Chapter 7 covers modeling and simulation. Chapter 7 and Chap. 9 explore all the major modeling techniques, and modeling and simulation, respectively.

Chapter 7 uses a formal language approach called Petri nets for solving the problems of biological processes. It demonstrates the effectiveness of this approach developing a software tool that can model and simulate any complex biological process using a hybrid functional Petri net with Extension (HFPNe). It is also a novel integrated approach that complements the system biotechnology approach explained in Chap. 6. A generic XML format is introduced to describe biological processes with HFPNe. The importance of visualization in the simulation of biological processes is also discussed in this chapter. This chapter covers computational modeling of biological processes with Petri net-based architectures. It also describes hybrid Petri nets and hybrid dynamic nets, hybrid functional Petri nets, implementation of HFPNe in genomic object nets, modeling of biological processes with HFPNe, and modeling from DNA to mRNA in eucaryotes and genomic object nets.

When the data to be analyzed is huge, the computational time required to analyze the data may run into days, or into months in some cases. Parallel computing alleviates this problem by making the processors efficiently use robust algorithms. Chapter 8 discusses parallel biological computing. The main components of intensive biological computing, namely, sequence assembly and sequence alignment, are discussed in this chapter. They have benefited a lot from parallel computing and will benefit more from the further research on parallel biological computing. This chapter introduces recent research on parallel sequence assembly and alignment. This chapter also provides good coverage of the main methods used in sequence assembly and sequence alignment.

Modeling plays a major role in the advancement of science and technology in any field since a good model will eventually become automated in the computational process. Bioinformatics is no exception. Chapter 9 describes modeling in bioinformatics: any representation that simulates a model of biological process. This chapter deals with important modeling approaches used in bioinformatics, namely, hidden Markov models (HMM), comparative modeling, probabilistic modeling, and molecular modeling. HMM has already taken a strong root in bioinformatics after its widespread use in speech recognition. Comparative modeling does great service to drug discovery as it relates the structure and functions of the protein as well as the gene. This chapter provides a detailed discussion on comparative modeling of proteins and genes. The theory of probability has made inroads into bioinformatics as well. The main probabilistic modeling techniques, namely, (1) Bayesian networks, (2) stochastic context-free grammars, and (3) probabilistic Boolean networks, are discussed. In order to understand the biological processes properly, knowledge of the molecule and molecular interactions are very much needed so that the projected functionality of any new drug under development can be verified. Molecular modeling provides such knowledge in the form of the molecular structure in terms of structural attributes such as bond angle, bond length, torsion angle, and potential energy. Further, the simulation that comes out of this modeling paves a way for further research into the intricacies of the molecular dynamics.

In all the chapters we have so far discussed the techniques or modeling to retrieve information from the molecular sequences. Chapter 10 discusses how we can locate a particular segment of the sequence, known as the motif or pattern, which is responsible for a particular manifestation such as a disease. This chapter deals with pattern matching and motif discovery. The major computational approaches used to find motifs are clearly described.

Knowledge of the spatial geometry sheds light on molecular structure. Fractal theory deals with such spatial geometry. It provides a mathematical formalism to describe any complex spatial and dynamic structure. It has been successfully applied to the study of many problems in science and engineering. Application of fractal theory on the structure of DNA and proteins is expected to solve complex problems that seem incomprehensible at the moment. Chapter 11 presents some tools built on the theory of fractal geometry that may play a useful role in solving biological problems. This chapter discusses the popular multifractal analysis used to characterize the spatial heterogeneity of both theoretical and experimental fractal patterns in DNA and protein sequences.

As we are aware, DNA contains numerous genes. The functions of each gene are not fully explored. Using traditional methods, several experiments need to be conducted to find out the functions of a single gene alone. However, modern technologies create opportunities to conduct experiments to find out the locations and the functions of genes simultaneously, using a technique called a microarray. Thousands of DNA samples are coated with glass or nylon in the form of a two-dimensional array, and encapsulated in a microchip for spectroscopic analysis. Chapter 12 deals with the microarray technique and microarray data analysis. It also explains knowledge discovery, data mining, clustering, and classification. Techniques on protein information resources and DNA sequence analysis are also covered.

References

Attwood, T.K. and Parry-Smith, D.J. (1999) Introduction to Bioinformatics, Prentice Hall.

Baldi, P. and Brunak, S. (2001) "Bioinformatics The Machine Learning Approach", The MIT Press.

Baxevanis, A.D. and Ouellette, B.F.F. (2001) Bioinformatics: A Practical Guide to the Analysis of Genes and Proteins, 2nd ed. New York: Wiley-Interscience, 2001.

Benson, D.A., Karsch-Mizrachi, I., Lipman, D.J., Ostell, J., Rapp, B.A. and Wheeler, D.L. (2002) "GenBank," Nucleic Acids Res., vol. 28, pp. 15-18, 2002.

Han, J. and Kamber, M. (2001) "Data Mining: Concepts and Techniques". San Francisco, Calif.: Morgan Kaufmann, 2001.

Jagota, A. (2000) "Data Analysis and Classification for Bioinformatics". California: Bay Press, 2000.

Kuonen, D. (2003) "Challenges in bioinformatics for statistical data miners", Bulletin of the Swiss Statistical Society, vol. 46, pp. 10-17.

Narayanan, A., Keedwell, E.C. and Olsson, B. (2002) "Artificial Intelligence Techniques for Bioinformatics," Applied Bioinformatics, vol. 1, pp. 191-222.

Ng, S.K. and Wong, L. (2004) "Accomplishments and challenges in bioinformatics", IT Professional, 2004, vol 6, issue: 1, pp. 44- 50.

Ohno-Machado, L., Vinterbo, S., Weber, G. (2002) "Classification of gene expression data using fuzzy logic", Journal of Intelligent and Fuzzy Systems, vol. 12, pp. 19-24.

Perry, L.M. (2000) "Focus on interactions with bioinformatics", Journal of the American Medical Informatics Association, vol. 7, no. 5, pp. 431-438.

Westhead, D.R., Parish, J.H. and Twyman, R.M. (2002) "Bioinformatics", Instant Notes in Bioinformatics, BIOS Scientific Publishing.

Wong, L. (2002) "Technologies for integrating biological data", Briefings in Bioinformatics, vol. 3, pp. 389-404.

Wong, L. (2000) "Kleisli, a functional query system", Journal of Functional Programming, vol. 10, pp. 19-56.

2 Overview of Structural Bioinformatics

Qing Zhang, Stella Veretnik, Philip E. Bourne

University of California San Diego, USA
9500 Gilman Drive La Jolla CA 92093-0537

2.1 Introduction

If we define bioinformatics as the development of algorithms and databases for understanding biological systems, then structural bioinformatics represents the subset that deals, directly or indirectly, with the structure of macromolecules. Structural bioinformatics includes study of the structures of DNA, RNA, and proteins. In this chapter we will be focusing primarily on the resources associated with protein structures. Knowledge of the protein structure allows us to investigate biological processes more directly and with much higher resolution and finer detail. For example, strikingly more details of protein-protein interactions can be obtained from the structure of the protein complex than from that of yeast two-hybrid assay. However, determination of protein structures is experimentally expensive and time consuming; this may explain why at the present time scientists are largely dependent on sequence rather than structure to infer the function of the protein. With the advent of structural genomics, we expect to systematically and rapidly solve a large number of macromolecular structures.

Knowledge of a large number of protein structures gives us a bird's-eye view of protein fold space, as can be seen from Fig. 2.1, and is helpful to understand the evolutionary principles behind structure, which architectures and topologies are observed (and why), which topologies are prevalent or avoided, and how the structure of the protein affects its function. A well populated protein universe might be the most important resource for assigning structures to sequences without solving them crystallographically, rather than by using predictive methods. As structure determination will be lagging far behind genomic sequencing for considerable time, the predicting protein structures will remain an important and valuable ability. At present, structural bioinformatics is in its renaissance, with large amounts of structural data, and well developed (and ever increasing) arsenal of algorithms, applications and databases. Its contribution to the advancement of understanding biological systems can hardly be overestimated.

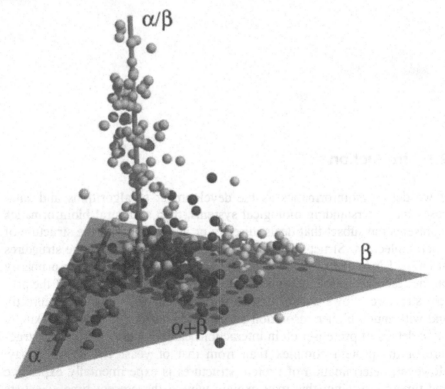

Fig. 2.1. A 3D representation of protein fold space measured in terms of structural similarities. Each sphere represents a protein family; proteins are characterized on the most global level as yellow (all β), red (all α), blue (α+β), and cyan (α/β). The Figure is reprinted with permission from Hoy J et al. (2003)

2.2 Organization of Structural Bioinformatics

It can be useful to organize the resources in structural bioinformatics along the following lines. The structural information about molecules – the 3-dimentional atomic coordinates of structures – is the core from which all the other details are derived (Fig. 2.2); it is a primary resource of structural data and is central to everything else. The files containing atomic coordinates are uninformative to the majority of structural biologists; thus, there are algorithmic tools (applications) that transform, classify, analyze, and model this primary data. The results of the data analysis are often (but not always) stored in other databases, considered to be secondary resources, since they contain value-added information. The overall schema starts with a primary resource to which various algorithms are applied to generate multiple secondary resources. Protein Data Bank (PDB) is an example of a primary resource; CE (combinatorial extension, structural comparison of proteins) is an example of an algorithm applied to the primary data, whose results the structural alignments of proteins are captured in the secondary resource. Algorithmic tools and the secondary resources can be divided into several broad categories: visualization, structural classification, structural alignment/structure modeling, structure prediction, and protein-protein/protein-ligand interactions.

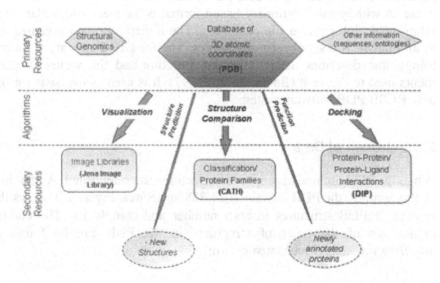

Fig. 2.2. Conceptual organization of resources in structural bioinformatics

2.3 Primary Resource: Protein Data Bank

Protein Data Bank (PDB), at http//www.pdb.org) (Bernstein et al., 1977, and Berman et al., 2000), the first biological database, was established in 1971 to store 3D biological macromolecular structures. Originally housed at Brookhaven National Laboratories, USA, it is now managed and maintained by the Research Collaboratory for Structural Bioinformatics (RCSB), which is a collaborative effort involving scientists at the San Diego Supercomputer Center, Rutgers University, and the National Institute of Standards and Technology. The PDB contains publicly available 3D structures of proteins, nucleic acids, and a variety of other complex biomolecules experimentally determined by X-ray crystallography, NMR spectroscopy, and, most recently, cryoelectron microscopy.

2.3.1 Data Format

The historical format used by PDB is the PDB format. It consists of a collection of fixed format records that describe the atomic coordinates, chemical and biochemical features, experimental details of the structure determination, and some structural features such as hydrogen bonds and secondary structure assignments. The exact PDB format specification is available through the PDB Website. In recent years, dictionary-based representations emerged to give data a consistent interface, making it easier to parse. A widely used dictionary-based format is the macromolecular crystallographic information file (mmCIF). The underlying data organization in an mmCIF is a set of relational tables. The mmCIF dictionary is an ontology that describes macromolecular structure and the various experiments used to derive it (Bourne et al., 1997). It is used as the basis for the new RCSB PDB software system.

2.3.2 Growth of Data

When the PDB archive began, seven structures were deposited. At the time of this writing, the PDB contained 24,358 structures. Figure 2.3 shows the growth of PDB structures in both number and complexity. The current breakdown of the types of structures in the PDB can be found at http://www.rcsb.org/pdb/statistics.html.

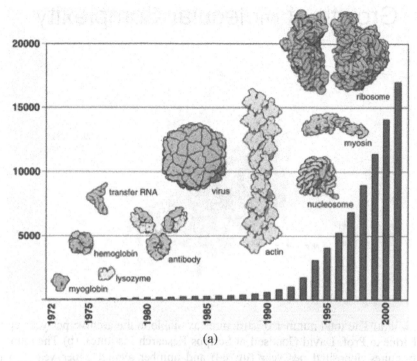

(a)

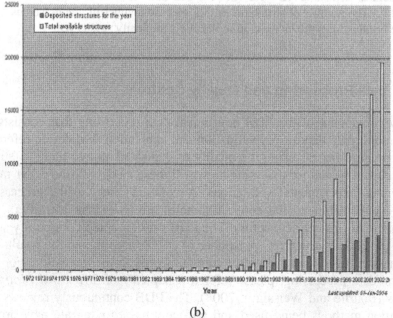

(b)

Growth of Molecular Complexity

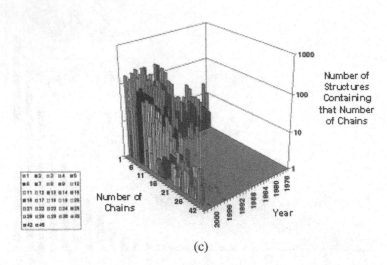

(c)

Fig. 2.3. (a) The total number of structures available in the archive per year up to 2001 (due to Prof. David Goodsell at Scripps Research Institute). (b) The number of structures deposited per year (in red) and number available per year (up to 2003). (c) The number of structures with a specific number of chains versus year. Figure (c) illustrates the increase in molecular complexity versus year

2.3.3 Data Processing and Quality Control

A key component of the PDB is efficient data processing that consists of three steps: data deposition, validation and annotation. Validation refers to the procedure for assessing the quality of deposited atomic models (structure validation) and for assessing how well these models fit the experimental results (experimental validation). Annotation refers to the process of adding information to the entry. Examples are SwissProt identifiers and consistent functional descriptors. The PDB uses accepted community standards to validate structures. A number of checks are run and the results are summarized in an email directly communicated to the depositor. For details on data processing, please refer to Chapter 9 of *Structural Bioinformatics* (Bourne and Weissigm, 2003). The PDB continuously reviews the validation methods being used and will continue to integrate new procedures as they are accepted as community standards.

2.3.4 The Future of the PDB

The RCSB PDB is currently reengineering its site and databases, and the new site is expected before the end of 2004. The new system (Bourne, et al., 2004) uses an Enterprise Java framework and is based on the MVC (Model, View, Controller) design pattern. Extensive efforts have been made to redesign a relational database built entirely from the curated mmCIF files, which will allow improved query access to the unified data. As a primary data source, PDB has been referred to by many secondary data sources. In the new system, PDB will include secondary information back into the PDB in a feedback loop. Examples are details of various structure classification schemes, gene ontology terms describing molecular function, involvement in biochemical processes, and cellular location, and specificity of disease.

2.3.5 Visualization

Visualization is important to help users interpret scientific data in many areas of bioinformatics. It is particularly important in structural bioinformatics since the foundation of this field is the 3D structure of biological macromolecules, which can only be interpreted using a molecular graphics program. Historically, to run a visualization program, a user needed to install and configure the program locally. With the advent of the World Wide Web, users can run increasingly complex applications without having to explicitly download them, relying instead on the Web page's delivery with a single mouse click. Table 2.1 lists a few examples of free structure visualization tools; for a more complete list, please see page 150 of Chapter 7 in *Structural Bioinformatics* (Bourne and Weissig 2003).

Table 2.1. A Subset of free structure visualization tools

Name	Description	URL
MICE	Collaborative visualization tool	http://mice.sdsc.edu/site/project.html
MolScript	Command-driven, OpenGL based tool	http://www.avatar.se/molscript/
PyMOL	Python-based visulization tool	http://pymol.sourceforge.net/
Rasmol	Lightweight interactive structure viewer	http://www.umass.edu/microbio/rasmol/
WebMol	Web deliverable java applet program	http://www.cmpharm.ucsf.edu/~walther/webmol.html

Most visualization applications are distributed as individual programs, and the users have to accept the deliverables determined by the author. Changes and enhancements are usually under the immediate control of the author of a given package. A more efficient solution is to provide users with high-level toolkits from which they can quickly develop custom applications and have all the flexibility to change and enhance these programs. The Molecular Biology ToolKit (MBT) (http://mbt.sdsc.edu), written in Java and Java3D and the MGL project (http://www.scripps.edu/pub/olson-web/), written in Python, stand out.

2.4 Secondary Resources and Applications

Secondary resources are value-added structural databases; they are frequently the result of data reduction by using algorithms or human expertise. Secondary resources and associated algorithms/methods are grouped based on type, namely, structural classification, structure prediction, functional assignments, protein-protein interactions, and protein-ligand interactions.

2.4.1 Structural Classification

Structural classification is a process of grouping proteins together by their level of 3D and sequence similarity. Clustering proteins by structural similarity is fundamental for the conceptual organization of the protein space, as well as for understanding evolutionary relationships among proteins. Structural classification is based on the striking observation made in early days of structural biology that structure is far more highly conserved than sequence. In short, protein fold space is limited (Levitt and Chothia, 1976, and Lesk and Chothia, 1980). This intriguing property is the result of physico chemical principles guiding the behavior of macromolecules and of evolutionary constraints. Proteins can diverge so that their sequence relationship is undetectable, but their folds remain the same. Alternatively, and less frequently, different functional proteins can converge to the same stable fold.

Structural classification is initially built by cross-comparison of known protein structures ("all-against-all" comparison) either manually by experts of using structural alignment algorithms. Hierarchy within classification (going from similarity on a very general level toward the level of detailed similarity in the architecture and topology) is achieved by repeating structural cross-comparison based on different alignment criteria. Classification can be done by comparing structures of the entire protein or, more frequently, by comparing structures of individual domains comprising the protein: both approaches exist in today's classifications, as is described below. A domain is regarded as a discrete folding unit that can be observed in different proteins.

Structural comparisons (alignments)

Structural alignment refers to the comparison of two structures without a priori knowledge of any equivalent residues (as opposed to structure superimposition, where some residues in two structures are defined as equivalent and the distances between corresponding residues are minimized). The majority of structure alignments are pairwise comparisons. The comparison process can be divided into three major steps: (1) representation of two structures in coordinate-independent space, (2) comparison and optimization, and (3) measuring the statistical significance of alignment against a random set of structures. Different alignment methods use different techniques as shown in Table 2.2. In general, there is a tradeoff between geometric alignment quality and its biological significance. It is possible to get highly aligned segments, but such segments are usually short, and are not biologically meaningful. On the other hand, longer regions of the structure will frequently have lower alignment resolution and consequently lower statistical significance. It is not simple to strike a balance between these two requirements. In the majority of implementations, the structures are compared as rigid bodies – no movement within the structure is allowed (Taylor and Orengo, 1989; Alexandrov et al., 1992; Holm and Sander 1993, Gibrat et al., 1996; and Shindyalov and Bourne, 2001). One deviation from this assumption is flexible alignment in which a limited number of motions in one structure is allowed in order to optimize the alignment (Shatsky et al., 2002, and Ye and Godzik, 2003).

Multiple alignments of structures are potentially more valuable, yet more difficult to accomplish algorithmically. A trivial approach is a progressive alignment, in which each of the structures are aligned one at a time to the template; superimposition of all the structures is the final result. This approach is heavily biased toward the structure chosen as a template and in reality, does not consider information simultaneously from multiple structures. Some improvements can be obtained by finding a median structure in the group and aligning all other structures to it (Gerstein and Levitt, 1996). A true multiple alignment attempts to provide the best consensus among all the structures. One approach is to start with a progressive alignment and proceed through a set of random moves in an attempt to optimize the multiple alignment (Shindyalov and Bourne, 1998). Each move is scored and accepted with a certain level of probability; the process continues until convergence. Aligning individual secondary structure elements without regard to their position within molecules is yet another approach (Dror et al., 2003). Multiple structural alignments can then be similarly used to define sequence profiles and may be a powerful tool for identifying remote family members in which some structural similarity is retained, but sequence similarity is too weak to detect. Multiple structural alignment is still in its infancy, with the most successful alignments being constructed by hand (Sowdhamini et al. 1998).

Table 2.2. Structure comparison resources.

Method for structure comparison	Description
	Pairwise rigid structural alignment
CE	Combinatorial Extension of the optimum path (Shindyalov and Bourne, 2001). Uses C_α distance matrix for optimal alignment of octameric fragments. Alignments are progressively extended in three consecutive decision-making steps; empirical thresholds are used at each step. http://cl.sdsc.edu/ce.html
COMPARER	Examines residues' and segments' properties; finds the best combinations using a combinatorial simulated annealing technique (Sali and Blundell, 1990). http://www-cryst.bioc.cam.ac.uk/COMPARER/
DALI	Distance matrix ALIgnment (Holm and Sander, 1993). Regions of structural overlap are identified using distance matrices based on C_α coordinates. Overlapping regions are later stitched together. http://www.ebi.ac.uk/dali/
GRATH	GRAfical meTHod for identifying folds (Orengo et al., 2003). Vector-based comparison of secondary structure elements, using orientation, tilt, and rotation of elements, Fast and suitable for large-scale structure comparisons. http://www.biochem.ucl.ac.uk/cgi-bin/cath/Grath.pl
SARF2	Spatial Arrangement of backbone Fragments (Alexandrov et al., 1992). Uses relative positioning of secondary structure elements in order to identify largest common ensembles. ttp://123d.ncifcrf.gov/sarf2.html
SSAP	Sequence Structure Alignment Program (Taylor and Orengo, 1989). Uses double dynamic programming for optimal structure alignment based on C^β- C^β distances among selected positions. http://www.biochem.ucl.ac.uk/cgi-bin/cath/GetSsapRasmol.pl

VAST	Vector Alignment Search Tool (Gibrat et al., 1996). Aligns secondary structure elements of the molecules. http://www.ncbi.nlm.nih.gov/Structure/VAST/vast.shtml
Pairwise flexible structural alignment	
FATCAT	Flexible Structure AlignmenT by Chaining fragment pairs Allowing Twist (Ye and Godzik, 2003). Optimizing the alignment and minimizing the number of rigid body movements around the pivotal points. http://ffas.ljcrf.edu/fatcat
FLEXPROT	Aligns two structures by allowing movement of the substructures (around identified hinges) (Shatsky et al., 2002). http://bioinfo3d.cs.tau.ac.il/Software/Align/FlexProt/flexprot.html
Multiple rigid alignment	
CE-MC	CE for multiple structure alignment using a Monte Carlo Method. http://cl.sdsc.edu/mc/mc.html
MUSTA	Determines short regions common to all structures, extends the structures by combinatorial clustering of superpositions (Leibowitz et al., 2001). http://bioinfo3d.cs.tau.ac.il/Software/Align/Musta/musta.html
MULTI-PROT	Finds the common geometric core between input structures (Shatsky et al., 2002). http://bioinfo3d.cs.tau.ac.il/MultiProt/
MASS	Multiple Alignment of Secondary Structures(Dror et al., 2003). Uses secondary structure representation, disregards sequential order of the elements. http://pc-gamba.math.tau.ac.il/MASS/

Structural domains

Structural domains in proteins can be broadly defined as semi-independent structural units that have a hydrophobic core, are capable of folding independently in the absence of the rest of the protein, and have an identifiable function. The typical size of domains is in the range of 60 to 400 residues. It is possible to view the protein universe from the perspective of structural domains: each protein is characterized as a single domain or a combination of two or more domains. Classification of protein structures can then be reduced to the classification of all structural domains found in proteins, for example, SCOP, as discussed subsequently. The numbers and boundaries of structural domains are frequently ambiguous, and some protein structures can have more than one reasonable partitioning into structural domains. This is exactly what one observes when one compares three different protein classifications: CATH, DALI, and SCOP. In about 20% of the cases, the same proteins have different numbers of domains in different classifications (Fig. 2.4). This inconsistency reflects immaturity in the field of structural bioinformatics. Domain definition methods are summarized in Table 2.3.

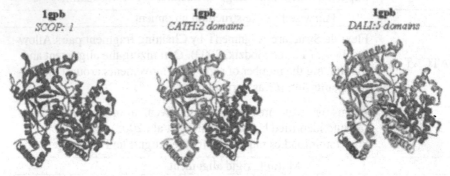

1gpb
SCOP: 1

1gpb
CATH:2 domains

1gpb
DALI:5 domains

Fig. 2.4. A typical case that show differences between classifications. The same protein 1gpb (glycogen phosphorylase B) is treated as one-, two- or five-domain protein in different classifications schemes

Examples of structural classifications

The three best known comprehensive structural classifications of proteins are CATH (Orengo et al., 1997), DaliDomainDictionary (Holm, 1998) and SCOP (Murzin et al., 1995). They represent different approaches to making a classification: SCOP is based on visual inspection and classification by human experts; the Dali Domain Dictionary uses completely automated classification, while CATH employs both algorithms and human expertise in its structural assignments.

SCOP is maintained by Murzin et al. (1995) and classifies protein structures into 4 hierarchical levels: Class (most general), Fold, Superfamily and Family. The structure is first partitioned into structural domains and then characterization is carried out on each individual domain. At the top level of the hierarchy, there are four major classes. They are defined in terms of secondary structures that contain: all α, all β, α/β, and $\alpha+\beta$, and sevenminor classes. In $\alpha+\beta$ class α-helices and β-sheets are largely separated in sequence and in 3D-dimentional space, while in α/β class, β-sheets are packed close to α-helices, often β-sheets and α-helices alternate.

Fold is the second level of classification and contains proteins that have the same major secondary structures in the same arrangements with the same topology. The overall structural similarities within fold are not always due to evolutionary relatedness of the proteins, but can be also due to physicochemical properties favoring certain packing arrangements. Thus, both functional diversion and functional conversion can be reasons for proteins sharing the same fold.

Proteins are further characterized into families. Proteins within the same family have the same fold, a clear evolutionary relationship, and a common function. Finally, proteins that belong to the same superfamily have also the same fold; although the homologous relationship is more tenuous, yet believed to exist.

Table 2.3. Structural domain resources

Resource	Description
SCOP	Manually curated hierarchical database of protein structures (Murzin et al., 1995). Purely structural classification of domains. http://scop.berkeley.edu
SUPERFAMILY	SCOP-defined superfamilies are represented by Hidden Markov Model (Gough, Karplus et al. 2001). http://supfam.mrc-lmb.cam.ac.uk/SUPERFAMILY/
CATH	Semi-automatically hierarchically constructed database of protein structures (Orengo et al., 1997). Defines domains based purely on structure. http://www.biochem.ucl.ac.uk/bsm/cath/
Dali Domain Dictionary	Automatically constructed database of domains based on structural definition of domain (Holm, 1998). http://www.ebi.ac.uk/dali/domain/3.1beta/
CDD	Domains as defined in SMART, PFAM and COG, e.g. a mixture of structure and sequence analysis (Marchler-Bauer et al., 2003). http://www.ncbi.nlm.nih.gov/Structure/cdd/cdd.shtml
SMART	Focuses on domains found in extracellular, signaling and chromatin-associated proteins (Schultz et al., 1998). Uses combination of sequence and structure analysis. http://smart.embl-heidelberg.de/
PFAM	A collection of multiple sequence alignments with inclusion of structural data (from SCOP) where possible (Bateman et al., 2004). A combination of sequence and structure analysis. http://www.sanger.ac.uk/Software/Pfam/

CATH classification is maintained by Orengo et al. (1997) and is organized into four hierarchical levels: class, architecture, topology, and homology, and is not fundamentally different from SCOP, but is different in the details. Again, the classification is performed on the level of structural domains, but unlike SCOP, CATH utilizes an array of algorithmic methods (augmented by human expertise), first to determine protein domains and then to find structural similarities. A consensus approach is applied during the domain assignment step, in which three different algorithmic applications, PUU (Holm and Sander, 1994), Domak (Siddiqui and Barton, 1995) and DETECTIVE (Sowdhamini et al., 1998) are called to assign a domain to a given structure. The automatic domain partitioning is accepted if all three methods produce similar domain assignments, which happens in approximately 50% of the cases. In the other 50%, the algorithms disagree and the domain assignment is performed by a human expert. A recent development is the application of GRaphical meTHthod for identifying folds (GRATH), which is a sequence comparison program. GRATH is employed to identify domains within the proteins by scanning a given protein against a library of known structural domains.

Dali Domain Dictionary classification is a completely automated classification from Holm and Sander (1998). In the case of DALI structure comparison, the algorithm was applied on the level of the entire protein to create a "protein universe" populated with clusters of folds. The FSSP resource is now being phased out and replaced by the Dali Domain Dictionary classification of protein space on the level of structural domains. Dali Domains are defined automatically using the principles of structure compactness and structure recurrence.

2.4.2 Structure Prediction

It is commonly accepted that the structure of a protein is uniquely determined by its sequence; hence, knowing the sequence should, in principle, be sufficient to obtain the structure. This would be very valuable in understanding protein functions of a wide variety of proteins, particularly since experimental methods (X-ray and NMR, primarily) remain slow and costly relative to sequence determination. Homology modeling, fold recognition and ab initio methods are presently the three major approaches in structure prediction.

Although gene prediction is common in bioinformatics and computational biology, only the progress of structure prediction is measured in a quantitative way, by the Critical Assessment of Structure Prediction (CASP) and the Critical Assessment of Fully Automated Structure Prediction (CAFASP) experiments. As an aside, CAPRI (Critical Assessment of Predicted Interactions) is the latest CASP-like experiment that focuses on the prediction of the detailed docking of pairs of protein molecules. A special issue has been published on the first rounds of results(Janin et al., 2003), with predictions on seven targets from 20 groups. The results indicate a need for better scoring functions and better techniques to handle conformational changes that occur in some cases of protein complexes.

CASP The primary goals of the CASP experiment are to establish the capabilities and limitations of different structure prediction approaches, and to determine where progress is being made and where the field is held back by specific bottlenecks. A high level of participation from the prediction community is critical to the success of the experiment. The overall participation has steadily increased from 34 groups in CASP1, to 70, 98, 163, and in CASP5, 216 (Moult et al., 2003). The evaluation from CASP5 of each major prediction is presented in the following paragraphs. In CASP5, the prediction of disorder in protein structures was included for the first time.

Homology Modeling (comparative modeling) is based on the observation that the structure changes much more slowly than the associated sequence during evolution. It can be used when there is strong similarity in the sequence of a protein of unknown structure to that of a different protein of known structure, most likely found in PDB. Homology modeling is the easiest approach; however, it requires a sequence close enough to the known structures. The process of homology modeling can be summarized in seven steps: template recognition and initial alignment, alignment correction, backbone generation, loop modeling, side-chain modeling, model optimization, and model validation. The assessment from CASP5 concluded that homology modeling is able to produce models, though only partially accurate, for proteins having very distant relationships with proteins of known structure (Tramontano and Morea, 2003).

Fold Recognition finds structural similarities when sequence similarity is low. A successful structure prediction in this category produces a model that can be inferred to have structural similarity to a known fold, but no immediately obvious sequence similarity. Fold recognition methods depend on advanced sequence alignment methods, comparisons of secondary structures, and the threading of sequences into a variety of templates in order to find a favorable hit. The conclusions from CASP5is that the template-based methods and fragment assembly-based methods perform well in protein structure prediction, but the correct prediction of multiple-domain proteins in general remains a challenge (Kinch et al., 2003).

Ab initio Methods (renamed new fold recognition methods at CASP4) seek to predict the native conformation of a protein from its sequence alone. They rely only on general physical principles and not on any existing structure on sequence data. David Baker's group developed a method to build structures from protein fragments. This method is based on a model of folding in which short segments (nine residues long) of the protein chain flicker between different local structures, consistent with their local sequence, and folding to the native state occurs when these local segments are oriented such that low free energy interactions are achieved throughout the protein(Simons et al., 1997). The conclusions from CASP5 in this category were:

- The quality of the best predictions was very good; for nearly every target, at least one group predicted a structure close to the correct one.
- Predictions for secondary structure showed, at best, limited progress since CASP4. For contact predictions, accuracies were still low, although there were several instances of accurate and useful contacts predicted de novo (Aloy et al., 203).

Prediction of Disordered Regions in Proteins Proteins are flexible and pliable molecules; often specific regions within proteins are intrinsically unordered, i.e., they exist in many different conformations to function. Disordered regions in proteins can be predicted from sequence, based on properties such as hydrophobicity, sequence complexity, charge and sequence composition. Several models have been proposed (Jones and Ward, 2003, and Obradovic et al., 2003) and a separate session at CASP5 was dedicated to the prediction of disordered regions in protein (Melamud and Moult, 2003).

As prediction methods have advanced, the distinctions between homology modeling, fold recognition and ab initio methods have blurred. The CASP and CAFASP experiments move the structure prediction field forward. The increasing need for targets to test predictions has been partially met by the PDB, where, with approval from depositors, sequences are released prior to structures. The recent development in structural genomics also provides a large pool of targets for structure prediction (see http://spam.sdsc.edu/sgtdb for targets and predictions).

2.4.3 Functional Assignments in Structural Genomics

What exactly a protein does, and how; when and where in the cell is it active; how is it regulated; and what are its interacting partners? These questions are traditionally answered by a battery of biochemical and genetic assays, most of which are complex and time consuming. It is, therefore, enticing to consider bypassing the traditional experimental methodologies, or at least supplementing them, and being able to assign a function to the protein simply from its sequence or structure.

The principal assumption underlying functional assignment is that proteins with similar sequences have similar functions. Thus, we can transfer what we know about the function of one protein to the other, as long as they share a reasonable level of sequence similarity. Very roughly, proteins that have greater than 40% sequence identity can be confidently assumed to have the same or similar structure, and most likely share the same function. It is important to verify that sequence conservation extends to functional site residues. However, even then there are exceptions, cases in which homologous proteins have different functions, as with lysozyme and α-lactalbumin (Acharya, Ren et al. 1991). When sequence identity falls below 30% (the 20 to 30% range is referred to as "twilight zone", and below it is a "midnight zone"), functional prediction from the sequence alone becomes inconclusive. At this point, structure becomes an important tool to facilitate functional prediction.

Table 2.4. Resources for functional assignment from structure

Function prediction resource	Description
PROCAT	Provides 3D enzyme active site templates. http://www.biochem.ucl.ac.uk/bsm/PROCAT/PROCAT.html
FFF	Fuzzy Functional Form Describes active sites in proteins in terms of a-carbon positions (Fetrow et al., 2001).
SPASM	Spatial Arrangement of Side-chain and Main-chain (http://xray.bmc.uu.se/usf/spasm.html)
Molecular Recognition	Identifies spatial arrangements of atoms around a particular chemical moiety (Kobayashi and Go, 1997)
Side-chain patterns	Detects active sites in proteins through the pattern of side-chain arrangement and sequence conservation (Russell, 1998).

As high throughput structural genomics progresses, the number of solved structures about which we know nothing is growing. The ability to assign functions to these structures will depend directly on the quality of our predictive methods. Several general approaches can be used in functional prediction. If we can identify proteins with similar sequences that have functional annotation, the annotation can, in general, be safely transferred. If there is no protein with similar sequence, functional annotation can be transferred from a protein with a similar structure (see above on structure comparison). Similarity of overall structure (fold) is a poor predictor of function, particularly for enzymes, as some folds are involved in many different types of reactions (Hegyi and Gerstein, 1999). Comparing spatial positioning of functional residues (in addition to the overall fold) is a more successful approach to identifying structures with similar function (see Table 2.4). Finally, if no similar structures exist, a rough ab initio prediction can be made, by looking for clefts in the structure, as active sites are often situated in the largest cleft (Laskowski et al., 1996).

It should be noted that the transfer of functional annotation based on structure similarity is mired with problems such as multifunctional proteins, proteins with very similar active sites butdifferent functions, and proteins with different folds and similar functions. Most of them reflect our incomplete understanding of structure-function relationships. Additional information is often sought to increase the confidence of prediction based on protein structure; identifying interacting partners of the protein is one such approach.

2.4.4 Protein-Protein Interactions

Proteins rarely function in isolation: rather, they form complexes. Existence of protein complexes might be unavoidable in the cell since "proteins bump into each other all the time" (Nooren and Thornton, 2003). Forming protein complexes may help increase structural stability; it is also a handy way to regulate protein activity. An increase in the complexity of the organism is achieved by increasing the complexity of its parts (regulatory and structural), which, in turn, is done by combinatorially assembling proteins into protein complexes. Because protein-protein interactions are directly involved in regulation of cellular processes, they are a central part of systems biology, whose approach is to bring together various types of data (sometimes contradictory) to get as complete and comprehensive a view of the biological system as possible. This understanding is often formalized in the network of interacting components within the cell; discovering interacting partners of the proteins is therefore part of this scheme.

Protein complexes can be transient or permanent, obligate (always existing in a complex) or non-obligate, homo- or hetero-oligomeric (Nooren and Thornton 2003). There are several ways to discover interacting partners of the protein. The most reliable and informative method is to solve the crystal structure of the protein complex; this, however, will remain a minor contributor due to the complexity of the process. The majority of the knowledge about protein-protein interactions (Table 2.5) will come from high throughput experimental approaches (such as yeast two-hybrid assay and mass spectrometry) and from theoretical prediction methods.

Table 2.5. Examples of the databases containing information on protein-protein interactions

Database	Description
GenomeWeb	Contains links to protein interaction databases (currently 11 sites are listed) http://www.hgmp.mrc.ac.uk/GenomeWeb/prot-interaction.html
DIP	Database of Interacting Proteins; contains experimentally determined interacting proteins; curated human experts and automated methods. http://www. doe-mbi.ucla.edu
BIND	Biomolecular Interaction Network Database; documents molecular interactions (proteins, DNA, RNA, ligands, etc). Information comes from high throughput experiments as well as from hand-curated data. http://blueprint.org/bind
InterDom	A database of putative interactive protein domains; derived from multiple sources http://interdom.i2r.a-star.edu.sg
SPIN-PP	Surface Properties of Interfaces – Protein-Protein; database of all protein-protein interactions present in PDB http://honiglab.cpmc.columbia.edu/SPIN
InterPreTS	Interaction Prediction through tertiary structure(Aloy and Russell 2003). Pairs of sequences homologous to interacting pairs (from DBID) are evaluated for preserving atomic contacts at the interaction interface. http://russlee.embl.de/interprets

Predictive methods use a combination of sequence conservation and structural analysis (Table 2.6). In multiple sequence alignments, where certain residues are conserved across the family, but different residue types are conserved within each subfamily, these are likely to be involved in interactions. Each subfamily interacts with a different partner and has a somewhat different nature of contacts (Lichtarge et al., 1996). Another way to use sequence conservation is to correlate inter-protein mutations: this can point to the regions oftwo proteins involved in interactions (Pazos et al., 1997). Correlated mutations are particularly useful when structures of each of the proteins exist in the apo form. Interactions between proteins can also be indirectly inferred from phylogenetic profiles, gene fusion, and gene neighborhoods. If two proteins are both present or both missing from the genomes of different species, they are likely to be involved in functional interactions (Pellegrini et al., 1999). Species that are missing two individual genes may have them as a single fused gene, which can be found in whole genome comparison (Marcotte et al., 1999). The length of the branches and the structure of phylogenetic trees offer further help (Pazos and Valencia, 2001). Interacting genes frequently are positioned closely within the genome; thus, a correlation of gene positions within distantly related genomes may serve as an additional clue to their interaction (Overbeek et al., 1999). Finally, there are applications that predict protein-protein binding surfaces based on sequence information (Zhou and Shan, 2001). These applications are trained on the protein complexes where precise contacts in the protein-protein interaction are known; thus, they learn to identify the sequence signal in the patches that are involved in binding.

Table 2.6. Computational approaches used for inferring protein-protein interactions

Computational approach	References
Family-depended conservation	Casari et al. 1995, Lichtarge et al. 1996, and Pereira-Leal and Seabra 2001
Correlated mutations	Pazos et al. 1997
Phylogenetic profiles	Pellegrini et al. 1999, and Ragan and Gaasterland 1998
Similarity of phylogenetic trees	Pazos and Valencia 2001, and Goh et al. 2000)
Conservation of gene neighbors	Tamames et al. 1997, and Overbeek et al. 1999
Gene Fusion	Marcotte et al. 1999
Protein-protein docking	Halperin et al. 2002, and Smith and Sternberg 2002
Prediction of binding surfaces	Zhou and Shan 2001, Fariselli et al. 2002

2.4.5 Protein-Ligand Interactions

An essential goal of structural bioinformatics is to facilitate the discovery of new chemical entities. These can range from drugs and biological probes to biomaterials. These chemicals function by binding to a target, often a protein, DNA, or RNA, through non-covalent interactions. We call these chemicals ligands.

Until recently, most drugs inthe market came from the lead compounds that are discovered by screening of natural compounds; but now computational methods have begun to play a major role in drug discovery. The computational ligand design can be divided into two strategies: ligand-based (analog-based) and target-based (structure-based) designs. These two strategies can be used individually or combined.

The ligand-based design uses pharmacophore (Guener, 2000) and quantitative structure-activity relationships (QSAR) (Hansch et al., 1995) to identify or modify a lead in the absence of a known 3D structure of the target. The success of this type of design depends on known affinities and molecular properties of a set of active compounds, for which the chemical structures are available.

The target-based design uses the 3D structure of the target molecule, determined primarily by X-ray and NMR, or by structure prediction. A critical issue in structural-based design is conformational analysis. Of interest are the lowest energy conformations for a ligand when it is free in solution and when it is bound to the target. A variety of conformational search tools have been developed to obtain multiple low-energy conformations (Leach, 1997).

The site-directed ligand can be generated using two approaches: docking and building. Docking methods search existing databases for matches to an active site, while building seeks to generate new ligands by connecting atoms of molecular fragments specifically chosen for a receptor. The aim of docking is to optimize the feasible binding geometries of a putative ligand with a target of known 3D structure. The docking procedure characterizes the binding site, positions the ligand into this site, and evaluates the strength of interactions for a specific ligand-target complex. A variety of algorithms have been developed for docking (Kuntz et al., 1982; Katchalski-Katzir et al., 1992; Lawrence and Davis, 1992; Bohacek and McMartin, 1994; Vakser, 1995; Rayer et al., 1996, Welch et al., 1996; Ewing and Kuntz, 1997; Gabb et al., 1997; Morris et al., 1998; Sandak et al., 1998; Liu and Wang, 1999; and David et al., 2001).

The development of computational methods has also made possible virtual library design (Lauri and Barlett, 1994; Sun et al., 1998; and Leach and Hann, 2000). It is faster to make many compounds computationally than experimentally. Virtual screening is therefore used to experimentally prioritize efforts to make the best use of chemical and screening resources.

With the advent of structural genomics, we rapidly gain knowledge of new protein structures. At the same time, the number of available ligands in both real and virtual libraries and the number of libraries are rapidly increasing. It has become necessary to efficiently manage these structures in the ligand-design context for instance, by searching a particular ligand and its potential targets and visualizing the protein-ligand interactions. An example of a protein-ligand database is relibase (http://relibase.ccdc. cam.ac.uk/), which contains experimental PDB structures with ligands and structures where only the ligand-binding partners were modeled into the structure (Hendlich, 1998). An approach (Su et al., 2001) was developed to organize ligand databases into families. The new vesion of PDB includes ligand search capability, using SMILES strings (http://www.daylight.com/ smiles/) and visualization of the 2D structure of the ligand using MARVIN (http://www.chemaxon. com/marvin/) and an interactive viewer developed by us that specifically to examine 3D ligand interactions with its target and ordered H_2O (Fig. 2.5).

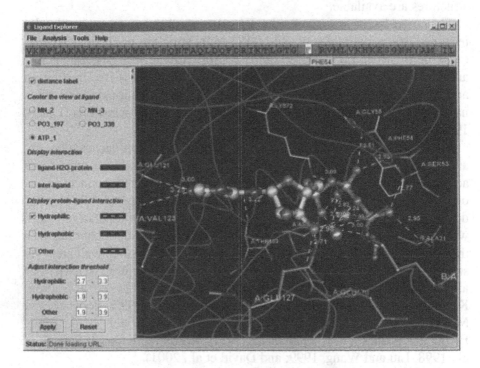

Fig. 2.5. This default view shows the binding site of a protein kinase complexed with MnATP and a peptide inhibitor (pdb id 1ATP). The ligands are shown in ball and stick. The backbones of the protein chains are shown as trace lines. The sequences are shown on the top in the sequence viewer, with residues highlighted in red that indicate the protein residues involved in a selected type of interaction. Only the protein residues involved in the selected interaction are displayed (in thin lines) in the structure viewer

2.5 Using Structural Bioinformatics Approaches in Drug Design

In recent years, there has been successful drug design using a variety of computational approaches, from QSAR to computer-aided drug design (CADD) (Leach, 2001) and structure-based drug design. An example is the structure-based drug discovery of HIV protease inhibitors (Rutenber, 1993). Structural bioinformatics bridges and builds on resources in bioinformatics, structural biology, and structure-based drug design. It can accelerate the quest of deriving a high-potency inhibitor from the chemical lead, while optimizing its physicochemical properties to maximize its chances for success as a drug (Fig. 2.6).

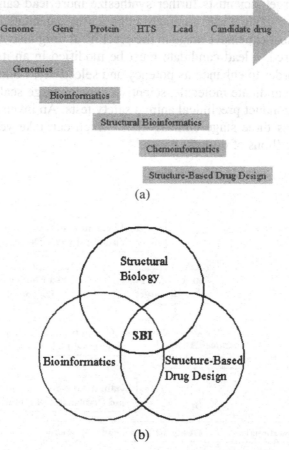

(a)

(b)

Fig. 2.6. (a) shows the roles informatics plays in the postgenomic drug discovery. (b) shows the relationship between structural bioinformatics and other disciplines in drug discovery

Presently, most pharmaceutical drug discovery programs begin with a known macromolecule target, and seek to discover a small organic molecule ligand that binds with high affinity and specificity. A genetic construct that encodes the entire length of the protein is not necessarily the ideal target for screening or structural studies; the full length protein may contain domains that are not relevant to the studies being performed, and the protein may express poorly, be insoluble, or fail to crystallize. To avoid these problems, structural bioinformatics, in particular, computational domain detection combined with experimental domain assignments, can be used to design suitable constructs. These constructs can then be evaluated for their expression levels, solubility, activity, and ability to crystallize.

The virtual screening and library design defines a group of lead candidates. By using the hints from examining the structure of lead compounds bound to a target, scientists further synthesize more lead candidates. The process of optimizing a lead compound into a drug candidate is usually the longest and most expensive stage in the preclinical drug discovery process. Once discovered, a lead candidate must be modified in an iterative cycle (Fig. 2.7) in order to enhance its potency and selectivity. Following the selection of the candidate molecule, scientists develop large-scale production methods and conduct preclinical animal safety tests. An invention of a new drug must pass three stage clinical trials, which can take years and cost hundreds of millions of dollars.

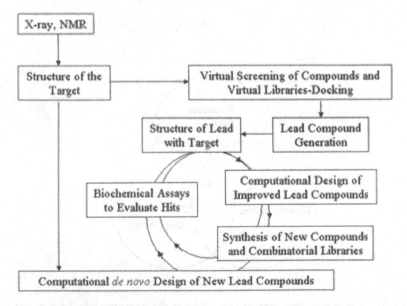

Fig. 2.7. de novo drug design cycles. (based on Krumrine J.'s figure on pp445 in Chapter 9 of Structural Bioinformatics (Bourne and Weissig, 2003))

Many drug discovery projects have failed simply because the binding pocket of the target did not have the required physicochemical properties for binding a small potent molecule. Thus, the initial analysis using structural bioinformatics approaches can provide a significant guide for the ultimate success of the target. With the advent of the genome era and the expected increase of available 3D protein structures from structural genomics, it is likely that in the near future most drug discovery programs will begin with structure-based approaches.

2.6 The Future

2.6.1 Integration over Multiple Resources

As an emerging new field, structural bioinformatics has already started providing many resources and databases to a wide community of scientists. Most resources available today on the Web provide a good number of cross-links to other resources with relevant information. However, in our opinion, what is still lacking is an integrated view that provides complete coverage of structure information through a single entry point. Integrating over multiple resources is a challenging task; many efforts have been made in this area (Williams, 1997), and we expect significant improvement in the next decade with the use of new technologies like Web services.

2.6.2 The Impact of Structural Genomics

Structural gemomics (Bourne, 1999, and Burley et al., 1999) is an effort to employ high throughput structure determination for several purposes, including the determination of as many protein structures as possible from a given genome, filling in protein fold space to facilitate comparative modeling, or the furthering of our understanding of basic biological functions.

2.6.3 The Role of Structural Bioinformatics in Systems Biology

The twenty-first century is a biology century. In order to understand systems biology, people carry out microarray experiments, comparing sequence similarities, and building biological networks. Currently, very few people exmine the role of structures when building these networks. Can structure be bypassed? Our somewhat biased answer is no: the devil is in the details, and structure often provides those details. Hence, in years to come we expect to see an increasing role for structural bioinformatics in system biology.

References

Acharya, K.R., Ren J.S., Stuart, D.I., Phillips, D.C. and Fenna, R.E. (1991). Crystal structure of human alpha-lactalbumin at 1.7 A resolution. J Mol Biol 221(2): 571-81.

Alexandrov, N.N., Takahashi, K., et al. (1992). Common spatial arrangements of backbone fragments in homologous and non-homologous proteins. J Mol Biol 225(1): 5-9.

Aloyand, P. and Russell, R.B. (2003). InterPreTS: protein interaction prediction through tertiary structure. Bioinformatics 19(1): 161-162.

Aloy, P., Stark, A., et al. (2003). Predictions without templates: new folds, secondary structure, and contacts in CASP5. proteins 53: 436-456.

Bateman, A., Coin, L., et al. (2004). The Pfam protein families database. Nucleic Acids Res 32 Database issue: D138-41.

Berman, H. M., Westbrook, J., et al. (2000). The Protein Data Bank. Nucleic Acids Res 28(1): 235-42.

Bernstein, F. C., Koetzle, T. F., et al. (1977). The Protein Data Bank: a computer-based archival file for macromolecular structures. J Mol Biol 112(3): 535-42.

Bohacek, R. S. and C. McMartin (1994). Multiple highly diverse structures complementary to enzyme binding sites: results of extensive application of de novo design method incorporating combinatorial grow. J Am Chem Soc 116: 5560-71.

Bourne, P. E. (1999). Bioinformatics 15: 715-6.

Bourne, P. E., Addess, K. J., ct al. (2004). The distribution and query systems of the RCSB Protein Data Bank. Nucleic Acids Res 32 Database issue: D223-5.

Bourne, P. E., Berman, H. M., et al. (1997). The macromolecular Crystallographic Information File (mmCIF).

Bourne, P. E. and Weissig, H. Eds. (2003). Structural Bioinformatics. Hoboken, NJ, Wiley-Liss, Inc.

Burley, S. K., Almo, S. C., et al. (1999). Structural genomics: beyond the human genome project. Nat Genet 23: 151-7.

Casari, G., Sander, C., et al. (1995). A method to predict functional residues in proteins. Nat Struct Biol 2(2): 171-8.

David, L., Luo, R., et al. (2001). Ligand-receptor docking with the Mining Minima optimizer. J Comput-Aided Mol Des 15: 157-71.

Dror, O., Benyamini, H., et al. (2003). MASS: multiple structural alignment by secondary structures. Bioinformatics 19 Suppl 1: I95-I104.

Ewing, T. J. A. and I. D. Kuntz (1997). Critical evaluation of search algorithms for automated molecular docking and database screening. J Comp Chem 18: 1175-89.

Fariselli, P., Pazos, F., et al. (2002). Prediction of protein--protein interaction sites in heterocomplexes with neural networks. Eur J Biochem 269(5): 1356-61.

Fetrow, J. S., Siew, N., et al. (2001). Genomic-scale comparison of sequence- and structure-based methods of function prediction: does structure provide additional insight? Protein Sci 10(5): 1005-14.

Gabb, H. A., Jackson, R. M., et al. (1997). Modeling protein docking using shape complementary, electrostatics, and biochemical information. J Mol Biol 272: 106-20.

Gerstein, M. and Levitt, M. (1996). Using iterative dynamic programming to obtain accurate pairwise and multiple alignments of protein structures. Proc Int Conf Intell Syst Mol Biol 4: 59-67.

Gibrat, J. F., Madej, T., et al. (1996). Surprising similarities in structure comparison. Curr Opin Struct Biol 6(3): 377-85.

Goh, C. S., Bogan, A. A., et al. (2000). Co-evolution of proteins with their interaction partners. J Mol Biol 299(2): 283-93.

Gough, J., Karplus, K., et al. (2001). Assignment of homology to genome sequences using a library of hidden Markov models that represent all proteins of known structure. J Mol Biol 313(4): 903-19.

Guener, O., Ed. (2000). Pharmacophore Perception, Developement, and Use in Drug Design. La Jolla, CA, International University Line USA.

Halperin, I., Ma, B., et al. (2002). Principles of docking: An overview of search algorithms and a guide to scoring functions. Proteins 47(4): 409-43.

Hansch, C., Leo, A., et al. (1995). Exploring QSAR. New York, Oxford University Press USA.

Hegyi, H. and Gerstein, M. (1999). The relationship between protein structure and function: a comprehensive survey with application to the yeast genome. J Mol Biol 288(1): 147-64.

Hendlich, M. (1998). Databases for protein-ligand complexes. Acta Crystallogr D 54: 1178-82.

Holm, L. and Sander, C. (1993). Protein structure comparison by alignment of distance matrices. J Mol Biol 233(1): 123-38.

Holm, L. and Sander, C. (1994). Parser for protein folding units. Proteins 19(3): 256-68.

Holm, L. and Sander, C. (1998). Dictionary of Recurrent Domains in Protein Structures. Proteins 1998(33): 88-96.

Hoy J et al. (2003). "A global representation of protein fold space" Proc. Nat. Acad. Sci.:100; 2386-2390.

Janin, J., Henrick, K., et al. (2003). CAPRI: a critical assessment of predicted interactions. Proteins 52: 2-9.

Jones, D. T. and Ward, J. J. (2003). Prediction of Disordered Regions in Proteins From Position Specific Score Matrices. Proteins 53: 573-578.

Katchalski-Katzir, Shariv, E., I., et al. (1992). Molecular surface recognition: determination of geometric fit between proteins and their ligands by correlation techniques. Proc Natl Acad Sci U S A 89: 2195-9.

Kinch, L. N., Wrabl, J. O., et al. (2003). CASP5 assessment of fold recognition target predictions. Proteins 53: 395-409.

Kobayashi, N. and Go, N. (1997). A method to search for similar protein local structures at ligand binding sites and its application to adenine recognition. Eur Biophys J **26**(2): 135-44.

Kuntz, I. D., Blaney, J. M., et al. (1982). A geometric approach to macromolecular-ligand interactions. J Mol Biol **161**: 269-88.

Laskowski, R. A., Luscombe, N. M., et al. (1996). Protein clefts in molecular recognition and function. Protein Sci **5**(12): 2438-52.

Lauri, G. and P. A. Barlett (1994). CAVEAT: a program to faciliate the design of organic molecules. J Comput-Aided Mol Des **8**(1): 51-66.

Lawrence, M. C. and Davis, P. C. (1992). CLIX: A search algorithm for finding novel ligands capable of binding proteins of known three-dimensional structure. Proteins **12**: 31-41.

Leach, A. R. (1997). A survey of methods for searching the conformational space of small and medium-sized molecules. New York, Wiley-VCH.

Leach, A. R. (2001). Molecular Modeling: Principles and Applications. Englewood Cliffs, NJ, Prentice Hall.

Leach, A. R. and Hann, M. M. (2000). The in silico world of virtual libraries. Drug Discovery Today **5**(8): 326-36.

Leibowitz, N., Nussinov, R., et al. (2001). MUSTA--a general, efficient, automated method for multiple structure alignment and detection of common motifs: application to proteins. J Comput Biol **8**(2): 93-121.

Lesk, A. M. and Chothia, C. (1980). How different amino acid sequences determine similar protein structures: the structure and evolutionary dynamics of the globins. J Mol Biol **136**(3): 225-70.

Levitt, M. and Chothia, C. (1976). Structural patterns in globular proteins. Nature **261**(5561): 552-8.

Lichtarge, O., Bourne, H. R., et al. (1996). An evolutionary trace method defines binding surfaces common to protein families. J Mol Biol **257**(2): 342-58.

Liu, M. and Wang, S. M. (1999). MCDOCK: A Monte Carlo simulation approach to the molecular docking problem. J Comput-Aided Mol Des **13**(5): 435-51.

Marchler-Bauer, A., Anderson, J. B., et al. (2003). CDD: a curated Entrez database of conserved domain alignments. Nucleic Acids Res **31**(1): 383-7.

Marcotte, E. M., Pellegrini, M., et al. (1999). Detecting protein function and protein-protein interactions from genome sequences. Science **285**(5428): 751-3.

Melamud, E. and Moult, J. (2003). Evaluation of disorder preditions in CASP5. Proteins **53**: 561-565.

Morris, G. M., Goodsell, D. S., et al. (1998). Automated docking using a lamarckian genetic algorithm and an impirical binding free energy function. J Comp Chem **19**: 1639-62.

Moult, J., Fidelis, K., et al. (2003). Critical Assessment of Methods of Protein Structure Prediction (CASP)-Round V. Proteins **53**: 334-339.

Murzin, A. G., Brenner, S. E., et al. (1995). SCOP: a structural classification of proteins database for the investigation of sequences and structures. J Mol Biol **247**(4): 536-40.

Nooren, I. M. and Thornton, J. M. (2003). Diversity of protein-protein interactions. Embo J **22**(14): 3486-92.

Obradovic, Z., Peng, K., et al. (2003). Predicting Intrinsic Disorder From Amino Acid Sequence. Proteins.

Orengo, C. A., Michie, A. D., et al. (1997). CATH--a hierarchic classification of protein domain structures. Structure 5(8): 1093-108.

Orengo, C. A., Pearl, et al. (2003). The CATH Domain Structure Database. Structural Bioinformatincs. P. E. Bourne and H. Weissig, Willey & Sons publication: 249-272.

Overbeek, R., Fonstein, M., et al. (1999). Use of contiguity on the chromosome to predict functional coupling. In Silico Biol 1(2): 93-108.

Pazos, F., Helmer-Citterich, M., et al. (1997). Correlated mutations contain information about protein-protein interaction. J Mol Biol 271(4): 511-23.

Pazos, F. and Valencia, A. (2001). Similarity of phylogenetic trees as indicator of protein-protein interaction. Protein Eng 14(9): 609-14.

Pellegrini, M., Marcotte, E. M., et al. (1999). Assigning protein functions by comparative genome analysis: protein phylogenetic profiles. Proc Natl Acad Sci U S A 96(8): 4285-8.

Pereira-Leal, J. B. and Seabra, M. C. (2001). Evolution of the Rab family of small GTP-binding proteins. J Mol Biol 313(4): 889-901.

Ragan, M. A. and Gaasterland, T. (1998). Microbial genescapes: a prokaryotic view of the yeast genome. Microb Comp Genomics 3(4): 219-35.

Rayer, M., Wefing, S., et al. (1996). Placement of medium-sized molecular fragments into active sites of proteins. 10: 41-54.

Russell, R. B. (1998). Detection of protein three-dimensional side-chain patterns: new examples of convergent evolution. J Mol Biol 279(5): 1211-27.

Rutenber, E., Fauman, E. B., et al. (1993). Structure of a non-peptide inhibitor complexed with HIV-1 protease. Developing a cycle of structure-based drug design. J Biol Chem 268(21): 15343-6.

Sali, A. and Blundell, T. L. (1990). Definition of general topological equivalence in protein structures. A procedure involving comparison of properties and relationships through simulated annealing and dynamic programming. J Mol Biol 212(2): 403-28.

Sandak, B., Wolfson, H. J., et al. (1998). Flexible docking allowing induced fit in proteins: Insights from an open to closed conformational isomers. Proteins 32: 159-74.

Schultz, J., Milpetz, F., et al. (1998). SMART, a simple modular architecture research tool: identification of signaling domains. Proc Natl Acad Sci U S A 95(11): 5857-64.

Shatsky, M., Nussinov, R., et al. (2002). MultiProt - aMultiple Protein Structural Alignment Algorithm. Workshop on algorithms in bioinformatics, Springer Verlag. 2452: 235-250.

Shatsky, M., Nussinov, R., et al. (2002). Flexible protein alignment and hinge detection. Proteins 48(2): 242-56.

Shindyalov, I. N. and Bourne, P. E. (1998). Protein structure alignment by incremental combinatorial extension (CE) of the optimal path. Protein Eng 11(9): 739-47.

Shindyalov, I. N. and Bourne, P. E. (2001). A database and tools for 3-D protein structure comparison and alignment using the Combinatorial Extension (CE) algorithm. Nucleic Acids Res **29**(1): 228-9.

Siddiqui, A. S. and Barton, G. J. (1995). Continuous and discontinuous domains: an algorithm for the automatic generation of reliable protein domain definitions. Protein Sci **4**(5): 872-84.

Simons, K. T., Kooperberg, C., et al. (1997). Assembly of protein tertiary structures from fragments with similar local sequences using simulated annealing and Bayesian scoring functions. J Mol Biol **268**(1): 209-25.

Smith, G. R. and Sternberg, M. J. (2002). Prediction of protein-protein interactions by docking methods. Curr Opin Struct Biol **12**(1): 28-35.

Sowdhamini, R., Burke, D. F., et al. (1998). Protein three-dimensional structural databases: domains, structurally aligned homologues and superfamilies. Acta Crystallogr D Biol Crystallogr **54**(Pt 6 Pt 1): 1168-77.

Su, A. I., Lorber, D. M., et al. (2001). Docking molecules by families to increase the diversity of hits in database screens: computational strategy and experimental evaluation. Proteins **42**: 279-93.

Sun, Y., T. J. A. Ewing, et al. (1998). CombiDOCK: structure-based combinatorial docking and library design. J Comput-Aided Mol Des **12**: 597-604.

Tamames, J., Casari, G., et al. (1997). Conserved clusters of functionally related genes in two bacterial genomes. J Mol Evol **44**(1): 66-73.

Taylor, W. R. and Orengo, C. A. (1989). Protein structure alignment. J Mol Biol **208**(1): 1-22.

Tramontano, A. and Morea, V. (2003). Assessment of homology-based predictions in CASP5. Proteins **53**: 352-368.

Vakser, I. A. (1995). Protein docking for low-resolution structures. Protein Eng **8**: 371-7.

Welch, W., Ruppert, J., et al. (1996). HAMMERHEAD: fast, fully automated docking of flexible ligands to protein binding sites. Chem Biol **3**: 449-63.

Williams, N. (1997). Bioinformatics: how to get databases talking the same language. Science **275**: 301-2.

Ye, Y. and Godzik, A. (2003). Flexible structure alignment by chaining aligned fragment pairs allowing twists. Bioinformatics **19 Suppl 2**: II246-II255.

Zhou, H. X. and Shan, Y. (2001). Prediction of protein interaction sites from sequence profile and residue neighbor list. Proteins **44**(3): 336-43.

3 Database Warehousing in Bioinformatics

Judice LY Koh and Vladimir Brusic

Institute for Infocomm Research
21 Heng Mui Keng Terrace, Singapore 119613
Email: vladimir@i2r.a-star.edu.sg, judice@i2r.a-star.edu.sg,

3.1 Introduction

The applications of computer technology in biology date as early as the 1960s, progressing rapidly in the last decade and evolving into the emergence of new field of bioinformatics. Bioinformatics combines the elements of biological sciences, biotechnology, computer science, and mathematics. Recent advances in biotechnology have enabled measurement of biological systems on a massive scale. Newly developed methods and instrumentation, such as high throughput sequencing and automation in genomics and proteomics, generate volumes of raw biological data at an explosive rate. In parallel with the growth of data, numerous computational tools for improved data analysis and management have emerged. These tools help extract relevant parts of the data (data reduction), establish correlations between different views of data (correlation analysis), and convert the information to knowledge discoveries (data mining). In addition, recent research has expanded into data storage and data management focusing on structure of the databases (data modeling), storage media (relational, flat file-based, XML, and others), and quality assurance of data.

The knowledge-based era of modern biological research seeks to combine data management systems with sophisticated data analysis tools, thus defining some of the major current activities in bioinformatics.

Molecular biology data management systems usually take the form of publicly accessible biological databases. A database is designed to manage a large amount of persistent, homogeneous, and structured data that is-shared among distributed users and processes (Bressan, 2002). When a dataset is organized in the form of a database, it must remain manageable and usable, supporting both data growth and increase in the number of database queries. In bioinformatics, the development of databases has been driven by an explosive growth of data as well as increasing user access to this data. For example, the number of entries in SWISS-Prot (www.expasy. org), a major public protein database and in DNA Data Bank of Japan (www.ddbj.nic.ac.jp), a major web accessible DNA databank, has grown rapidly from 999 to 2003. The number of accesses to Swiss-Prot has grown by approximately one million added connections per year (Tables 3.1 and 3.2).

Table 3.1. Number of monthly web access example

SWISS-Prot release version	Month/Year	No. of entries	No. of access in the month
38.0	07/1999	80,000	2,040,437
39.0	05/2000	86,593	3,162,154
40.0	10/2001	101,602	5,642,523
41.0	02/2003	122,564	8,018,544
42.0	10/2003	135,850	9,510,337

The number of entries in SWISS-Prot and the number of monthly web accesses to SWISS-Prot from 1999 to 2003.

The growth of biological data resulted mainly from the large volume of nucleotide sequences generated from the genome sequencing projects. The first viral genome, bacteriophage FX-174, containing 5,386 base pairs (bps) was sequenced in 1978 (Sanger et al., 1978). More than a decade later, the first free-living organism, Haemophilus influenzae, containing 1.8 million base pairs, was sequenced (Fleischmann et al., 1995). The human genome of some 3.5 billion bp was published in 2001 (Lander et al. 2001), followed by the publication of mouse genome a year later (Waterston et al., 2002). Today, more than 1,500 viral genomes, 110 bacterial and archaea genomes and 20 eukaryotic genomes have been sequenced. Because of the alternative splicing of the messenger RNA (Fields, 2001) it is estimated that some 30,000 human genes encode as much as ten times more proteins. Rapid accumulation of genomic sequences, followed by a mounting pool of protein sequences, and three-dimensional (3D) structures will continue to fuel the development of database technologies for managing these data.

Table 3.2. Number of monthly web access example

DDBJ release version	Month/Year	No. of entries
38	07/1999	4,294,369
41	04/2000	5,962,608
47	10/2001	13,266,610
53	03/2003	23,250,813
56	12/2003	30,405,173

The number of entries in DDBJ from 1999 to 2003.

Numerous databases have been created to store and manage the nucleotide sequences and related views of the same data, such as 3D biological macromolecular structures, protein sequences, physical maps, and structural or functional domains. Among the most significant DNA databases are DDBJ, GenBank (www.ncbi.nlm.nih.gov/Genbank), and EMBL (www.ebi.ac.uk/Databases). Major protein databases are Swiss-Prot, TrEMBL (www.ebi.ac.uk/trembl), PIR (pir.georgetown.edu/pirwww/pir home3.shtml), and Protein Data Bank (www.pdb.org). Each of these databases usually provides a single specific view of the data. For example, PDB contains 3D biological macromolecular structures. However, researchers typically utilize diverse information from multiple databases to support planning of experiments or analysis and interpretation of results. The common practice of manually accessing and compiling extracted data of dissimilar views can be very costly and time consuming. The concept of data warehousing, a convenient solution to managing different views of data and ensuring data interoperability, has been recently applied in bioinformatics. A biological data warehouse is a subject-oriented, integrated, non-volatile, expert interpreted collection of data in support of biological data analyses and knowledge discovery (Schönbach et al., 2000). This definition suggests that a data warehouse is organized around specific subject. The goal of constructing a data warehouse is to facilitate high-level analysis, summarization of information, and extraction of new knowledge hidden in the data. We refer to the databases that provide raw data for the data warehouse as data sources.

In this chapter, we introduce the basic concepts of data warehousing and discuss the role of data warehousing for improved data analysis and data management. We present several case studies and discuss the lessons learned. This chapter focuses on a) describing the nature of biological data and problems frequently encountered in managing them, b) transforming data into knowledge using data warehousing, c) data warehousing principles and the basic architecture of a biological data warehouse, and d) data quality.

3.2 Bioinformatics Data

Bioinformatics data consists of different views of biological information. Bioinformatics databases are diverse in their data formats, and are highly redundant. The bioinformatics data views include biological sequences (DNA, RNA, and proteins), gene or protein expression, functional properties, molecular interactions, clinical data, system descriptions, and related publications. The data appear as sequences, sequence annotations, structural models, physical maps, clinical records, interaction pathways, gene and protein expressions, protein-protein interactions, and other forms in data sources such as databases, private data collections, and related publications. The types of bioinformatics databases are summarized in the two major catalogues of molecular databases: the annual database issue of Nucleic Acid Research (Baxevanis, 2003), and the DBCAT, a catalog of public databases at Infobiogen (www.infobiogen.fr/services/dbcat). In August 2003, NAR listed a total of 399 databases classified into 17 categories and DBCAT listed 511 databases classified into seven categories (Table 3.3).

There is substantial diversity and variation in bioinformatics data, even among databases containing data of the same view (the same type of data). Each database has its own infrastructure and proprietary data format (common data standards and data exchange formats are not established in this field). For example, sequence entries are described in different formats in GenBank, Swiss-Prot, and EMBL. GenBank developed the ASN.1 (Abstract Syntax Notation One) format while Swiss-Prot designed its own format. The Swiss-Prot data format differs slightly from that of the EMBL database. Recent introduction of XML (Extensible Markup Language) as the generic data exchange format has also given rise to several variants of the XML representations of bioinformatics data. In addition to ASN.1, GenBank uses the GBSeq XML (www.ncbi.nlm.nih.gov/IEB/ToolBox/C_DOC/lxr/source/asn/gbseq.asn) format and enables the conversion of ASN.1 data to GBSeq XML. SwissProt has developed its own XML, known as SPTr-XML (www.ebi.ac.uk/swissprot/SP-ML/mapping-guide.html), and EMBL has developed the XEMBL (www.ebi.ac.uk/ xembl). The XML formats for other bioinformatics data include the Gene Expression markup language GEML (www.rosettabio.com/tech/geml/ default.htm), MicroArray and Gene markup language MAGE-ML (www.mged.org/Workgroups/MAGE/mage.html), and CellML (www. cellml.org). Despite a variety of available data formats, a universal protocol for data exchange has not been established, contributing to the complication of bioinformatics data management.

Table 3.3. Number of individual database

NAR	Number	DBCAT	Number
Major Sequence Repositories	9	DNA	87
Comparative Genomics	4		
Gene Expression	19		
Gene Identification and Structure	27		
Genetic and Physical Maps	12	Mapping	29
Genomic Databases	52	Genomics	58
Intermolecular Interactions	7		
Metabolic Pathways/Cellular Regulation	11		
Mutation Databases	31		
Pathology	7		
Protein Databases	56	Protein	94
Protein Sequence Motifs	20		
Proteome Resources	6		
RNA Sequences	26	RNA sequences	29
Retrieval Systems and Database Structure	3		
Structure	34	Protein structure	18
Transgenics	2		
		Literature	43
Varied Biomedical Content	20	Miscellaneous	153
Total	399		511

Number of individual databases sorted by categories (as of September 2003) listed in the NAR and DBCAT catalogues.

Bioinformatics data across diverse databases is often highly redundant. Because benchmarking and quality control mechanisms are rudimentary, an entry can exist in different forms in more than one database. To address the problem of redundancy in the nucleotide sequences, EMBL (www.ebi. ac.uk/embl), GenBank and DDBJ established the agreement for data redistribution (Brunak et al., 2002). Any nucleotide sequence submitted to any of the three main repositories is redistributed to the others on a daily basis. Data structure and format differences are resolved by enforcing on a set of regulations on the three databases. In theory, this means that only one of these three databases needs to be searched for RNA and DNA sequences. However, an analysis of scorpion toxins done by our group indicates a much more complex situation. A number of problems surfaced at the data preparation stage of version 1.0 of SCORPION, a fully referenced database of scorpion toxins (Srinivasan et al., 2002). The entries compiled from the public databases GenBank, Swiss-Prot, EMBL, DDBJ, TrEMBL, and PDB were overlapping to various degrees (Table 3.4). From among the raw entries, we found 143 cases of replication (references to the same scorpion toxin) across two or more databases. Nearly half of the raw entries were incomplete and required enrichment with additional structural and functional annotations. One third of the entries contained errors or discrepancies (Table 3.5). To assure non-redundancy in our dataset, duplicate entries were deleted and redundant or partial entries were merged manually. Errors and discrepancies identified inside entries were corrected.

Table 3.4. Scorpion toxin entries

Databases	Number of toxins
GenBank, Swiss-Prot, EMBL, DDBJ, PDB	3
GenBank, Swiss-Prot, EMBL, DDBJ, PIR	10
GenBank, Swiss-Prot, EMBL, DDBJ	19
GenBank, Swiss-Prot, PIR, PDB	10
GenBank, EMBL, DDBJ, TrEMBL	17
GenBank, Swiss-Prot, PIR	36
GenBank, Swiss-Prot, PDB	5
GenBank, EMBL, DDBJ	16
GenBank, Swiss-Prot	9
GenBank, PIR	6
GenBank, PDB	2
GenBank, TrEMBL	2
Swiss-Prot, PDB	8
Total	143

Scorpion toxin entries replicated across multiple databases (from version 1.0 of the SCORPION database).

The bioinformatics data is characterized by enormous diversity matched by high redundancy, across both individual and multiple databases. Enabling interoperability of the data from different sources requires resolution of data disparity and transformation in the common form (data integration), and the removal of redundant data, errors, and discrepancies (data cleaning). Frequently encountered data redundancy issues are: (1) fragments and partial entries of the same item (e.g. sequence) may be stored in several source records; (2) databases update and cross-reference one another with a negative side effect of occasionally creating duplicates, redundant entries, and proliferating errors; (3) the same sequence may be submitted to more than one database without cross-referencing those records; and (4) the "owners" of the sequence record may submit a sequence more than once to the same database. To enable the extraction of knowledge in a data warehousing environment, these are rectified by data warehouse integration and data cleaning components.

Table 3.5. Error and discrepancies

Incomplete annotation	Number of entries
Value added information from journals	101
SwissProt links to PDB structure of poor homology	51
Errors/ Discrepancies	
Toxin names from journals not used in databases	30
No link between databases	23
Different sequence for the same toxin	15
Different names for the same sequence	11
Wrong links between databases	1

Errors and discrepancies in scorpion toxin entries (from version 1.0 of the SCORPION database).

3.3 Transforming Data to Knowledge

Transformation of data to knowledge, also known as knowledge discovery from databases (KDD), is a common goal for users of bioinformatics databases. KDD is the "non-trivial extraction of implicit, previously unknown, and potential useful information from data" (Frawley et al., 1991). The need for KDD arises from recent progress in biotechnology that has enabled identification of the raw DNA or protein sequences in large numbers (hundreds, or even thousands) from a single experiment. But, the refined information, such as physicochemical properties, the classification of a group of sequences, their 3D structures, or their functional properties is derived from the analysis and experimentation at a much slower rate. In this scenario, a minority of the raw data is subject to further research while a large portion is not analyzed further and the explicit knowledge remains hidden. From our experience with two projects aimed at enabling KDD, we established that the data preparation step is the slowest component of the data-to-knowledge conversion.

Figure 3.1 shows a knowledge discovery framework developed for the analysis of protein allergens (http://research.i2r.a-star.edu.sg/Templar/DB/

Allergen). This system comprises a set of well-defined and classified entries of allergens combined with bioinformatics tools for the prediction of allergenicity and the analysis of allergic cross-reactivity. If a new sequence has conserved regions having either sequence identity of six or more consecutive amino acids to any known allergens, or more than 35% identity over 80 or more amino acid regions, it represents a potential allergen. To construct the allergen discovery enabling database, we retrieved protein sequences distributed across multiple data sources, and further enriched the data by annotation from the literature. The annotated information was then cleaned for errors and discrepancies. In reality, the data preparation phase involves numerous steps of data conversions and data cleaning before the data is well organized and can be used for prediction or data mining tasks.

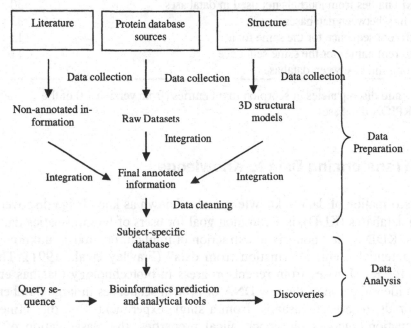

Fig. 3.1. A general KDD framework applied to the analysis of protein allergens

Figure 3.2 shows a structure of a data warehouse containing multiple views to data. The Functional Immunology Database FIMM (Schönbach et al., 2001), a data retrieval and analysis tools for the study of Human Leukocyte Antigen (HLA), provides a unique source of information for HLA-peptide interactions, HLA structures and ligands, T-cell epitopes, antigens, diseases, and HLA-disease associations. It is a data warehouse that has been constructed manually to support functional immunology. Each FIMM data dimension refers to data of a given view, so the different views of data that are integrated to FIMM include antigens, HLA, structures, peptides, diseases, and related references. Our experience in constructing FIMM is that it takes at least half a year of an expert annotator's effort for data preparation, integration of various dimensions, value adding from journal sources, and linking the dimensions.

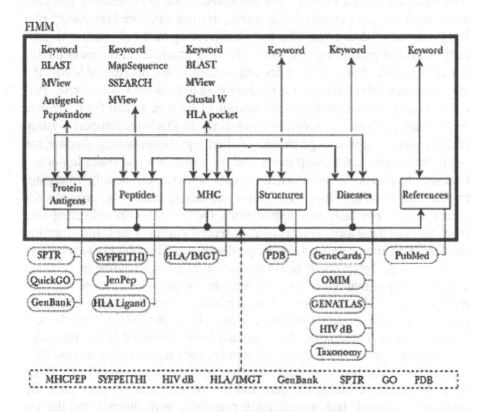

Fig. 3.2. Data views of FIMM, internal links, and links to external sources (research.i2r.a-star.edu.sg/fimm/information.html)

Transforming heterogeneous raw data to a form suitable for extraction of hidden knowledge is the goal of the KDD. This transformation process is highly dependent on data preparation, integration, and cleaning, which can be done manually or semi-automatically. A data warehouse provides an environment of reusable data integration mechanisms and data cleaning support to manage and organize assorted sets of specialized data for different data mining purposes.

3.4 Data Warehousing

Data warehousing emerged in the business domain in the 1990s as a solution for the "warehousing of information" at the beginning of the information explosion era. The steps involved in data warehousing processes are data integration, data cleaning (be discussed in the next section), and data analysis. A business-oriented data warehouse is a structured repository of a large volume of data integrated from different operational sources to support analytical processing (Inmon, 1996). For example, in business intelligence (Almeida et al., 1999), sales and customer data distributed across the enterprise are integrated into a read-only analytical data warehouse. Patterns such as the buying habits of customers are then mined from the data warehouse to formulate targeted marketing. In Decision Support System (DSS), a data warehouse generates detailed reports containing that are not relationships obvious to help users analyze a situation and make important business decisions. In bioinformatics, data warehousing is only emerging, but the effort can help biologists select and design critical experiments for their research. For biological applications, the task involves collecting data from various databases, resolving data record conflicts and, transforming data into a form usable for knowledge discovery. This process requires effective storage, integration, and organization of a large volume of data into a single, well-structured repository suitable for analytical processing. The maintenance of the database is a major issue, given the requirements for common schema, scalable database architecture, and mechanisms for updating the data. These issues have already been addressed in business data warehousing, providing a guide for general data warehousing issues. Biological data warehousing, however, has specific requirements resulting from the nature of biological data and the systems that generate data. By combining general data warehousing principles with domain-specific requirements, we can devise an efficient platform for data analysis using molecular biological data warehousing. This will contribute to more efficient knowledge discovery and support for biological research.

Currently, the application of data warehousing principles to bioinformatics data is not fully explored. The few examples of biological data warehouses are a gene expression data warehouse (Markowitz et al., 2001), GIMS, a genomic data warehouse (Cornell et al., 2003), and TMID, a test bed implementation of view maintenance of protein sequences (Engström et al., 2003). These data warehouses share two features:

1. Data extraction and integration from disparate sources, with alternative proposals for organizing the consolidated data.

2. Facilitation of data analysis, using one or more data mining techniques
for the discovery of new knowledge (patterns, explanations, concepts,
etc.) from the dataset.

Data integration focuses on achieving interoperability of different views
of the data, and several data integration solutions have been developed.
Data analysis depends largely on the objectives of the data warehouse. The
selection of data mining tools depends on the purpose of the data warehouse.

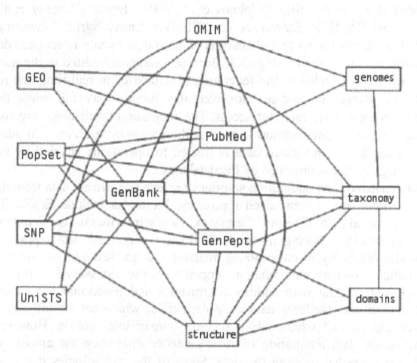

Fig. 3.3. The NCBI Entrez system and interface to a database collection
(www.ncbi.nih.gov/Database). Some of the Entrez databases are not shown in this
figure. The links show database connectivity. *GenBank* – nucleotide sequences;
PubMed – publication abstracts; *GenPept* – protein sequences; *OMIM* – Mende-
lian inheritance and genetic disorders in humans; *genomes* – various genomes;
taxonomy – names of organisms and taxonomic structure; *domains* – 3D structural
domains; structure – 3D macromolecular structures, including proteins and
polynucleotides; *UniSTS* – markers, or Sequence Tagged Sites (STS); *SNP* – single nucleotide polymorphism database; *PopSet* – DNA sequences selected for evolutionary studies; *GEO* – gene expression and hybridization array

Data integration systems for bioinformatics data adopt one of two approaches: virtual or materialized integration (Durand et al., 2003). Virtual integration systems (also known as federated databases) provide a software layer on top of multiple data sources that are independently maintained. The software layer is middleware that acts between the virtual warehouse and the data sources containing the physical data. Mediators, wrappers, or agents are used in the middleware, depending on the implementation strategy, to query the sources and extract relevant data into consolidated reports. The examples include DiscoveryLink (Haas et al., 2001), Kleisli (Chung et al., 1999), SRS (Zdobnov et al., 2002), Entrez (Wheeler et al., 2003), and TAMBIS (Stevens et al., 2000). The Entrez retrieval system at NCBI facilitates access to and analysis of more than twenty interlinked databases, as can be seen in Fig. 3.3. Because queries submitted to the middleware are channeled to the federation of databases in real-time, the results are always up-to-date. However, the queries may fail when the databases are not available for access. The integration mechanisms are also vulnerable to communication latency at the data source servers. In addition, analysis the integrated data is limited to operations enabled by the searching interfaces provided by the databases.

Materialized data integration solutions retrieve and extract data from the data sources into a centralized repository. Examples include EnsEMBL (Clamp et al., 2003) and GenoMax (www.informaxinc.com/content. cfm?pageid=19). Storing materialized data in a derived data repository provides flexibility in customizing analysis and queries, and in data manipulation. The data manipulation support tools are necessary for efficient enrichment of data with additional structural and functional annotation. These tools also facilitate data cleaning, part of which can be fully automated and part of which which requires human intervention. However, materialized data integration must take into consideration the amount of disk space needed to store the data. Some of the technologies that have been developed for integrating biological data have been summarized (Wong, 2002).

3.5 Data Warehouse Architecture

A bioinformatics data warehouse requires several components for operation: (1) retrieval of data from databases, (2) mechanism for cleaning data, (3) flexibility of manipulating the datasets, and (4) integrating and designing purposeful analysis tools that can be used jointly or independently. A

conceptual map linking these components in a data warehouse is given in
Fig. 3.4.

The major components of a data warehouse provide for initial and incremental data integration, data annotation, and data mining. Data integration also includes subcomponents for data retrieval, data cleaning, and data
transformation. These components enable compilation of raw data from
various databases. Data cleaning support tools are used for filtering of irrelevant and redundant records. To enable the interoperability of tools on
the heterogeneous datasets and for ease of data management, the data is
transformed into a common data format (records representing similar
views) or interoperable formats (for records representing different views).
Because information in databases is constantly updated, these steps of re-
trieving, cleaning, and transforming must be repeated for an incremental
data integration process.

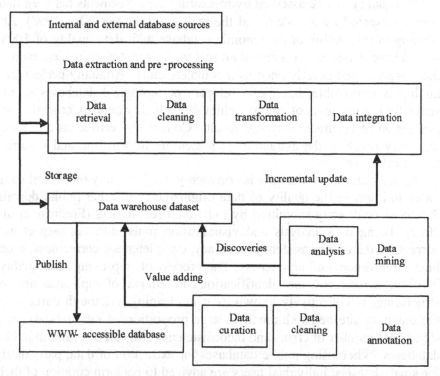

Fig. 3.4. Conceptual map of data warehousing process

Once the initial dataset is created, the annotation component enables the
addition of value-added information from experimental results or related
publications to the dataset. Data cleaning is also supported at the annotation stage, facilitating removal of erroneous data propagated from the data

sources. The analysis of data is enabled by incorporating general or specific data mining tools. The new knowledge extracted from these analyses is produced as an elaborate report.

3.6 Data Quality

Data quality is an essential aspect of databases. It generally refers to the "fitness" of the data in the databases. Data quality can be improved using data cleaning, the process of detecting and removing errors and discrepancies. Bioinformatics databases are usually cleaned manually, or with the use of proprietary programs due to the complexity of errors in bioinformatics data; we observed four sources of errors in bioinformatics datasets (details given in a later part of this section).

Data quality can be assessed by measuring the agreements between data views presented by a system and the real-world entities (Orr, 1998). According to this definition, a genomic database with data quality of 100% would have completely presented all real-world genetic sequences, each of them represented exactly once as a complete entry. Attaining perfect data quality is impossible, but the developers of biological databases should strive for highest level of quality achievable. Quality data are crucial to the generation of accurate analytical results. Conversely, erroneous and noisy data may result in the extraction of inaccurate information and incorrect analytical results.

Manual curation of the data is commonly used in many biological databases to improve the quality of data originated from other public domain databases or directly submitted by individual researchers (Fredman et al., 2002). Using data analysis and visualization tools, curators inspect and correct the data for consistency, accuracy, completeness, correctness, timeliness, relevance, and uniqueness. The process of improving data quality, involving error correction, identification and removal of duplicates, and restructuring, is collectively known as data cleaning. Although curation at the database site helps eliminate a large proportion of raw data errors, a significant number of errors and inconsistencies still can be found in public databases. When using public databases for extraction of data, particularly for small datasets, individual users are advised to perform curation of their data to assure the quality of data and results.

The use of a manual data cleaning process poses difficulties in sustaining data quality as the number of sequences continues to grow exponentially. Yet, an inspection of some of the discrepancies that can be found in biological data explains why data cleaning issues are too complicated to be fully automated. For instance, a pair of protein sequences differing by a few amino acids can represent either variants/isoforms (or the result of an incorrect entry of the sequence) or sequencing errors. It is not easy to differentiate between real variants and errors since functional annotations from submissions are not consistent. Curators need to cross-reference annotations to the publications in an attempt to standardize them and, if possible, to impose use of controlled vocabulary; but this is time consuming.

The focus on data quality improvement is seldom emphasized in biological databases, but there have been attempts to automate internal data cleaning. For example, the now discontinued Genomic Sequence Database (GSDB) identified the need of improved data quality (Harger C et al., 1998) and provided solutions for eliminating vector contamination errors contained in the sequences. They also suggested solutions for identification of assemblies of discontinuous sequences. By removing erroneous sequences and organizing sets of sequence fragments into more meaningful groupings, they achieved better quality of data used for gene level studies and genomic comparison studies.

Four sources of errors are observed in bioinformatics datasets: attribute, record, and single and multi-source levels. The attribute level errors in bioinformatics databases are incorrect values of individual fields (such as "0.9 gene" for gene name), misspellings, wrong abbreviations, or values placed in the wrong field (e.g., organism name inside the definition field). These errors occur most often because of the errors in the original data submission, or from automated systems for record processing. The record-level errors often result from conflicts between or misplacement of fields within a record. Examples include wrong accession or version numbers, features entered as comments, or non-functional links inside the database. Single-source database level errors refer to conflicting or duplicate (redundant) entries within a single database. Examples include exact or fragmentary duplicates having identical content across separate records. The multi-source database errors occur because of imperfect data integration and source synchronization problems (see the example in Table 3.4). The majority of data in current public databases lacks important functional and structural descriptions, although they may be available in the literature. At least five types of errors have been identified in the SCORPION databases (Table 3.5), plus numerous attribute level errors (data not shown). These results indicate high error rates in molecular databases.

With increasing data mining and analytical projects that are dependent on the use of databases, data quality is becoming an important factor in assessing their usability. A data warehouse contains data obtained from various sources, so it is vulnerable to all four sources of errors.

3.7 Concluding Remarks

Bioinformatics is a field where data grows at an exponential rate and knowledge grows only at linear rate. The ultimate challenge for the biological database community is to help close the gap between growth of data and knowledge. Recently developed KDD technologies address this issue. KDD depends to a large extent on the presence of a clean, up-to-date, and well organized dataset. In reality, this requires tedious data cleaning and integration efforts due to the diversity and distribution of the biological data. Data warehousing emerges in bioinformatics to support biological knowledge discovery.

Currently, not all data warehousing concepts have been applied to bioinformatics. For example, the dimensional data model, based on relational tables, is not widely seen in bioinformatics due to the complexity of the real data. Data warehousing has been historically developed using mainly relational databases systems, which are not as broadly used in bioinformatics.

The emergence of data warehousing in the business domain has resulted from the growth in size and complexity of business data, causing difficulty in the data management and analysis. Over the years, the data warehousing field evolved rapidly, and data warehousing concepts are now widely applied for business intelligence and for supporting important business decisions. A similar trend is emerging in bioinformatics. The continuing data growth will lead to an increasing need for a large-scale data management and analysis system in the near future. Currently, database developments largely use a flat file format. Future developments are likely to emerge as scalable relational-based management systems (with data dimensions for proteins, DNA, structures, references, among others). Data warehousing principles have also been successfully applied in medical/clinical domains.

The transfer of data warehousing experiences from other domains to bioinformatics is important for designing an organized environment for searching biological data (genes, proteins, and structures), manipulating subsets of the datasets and subjecting them to complex analyses. Substantial efforts are required to achieve management of bioinformatics data at the warehouse level, but the speed up in the efficiency of discovery will justify such investments.

Acknowledgements. The authors would like to thank Asif M. Khan for his insightful comments that helped improve the manuscript.

References

Almeida, M.S., Ishikawa M, Reinschmidt, J. and Roeber, T. (1999) Getting started with data warehouse and business intelligence. IBM redbooks.

Baxevanis, A.D. (2003) The Molecular Biology Database Collection: 2003 update. Nucleic Acids Res. 31:1-12.

Bressan, S. (2002) Introduction to database systems. McGraw-Hill Education.

Brunak, S., Danchin, A., Hattori, M., Nakamura, H., Shinozaki, K., Matise T. and Preus, D. (2002) Nucleotide Sequence Database Policies. Science 298 (5597):1333.

Chung, S.Y. and Wong, L. (1999) Kleisli: a new tool for data integration in biology. Trends Biotechnol. 17:351-355.

Clamp, M., Andrews, D., Barker, D., Bevan, P., Cameron, G., Chen, Y., Clark, L., Cox, T., Cuff, J., Curwen, V., Down,T., Durbin, R., Eyras, E., Gilbert, J., Hammond, M., Hubbard, T., Kasprzyk, A., Keefe, D., Lehvaslaiho, H, Iyer, V., Melsopp, C., Mongin, E., Pettett, R., Potter, S., Rust, A., Schmidt, E., Searle, S., Slater, G., Smith, J., Spooner, W., Stabenau, A., Stalker, J., Stupka, E., Ureta-Vidal, A., Vastrik, I. and Birney, E. (2003) Ensembl 2002: accommodating comparative genomics. Nucleic Acids Res. 31:38-42.

Cornell, M., Paton, N.W., Wu, S., Goble, C.A., Miller, C.J., Kirby, P., Eilbeck, K., Brass, A., Hayes, A. and Oliver, S.G. (2003) GIMS – an integrated data storage and analysis environment for genomic and functional data, Yeast 15:1291-1306.

Durand, P., Medigue, C., Morgat, A., Vandenbrouck, Y., Viari, A., Rechenmann, F. (2003) Integration of data and methods for genome analysis. Curr Opin Drug Discov Devel. 6:346-352.

Engström, H., Asthorsso, K. (2003) A Data Warehouse Approach to Maintenance of Integrated Biological Data. Workshop on Bioinformatics, in conjunction with ICDE 2003.

Fields, S. (2001) Proteomics in genomeland. Science 16; 291:1221-1224.

Fleischmann, R.D., Adams, M.D., White, O. and Clayton, R.A., Kirkness EF, Kerlavage AR, Bult CJ, Tomb JF, Dougherty BA, Merrick JM et al. (1995) Whole genome random sequencing and assembly of Haemophilus influenzae Rd. Science 269:496-512

Frawley, W.J., Piatetsky-Shapiro, G., Matheus, C. (1991) Knowledge Discovery In Databases: An Overview. In: Knowledge Discovery In Databases, eds. G. Piatetsky-Shapiro, and W. J. Frawley, AAAI Press/MIT Press, Cambridge, MA., 1991, pp 1-30.

Fredman, D., Siegfried, M., Yuan, Y.P., Bork, P., Lehvaslaiho, H., Brookes and A.J. (2002) HGVbase: a human sequence variation database emphasizing data quality and a broad spectrum of data sources. Nucleic Acids Res. 30:387-391.

Haas, L.M,, Schwartz, P.M., Kodali, P., Kotlar, E., Rice, J.E., Swope, W.C. (2001) DiscoveryLink: A system for integrated access to life sciences data sources. IBM Systems Journal 40:489-511.

Harger, C., Skupski, M., Bingham, J., Farmer, A., Hoisie, S., Hraber, P., Kiphart, D., Krakowski, L., McLeod, M., Schwertfeger, J. et al. (1998) The Genome Sequence DataBase (GSDB): improving data quality and data access. Nucleic Acids Res. 26:21–26.

Inmon, W.H. (1993) Building the Data Warehouse, Wiley-QED, New York.

Lander, E.S., Linton, L.M., Birren, B., Nusbaum, C., Zody, M.C., Baldwin, J., Devon, K., Dewar, K., Doyle, M., FitzHugh, W. et al. (2001) Initial sequencing and analysis of the human genome. Nature 409:860-921

Markowitz VM, Topaloglou T (2001) Applying Data Warehouse Concepts to Gene Expression Data Management, Proceedings of the 2nd IEEE International Symposium on Bioinformatics and Bioengineering (BIBE '01)

Orr, K. (1998) Data quality and systems theory. Communication of the ACM 41:66-71.

Sanger, F., Coulson, A.R., Friedmann, T., Air, G.M., Barrel, B.G., Brown, N.L., Fiddes, J.C., Hutchison, C.A., Slocombe, P.M. and Smit, M. (1978) The nucleotide sequence of bacteriophage phiX174. J Mol Biol. 125:225-246.

Schönbach, C., Kowalski-Saunders, P., Brusic, V. (2000) Data warehousing in molecular biology. Briefings in Bioinformatics 1:190-198.

Schönbach, C., Koh, J.L.Y., Flower, D.R., Wong, L., Brusic, V. (2002) FIMM, a database of functional molecular immunology - update 2001. Nucleic Acids Res. 30:226-229.

Srinivasan, K.N., Gopalakrishnakone, P., Tan, P.T., Chew, K.C., Cheng, B., Kini, R.M., Koh, J,L., Seah, S.H. and Brusic, V. (2002) SCORPION, a molecular database of scorpion toxins. Toxicon 40:23-31.

Stevens, R., Baker, P., Bechhofer, S., Ng, G., Jacoby, A., Paton, N.W., Goble, C.A. and Brass, A. (2000) TAMBIS: transparent access to multiple bioinformatics information sources. Bioinformatics 16:184-185.

Waterston, R.H., Lindblad-Toh, K., Birney, E., Rogers, J., Abril, J.F., Agarwal, P., Agarwala, R., Ainscough, R., Alexandersson, M., An, P. et al. (2002) Initial sequencing and comparative analysis of the mouse genome. Nature 420:520-562.

Wheeler, D.L., Church, D,M., Federhen, S., Lash, A.E., Madden, T.L., Pontius, J.U., Schuler, G.D., Schriml, L.M., Sequeira, E., Tatusova, T.A. and Wagner, L. (2003) Database resources of the National Center for Biotechnology. Nucleic Acids Res. 31:28-33.

Wong, L. (2002) Technologies for Integrating Biological Data. Briefings in Bioinformatics 3:389-404.

Zdobnov, E.M., Lopez, R., Apweiler, R. and Etzold, T. (2002) The EBI SRS server-new features. Bioinformatics 18:1149-1150.

4 Data Mining for Bioinformatics

A.W.-C. Liew[1], Hong Yan[1,2], and Mengsu Yang[3]

[1] Department of Computer Engineering and Information Technology
City University of Hong Kong, Tat Chee Avenue, Kowloon, Hong Kong
[2] School of Electrical and Information Engineering
University of Sydney, NSW 2006, Australia
[3] Department of Biology and Chemistry
City University of Hong Kong, Tat Chee Avenue, Kowloon, Hong Kong

4.1 Introduction

Biological data is exhaustively vast. Extracting any information from it is not an easy task. It is like mining a tiny bit of gold from the voluminous portion of ore taken from a gold mine. The word "mining" is taken from the mining industry, extracts precious metals from which ores. Data mining in bioinformatics implies extracting valuable information from a large amount of incomprehensible, biological data. In other words, it is a process that leads to knowledge discovery.

An intense effort worldwide by a large segment of the scientific community has focused an mining precious information from genetic data. Data mining in bioinformatics deals with different techniques and algorithms to gain knowledge from data of biological sequences, structures and microarrays.

In this chapter, we will discuss the analysis of biomedical, DNA, and protein data. A detailed discussion is made on the major databases, such as the nucleotide sequence database, the protein sequence database, and the gene expression database. In order to make use of the data from these databases, efficient software tools are needed to retrieve data, compare biological sequences, discover patterns, and visualize the discovered knowledge. The most widely used tools are also covered.

DNA is a very large molecule that contains amazingly complex information in the form of sequences and structures of amino acids. In order to extract such information, one has to understand the DNA sequences. After a brief discussion on the DNA sequences, the popular techniques and tools used to analyze the DNA sequence data are explained.

Finally, we will have to encounter the product that is based on the information stored in DNA, known as protein. The protein is a relatively large molecule that contains a combination of around 20 amino acids. An understanding of the amino acid sequence will help us probe into problems or events for which the protein is responsible. The basics of the protein sequences are briefly discussed. The techniques, algorithms and the associated tools to analyze the protein data are explained in detail in this chapter in the light of the latest developments.

Even though microarray forms an integral part of data-mining, this relatively mature area needs a separate chapter. We will discuss analysis of microarray data in Chapter 12.

4.2 Biomedical Data Analysis

Recent advances in molecular biology and genomic research, such as high throughput sequencing methods and cDNA microarray technology, have generated an unprecedented amount of data. Efficient analysis of this data by computational methods is becoming a major challenge. Many algorithms have been developed for classifying sequences, detecting weak similarities, separating protein coding regions from non-coding regions in DNA sequences, predicting protein structure and function, and reconstructing the underlying evolutionary history.

Biomedical data can exist in many different forms. We are mainly concerned with biomolecular data based on DNA sequence, protein sequence, and gene expression. A DNA sequence consists of four components, namely, adenine (A), cytosine (C), guanine (G) and thymine (T), specifying the genetic code of the organism. A protein sequence consists of 20 amino acids, coded from the coding region of a DNA sequence. Gene expression data measures the expression of a particular gene, whether up-regulated, down-regulated, or non-expressing, under specific conditions in a cell. A major challenge in bioinformatics research is predicting the structure and function of biosequences by analysis of different biomolecular data. The availability of comprehensive databases and powerful software tools has greatly facilitated research in these areas.

4.2.1 Major Nucleotide Sequence Database, Protein Sequence Database, and Gene Expression Database

To facilitate research and exchange of information in the fast evolving fields of genomics and bioinformatics, many public online databases have been created. These databases enable researchers to share their works or to access the works of others in the most up-to-date manner. In fact, computer access is the only method of getting up-to-date nucleic acid and protein sequence information today. In addition, several journals that publish sequencing research nowadays require researchers to deposit their sequences electronically into one of the major databases prior to publication of their works. It is therefore important to be acquainted with the major databases.

The three major DNA sequence databases that are in widespread use by the biological community are as follows:

- EMBL (http://www.ebi.ac.uk/embl/index.html) (Kulikova et al., 2004): The EMBL database is maintained by the European Bioinformatics Institute (EBI), an outstation of the European Molecular Biology Laboratory (EMBL) in Heidelberg, Germany, and is Europe's primary collection of nucleotide sequences. The EMBL database is updated quarterly. The current release is EMBL Release 77 (based on the database frozen on 26 November 2003), which contains 30.4 million sequence entries comprising 36.0 billion nucleotides.
- GenBank (http://www.ncbi.nlm.nih.gov/Genbank/) (Benson et al., 2003): The GenBank database is maintained by the National Center for Biotechnology Information (NCBI), a division of the National Library of Medicine (NLM), located on the campus of the US National Institutes of Health (NIH) in Bethesda, MD, USA. A new release is made every two months by GenBank, and the current release is Release 139 (based on the database frozen on 19 December 2003), which contains a similar number of sequence entry and nucleotide bases as EMBL.
- DDBJ (http://www.ddbj.nig.ac.jp/Welcome-e.html) (Tateno et al., 2002 and Miyazaki et al., 2003, 2004): The DDBJ database is maintained by the DNA Data Bank of Japan at the National Institute of Genetics (NIG) in Japan. A new release is made about every three months and the latest release in DDBJ is Release 56 (based on the database frozen on 26 No-

vember 2003), which contains 30.4 million sequence entries comprising 36.1 billion bases.

The three databases have collaborated to form the International Nucleotide Sequence Database Collaboration (http://www.ncbi.nlm.nih.gov/projects/collab/). Although the three databases have separate sites for data submission, they exchange data on a daily basis. So, apart from the variation in style and annotation format, the sequence information in these databases is virtually the same at any given time. An excellent description of the database formats and entries for these databases has been provided (Markel and Leon, 2003).

The three major databases for protein sequence are:

- Swiss-Prot (http://www.ebi.ac.uk/swissprot/index.html). The Swiss-Prot database, established in 1986, is considered to be the prime protein sequence database. It is maintained collaboratively by the Swiss Institute for Bioinformatics (SIB, http://www.isb-sib.ch/) and EBI. The current Swiss-Prot Release is version 42.10 (as of 16 February 2004), and contains 144,731 sequence entries comprising 53.36 million amino acids. The protein sequences in SWISS-PROT are nonredundant, annotated, and cross-referenced to many other databases, and are continually updated by a staff of scientists/curators.
- TrEMBL (http://www.ebi.ac.uk/trembl/index.html). The TrEMBL database, maintained by EBI, contains the translations of all coding sequences (CDS) present in the EMBL Nucleotide Sequence Database, that are not yet integrated into SWISS-PROT. TrEMBL is split into two main sections: SP-TrEMBL and REM-TrEMBL. SP-TrEMBL (Swiss-Prot TrEMBL) contains the entries that should eventually be incorporated into Swiss-Prot and that can be considered as a preliminary section of Swiss-Prot, since all SP-TrEMBL entries have been assigned Swiss-Prot accession numbers. REM-TrEMBL (REMaining TrEMBL) contains the entries that are not to be included in Swiss-Prot. REM-TrEMBL entries have no accession numbers. It includes immunoglobulins and T-cell receptors, synthetic sequences, patent application sequences, small fragments, and coding sequence translations where there is strong evidence to believe that the proteins are not real.
- PIR (http://pir.georgetown.edu/pirwww/). The Protein Information Resource (PIR), located at Georgetown University Medical Center, is an integrated public bioinformatics resource that supports genomic and proteomic research and scientific studies (Wu et al., 2003). It maintains several protein-related databases: (i) The PIR-PSD (PIR Protein Se-

quence Database), which is an annotated protein database currently containing over 283,366 sequences covering the entire taxonomic range (Release 78.03, 24 November 2003). The PIR-PSD database is nonredundant and annotated, and the protein sequences in the database are classified into protein families, protein superfamilies, and homology domains. (ii) The *i*ProClass database, an integrated resource that provides comprehensive family relationships and structural/functional features of proteins (Wu et al., 2001). It currently consists of non-redundant PIR and SwissProt/TrEMBL proteins organized with more than 36,300 PIR superfamilies, 145,300 families, 7,310 domains, 1,300 motifs, 280 post-translational modification sites, and links to over 50 biological databases. The protein information in *i*ProClass includes family relationships at both global (superfamily/family) and local (domain, motif, and site) levels, as well as structural and functional classifications and features of proteins. The *i*Proclass current release is 2.41 (16 February 2004) and contains 1.23 million entries. (iii) The PIR-NREF (PIR Nonredundant REFerence protein database), which contains all sequences in PIR-PSD, SwissProt, TrEMBL, RefSeq, GenPept, and PDB. Identical sequences from the same source of organism (species) reported in different databases are presented as a single NREF entry with protein IDs and names from each underlying database, in addition to protein sequence, taxonomy, and composite bibliography. Related sequences identified by all-against-all FASTA search are listed for each NREF entry. The Web site provides direct entry retrieval (based on protein IDs), text search (based on protein or species names), and sequence search (based on BLAST, peptide match, and pattern match) for full-scale and species-based protein identification. Species-based browsing and searching are supported for about 100 organisms, including over 70 complete genomes. The PIR-NREF current release is 1.41 (16 February 2004) and contains 1.48 million entries.

In October 2002, a collaboration was formed between EBI, SIB (Swiss Institute of Bioinformatics), and PIR produced a single worldwide database of protein sequence and function called UniProt (http://pir.georgetown.edu/uniprot/) by unifying the Swiss-Prot, TrEMBL, and PIR database activities.

Recent advances in cDNA microarray technology have also generated a great amount of microarray gene expression data. To facilitate storing and sharing of such data, several public gene expression databases have been recently established:

- The ArrayExpress at the EBI (http://www.ebi.ac.uk/arrayexpress /index.html) is a public repository for microarray data, which is aimed at storing well annotated data in accordance with MGED recommendations. The Microarray Gene Expression Data (MGED) Society (http://www.mged.org/index.html) is an international organization of biologists, computer scientists, and data analysts that aims to facilitate the sharing of microarray data generated by functional genomics and proteomics experiments (Stoeckert et al., 2002; Ball et al., 2002; and Brazma et al., 2001). The current focus of MGED is on establishing standards for microarray data annotation and exchange, facilitating the creation of microarray databases and related software implementing these standards, and promoting the sharing of high quality, well annotated data within the life sciences community.
- The Gene Expression Omnibus (http://www.ncbi.nlm.nih.gov/geo/) at NCBI is a gene expression and hybridization array data repository, as well as a curated, online resource for gene expression data browsing, query, and retrieval. GEO was the first fully public high throughput gene expression data repository, and became operational in July 2000.

Beside the major databases mentioned above, many research centers and institutes also put out Web sites that contain useful subsets of sequence data that are freely available to researchers. Special-purpose sets of sequences, such as transcription factor database, tumor gene database, restriction enzyme database, or even codon usage database, can be found in these Web sites (Williams, 1999 and Galperin, 2004). The major databases and these Web sites usually also include different data mining and analysis tools that can be used to analyze sequence data. A useful compilation of the various biological databases can be found in the special database issue (the first issue of each year) of the journal *Nucleic Acids Research*.

4.2.2 Software Tools for Bioinformatics Research

Due to the vast amount of available data, computer retrieval and analysis of biomedical data is becoming more important than ever. Many software tools have been developed for this purpose. The software tools that facilitate research in bioinformatics can be broadly categorized into four classes: (1) data retrieval tools, (2) sequence comparison and alignment tools, (3) pattern discovery tools, and (4) visualization tools.

A major tool for data retrieval is *Entrez* (Geer and Sayers, 2003). *Entrez* is a integrated data retrieval system developed by NCBI that provides integrated access to a wide range of data domains, including literature, nucleotide and protein sequences, complete genomes, 3D structures, and more. One can use *Entrez* to:

- Identify a representative, well annotated mRNA sequence record from the millions of sequences in the *Entrez* Nucleotide data domain.
- Retrieve associated literature and protein records.
- Identify conserved domains within the protein.
- Identify known mutations within the gene or protein.
- Find a resolved three-dimensional structure for the protein, or, in its absence, identify structures with homologous sequence.
- View the genomic context of the gene and download the sequence region.

Commonly used sequence comparison and alignment tools are BLAST (Basic Local Alignment Search Tool, available at http://www.ncbi.nlm. nih.gov/BLAST/) (Altschul et al., 1990, 1997) and FASTA (FAST Alignment, available at http://www.ebi.ac.uk/fasta33/) (Pearson and Lipman, 1988 and Pearson 1990). BLAST is used for comparing gene and protein sequences against others in public databases. It now comes in several flavors including PSI-BLAST, PHI-BLAST, and BLAST2. Specialized BLASTs are also available for human, microbial, malaria, and other genomes, as well as for vector contamination, immunoglobulins, and tentative human consensus sequences. FASTA can be used for a fast protein comparison or a fast nucleotide comparison. The program achieves a high level of sensitivity for similarity searching at high speed by performing optimized searches for local alignments using a substitution matrix. The high speed of this program is achieved by using the observed pattern of word hits to identify potential matches before attempting the more time consuming optimized search. For multiple sequence alignment, the tool available is ClustalW (available at http://www.ebi.ac.uk/clustalw/) (Thompson et al., 1994). ClustalW can be used to align DNA or protein sequences in order to elucidate their relationships as well as their evolutionary origin.

Pattern discovery tools are used to search for patterns or features in the data. An important pattern discovery tool is cluster analysis. It is used to find groupings in a given dataset such that objects in the same group are similar to each other while objects in different groups are dissimilar. Cluster analysis has been used extensively in gene expression data analysis (see http://rana.lbl.gov/EisenSoftware.htm). Another important application of pattern discovery tools is in sequence analysis. This class of tools uses advanced mathematical modeling and statistical inferences to find specific subsequences, functional sites, and structures, such as the prediction of genes, exon/introns, splice sites, transcription factor binding sites, promoters and 2/3D protein structure. Two useful integrated tools for pattern discovery are Expression Profiler (http://ep.ebi.ac.uk/EP/) (Vilo et al., 2003), and GeneQuiz (available at http://jura.ebi.ac.uk:8765/ext-genequiz/) (Andrade et al., 1999 and Hoersch et al., 2000). Expression Profiler is a set of tools for clustering, analysis, and visualization of gene expression and other genomic data. Tools in the Expression Profiler allow the user to perform cluster analysis, pattern discovery, and pattern visualization, to study and search gene ontology categories, and generate sequence logos, and extract regulatory sequences, to study protein interactions, and to link analysis results to external tools and databases. GeneQuiz is an integrated system for large-scale biological sequence analysis using a variety of search and analysis methods and up-to-date protein and DNA databases. It consists of four modules: (1) GQupdate (the database update), (2) GQsearch (the search system, which also includes many sequence analysis tools for functional analysis of protein sequence), (3) GQreason (the interpretation module), and (4) GQbrowse (the visualization and browsing system).

Visualization tools allow an interactive, graphical display of genomic data. Most major genome analysis packages, such as Expression Profiler, and GeneQuiz, have a visualization tool integrated in them. Besides, many visualization software packages are also available freely on the Internet or by request from the authors. Some examples are as follows:

- TreeView (available at http://rana.lbl.gov/EisenSoftware.htm), which provides a graphical display of clustering results and other analyses from the companion package Cluster, and supports tree-based and image-based browsing of hierarchical trees.
- BioViews (Helt et al., 1998), a Java-based genome browser applet which provides a three-level interconnected graphical view of genomic data: a physical map, an annotated sequence map, and a DNA sequence display.
- Genes_Graph (Serov et al., 1998), a Java applet that enables visualization of genetic network database in GeNet (Spirov and Samsonova, 1997).
- Protein Explorer (available at http://www.proteinexplorer.org) (Martz, 2003), which provides 3D protein structure visualization in an interactive manner.

In summary, with the wealth of information generated by technological advancement in biosciences, some familiarity with the various biomedical databases and computer tools is a basic prerequisite and would allow a researcher to benefit from the efforts and contributions of many biologists and scientists.

4.3 DNA Data Analysis

4.3.1 DNA Sequence

DNA is the basis of heredity (Alberts et al., 1989). It is a polymer made up of small molecules called nucleotides, which can be distinguished by the four bases: adenine (A), cytosine (C), guanine (G), and thymine (T). A DNA sequence is therefore specified completely by a sequence consisting of the four alphabets A, C, G, and T. DNA usually occurs in double strands, and the bases in the two strands are complementary to each other, i.e., A pairing with T and G pairing with C with hydrogen bonds. For example, a single strand of DNA (written in the 5 to 3 direction): 5 AACCGTACC 3 is paired to a complementary strand running in the opposite direction:

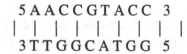

The double-stranded DNA forms a helical structure in space and we have the well known double helix (see Fig. 4.1). The pairing mechanism allows one strand of DNA to serve as template for producing the reverse complement strand, thus explaining how DNA can duplicate.

The DNA of an organism is determined by a process called sequencing. DNA sequencing involves the process of determining the exact order of the four nucleotides A, C, G, and T that make up the DNA sequence. A standard method for sequencing is based on separating DNA fragments by gel electrophoresis (Sanger et al., 1977). However, the method is extremely labor-intensive and expensive, which prevents its use in large-scale sequencing applications. Capillary electrophoresis (Dovichi and Zhang, 2001) is rapidly becoming the method of choice in large sequencing centers nowadays. The sequencing process generates a set of four traces of signal intensities corresponding to each of the four nucleotide bases. The actual sequence of nucleotides is then determined from the traces by a process called basecalling. A widely used noncommercial software package for basecalling is Phred, which is available from http://www.phrap.org/.

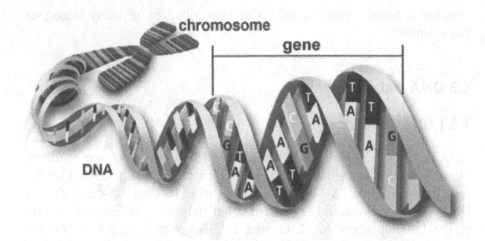

Fig. 4.1. The double helix of DNA sequence with a gene in the sequence delimited. Genes are specific sequences of bases that encode instructions on how to make proteins. (Courtesy of U. S. Department of Energy Human Genome Program, http://www.ornl.gov/hgmis)

DNA carries the genetic information required by an organism to function. The flow of information within a cell is summarized by the *Central Dogma of Molecular Biology*, as can be seen schematically in Fig. 4.2.

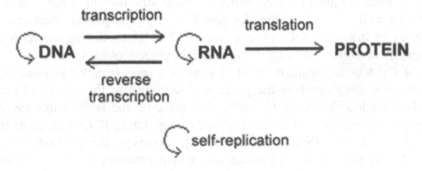

Fig. 4.2. Flow of information within a cell

An intermediate step from DNA to protein synthesis in Fig. 4.2 is called transcription. Transcription copies information in the DNA into copies called RNA. If a segment in the DNA sequence encodes a protein (i.e., corresponds to a coding region in the DNA sequence), the RNA is called messenger, or mRNA. However, the end products of some genes are simply RNA copies, not protein. Typically, these are transfer RNAs (tRNAs) and ribosomal RNAs (rRNAs), which are components of the translation apparatus. In transcription, the DNA nucleotides A, C, G, and T are respectively transcribed into RNA nucleotides U (uracil, U, replaces thymine, T, in RNA molecules), G, C, and A.

Transcription involves a three steps process: (1) INITIATION, where the enzyme called RNA polymerase binds to specific sequences upstream, such as a promoter, i.e., a TATA box, in a DNA sequence; (2) ELONGATION, where nucleotides U, G, C, and A are joined together in the 5 to 3 direction; and (3) TERMINATION, where the RNA polymerase reaches terminator sequences in the DNA and falls off, and transcription ceases. During transcription, the strands of the double helix DNA are first separated by breaking the hydrogen bonds between the base pairs. One strand of the DNA is then used as a template to make a single strand of RNA, which grows in the 5 to 3 direction.

Table 4.1. Twenty amino acids and their abbreviations.

AMINO ACID	ABBREVIATION
Alanine	Ala (A)
Arginine	Arg (R)
aspartic acid	Asp (D)
Asparginine	Asn (N)
Cystenine	Cys (C)
glutamic acid	Glu (E)
Glutamine	Gln (Q)
Glycine	Gly (G)
Histine	His (H)
Isoleucine	Ile (I)
Leucine	Leu (L)
Lysine	Lys (K)
Methionine	Met (M)
phenylalanine	Phe (F)
Praline	Pro (P)
Serine	Ser (S)
Threonine	Thr (T)
Tryptophan	Trp (W)
Tyrosine	Tyr (Y)
Valine	Val (V)

The transcription process is different in prokaryotes (i.e., simple bacteria) and eukaryotes (non-bacteria possessing a nucleus, e.g., fungi, unicellular paramecia, and all plants and animals). In prokaryotes, RNA polymerase produces an mRNA transcript directly from the DNA template. In eukaryotes, genes in a DNA sequence are not continuous, but instead are broken up into coding regions (exons, which code for proteins) and non-coding regions (introns). The RNA is transcribed in the nucleus and then undergoes posttranscriptional modification (i.e., pre-mRNA splicing), where the introns are spliced and the remaining exons are joined to form the final mRNA, which is used for protein synthesis during translation.

Table 4.2. The genetic code

	U	C	A	G	
	Phe	Ser	Tyr	Cys	U
	Phe	Ser	Tyr	Cys	C
U	Leu	Ser	Stop	Stop	A
	Leu	Ser	Stop	Trp	G
	Leu	Pro	His	Arg	U
	Leu	Pro	His	Arg	C
C	Leu	Pro	Gln	Arg	A
	Leu	Pro	Gln	Arg	G
	Ile	Thr	Asn	Ser	U
	Ile	Thr	Asn	Ser	C
A	Ile	Thr	Lys	Arg	A
	Met	Thr	Lys	Arg	G
	Val	Ala	Asp	Gly	U
	Val	Ala	Asp	Gly	C
G	Val	Ala	Glu	Gly	A
	Val	Ala	Glu	Gly	G

Thus, embedded within the DNA sequence are specific subsequences that control the initiation or termination of transcription. These subsequences, such as promoters, enhancers, silencers, and terminators, are regulators of gene expression. Other sequences of interest within a (eukaryotes) DNA sequence are coding regions (exons), non-coding regions (introns and intergenic regions), splice signals or splice sites, and the location of the open reading frames (ORFs). An active area of research in genomics and bioinformatics is the identification of these controlling elements or segments in a given DNA sequence, for applications such as gene prediction.

The final step of information flow shown in the schematic of Fig. 4.2 is the translation process. The information encoded in the mRNA is used to specify the precise ordering of the amino acids, which form proteins. Proteins are composed of 20 different amino acids (see Table 4.1 for the list of amino acids and their abbreviations). Since the DNA sequence dictates the eventual amino acid sequence, each of the 20 amino acids needs a minimum of three nucleotide bases to encode. With a triplet of contiguous nucleotides along the DNA or RNA chain coding one amino acid, there are 4^3 = 64 combinations. The genetic code is now known to be a triplet, comma-free code, where successive codons consisting of three successive RNA nucleotides encode one of the 20 amino acids or the signal to stop translation. Since there are 64 combinations, there is redundancy in the coding scheme. Table 4.2 lists the genetic code for the 20 amino acids. We see that the same amino acid can be encoded by several different codons that are synonyms. For example, the amino acid leucine (Leu) is encoded by six different codons. There are three codons, UAA, UAG, and UGA, that do not encode any amino acids. They are the stop codons that terminate the translation process.

---

5   ATGCCCAAGCTGAATAGCGTAGAGGGGTTTTCATCATTTGAGGACGATGTATAA   3

----

1)   ATG CCC AAG CTG AAT AGC GTA GAG GGG TTT TCA TCA TTT GAG GAC GAT
     GTA TAA
     Amino acids: M P K L N S V E G F S S F E D D V *
2)   TGC CCA AGC TGA ATA GCG TAG AGG GGT TTT CAT CAT TTG AGG ACG ATG
     TAT
     Amino acids: C P S * I A * R G F H H L R T M Y
3)   GCC CAA GCT GAA TAG CGT AGA GGG GTT TTC ATC ATT TGA GGA CGA TGT
     ATA
     Amino acids: A Q A E * R R G V F I I * G R C I

Fig. 4.3. The three possible reading frames of a DNA sequence in the forward direction. The longest open reading frame is in frame 1

Since codons of three nucleotides determine which amino acid will be added next in the growing protein chain, it is important then to decide with which nucleotide to start translation, and when to stop. This is called an open reading frame (ORF). Once a gene has been sequenced, it is important to determine the correct open reading frame. Every region of DNA has six possible reading frames, three in each direction. The reading frame that is used determines which amino acids would be encoded by a gene. Typically only one reading frame is used in translating a gene (in eukaryotes), and this is often the longest open reading frame. Once the open reading frame is known, the DNA sequence can be translated into its corresponding amino acid sequence. An open reading frame starts with an ATG (Met) in most species and ends with a stop codon (TAA, TAG, or TGA). For example, the sequence of DNA in Fig. 4.3 can be read in six reading frames, three in the forward direction and three in the reverse. The three reading frames in the forward direction are shown with the translated amino acids below each DNA sequence. Frame 1 start with the "A", Frame 2 with the "T" and Frame 3 with the "G". Stop codons are indicated by an "*" in the protein sequence. The longest ORF is in Frame 1. Determination of the correct reading frame is an important problem in genomics and bio-informatics.

4.3.2 DNA Data Analysis

Sequence Comparison and Alignment

After a new DNA sequence is obtained, the next step is to study the functional and structural information encoded in the sequence. One way to do this is by comparing the new sequence with sequences that have already being well studied and annotated. Sequences that are similar would probably have the same function, be it a functional role (i.e., ORFs coding for similar proteins), regulatory role (i.e., similar regulatory or biochemical pathways), or structural properties in the case of proteins. Additionally, if two sequences from different organisms are similar, there may be a common ancestor sequence, and the sequences are then said to be homologous. Relationship between homologous sequences has important implications in speciation study and phylogenetic analysis.

One method for sequence comparison is sequence alignment. Sequence alignment is the procedure of comparing two (pairwise alignment) or more (multiple sequence alignment) sequences by searching for a series of individual characters or character patterns that are in the same order in the sequences. For base-by-base comparison of two sequences, a rigorous alignment of the two sequences using string matching techniques is needed.

The standard pairwise alignment method is based on dynamic programming (Needleman and Wunsch, 1970, and Smith and Waterman, 1981a, b). The method compares every pairs of characters in the two sequences and generates an alignment and a score, which is dependent on the scoring scheme used (i.e., a scoring matrix for the different base-pair combinations, match and mismatch scores, and a scheme for insertion/deletion, gap, penalties). This alignment will include matched and mismatched characters and gaps in the two sequences that are positioned, so that the number of matches between identical characters is the maximum possible.

Sequence alignment can be either global (Needleman and Wunsch, 1970) or local (Smith and Waterman, 1981a, b). Global alignment tries to align the entire sequence in such a way as to maximize the degree of similarity between the two sequences. However, for most DNA sequence comparisons, one is usually more interested in finding conserved patterns or segments in two sequences by local alignment. In local alignment, the alignment stops at the ends of regions of strong similarity, and a much higher priority is given to finding these local regions than to extending the alignment to include more neighboring pairs. The Smith-Waterman algorithm finds a pair of segments, one from each of two long sequences, such that there is no other pair of segments with greater similarity. Both the Needleman-Wunsch algorithm and the Smith-Waterman algorithm for sequence alignment is available freely on EMBOSS (European Molecular Biology Open Software Suite, http://www.uk.embnet.org/Softwares/EMBOSS/) in programs called needle and water, respectively.

Although dynamic programming for sequence alignment is an efficient mathematical technique for optimum alignment, it is still too slow for comparing large numbers of bases. Typical DNA database today contains billions of bases, and the number is increasing rapidly. To allow sequence search and comparison to be performed at a reasonable time, fast heuristic local alignment algorithms have been developed. Although the resulting alignment is not guaranteed to be optimal anymore, the advantage of tremendous speed of the algorithms seems to far outweigh their potential shortcomings in optimality or sensitivity.

The most widely used heuristic database search tool is BLAST (Basic Local Alignment Search Tool) (Altschul et al., 1990, 1997), which runs one to two orders of magnitude faster than the Smith-Waterman algorithm. It has become the standard for sequence alignment and database searching. BLAST is freely available in many websites around the world, such as NCBI (National Center for Biotechnology Information, http://www.ncbi.nlm.nih.gov/BLAST) and the EBI (European Bioinformatics Institute, http://www.ebi.ad.uk/blastall). Many variants of BLAST have been developed to search for different type of databases and for different applications. For example, the NCBI website offers different types of BLAST database search that allow a user to search for protein sequence, DNA/RNA sequence, entire genome search, etc.

Sometimes it is necessary to align more than two sequences. Although the basic dynamic programming algorithm can be extended to multiple sequences to find optimum alignment, the complexity quickly gets out of hand to make the method impractical. Just three sequences of 1,000 bases each would require $1,000^3 = 1{\times}10^9$ comparisons, compared to $1,000^2 = 1{\times}10^6$ comparisons for two sequence alignment. A way to handle multiple

78   W.-C. Liew et al.

sequence alignment is to break down the problem into a series of pairwise matches which are then combined progressively in some way to obtain the final alignment. This is the technique used in *ClustalW* (Thompson et al., 1994, 1997) (available at http://www.ebi.ac.uk/clustalw/). Other algorithms for multiple sequence alignment are SAGA (Sequence Alignment by Genetic Algorithm, Notredame and Higgins, 1996, and Notredame and Higgins, 1996), MSASA (Multiple Sequence Alignment by Simulated Annealing, Kim et al., 1994), Hidden Markov Model-based methods such as SAM (Sequence Alignment and, Modeling software system, available at http://www.cse.ucsd.edu/research/compbio/sam.html, Hughey and Krogh 1996), and HMMER (http://hmmer.wustl.edu/, Eddy, 1998).

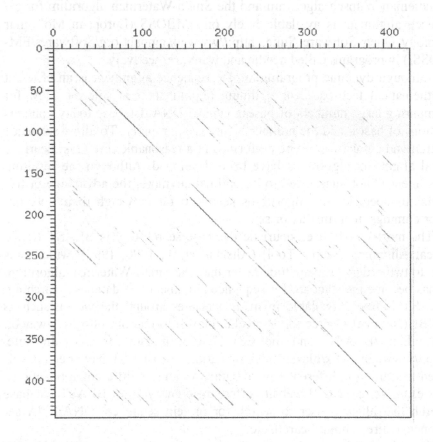

Fig. 4.4. Dot plot of two coding DNA sequences: the alpha chain of human hemoglobin is assigned to the horizontal axis and the beta chain of human hemoglobin is assigned to the vertical axis

Table 4.3. DNA sequences of the first exons of beta-globin genes for eight different species.

A	Human beta-globin	92 Bases

ATGGTGCACCTGACTCCTGAGGAGAAGTCTGCCGTTACTGCCCTGTGGGGC
AAGGTGAACGTGGATTAAGTTGGTGGTGAGGCCCTGGGCAG

B	Goat alanine beta-globin	86 Bases

ATGCTGACTGCTGAGGAGAAGGCTGCCGTCACCGGCTTCTGGGGCAAGGTG
AAAGTGGATGAAGTTGGTGCTGAGGCCCTGGGCAG

C	Opossum beta-hemoglobin beta-M-gene	92 Bases

ATGGTGCACTTGACTTCTGAGGAGAAGAACTGCATCACTACCATCTGGTCTA
AGGTGCAGGTTGACCAGACTGGTGGTGAGGCCCTTGGCAG

D	Gallus gallus beta-globin	92 Bases

ATGGTGCACTGGACTGCTGAGGAGAAGCAGCTCATCACCGGCCTCTGGGGC
AAGGTCAATGTGGCCGAATGTGGGGCCGAAGCCCTGGCCAG

E	Lemur beta-globin	92 Bases

ATGACTTTGCTGAGTGCTGAGGAGAATGCTCATGTCACCTCTCTGTGGGGCA
AGGTGGATGTAGAGAAAGTTGGTGGCGAGGCCTTGGGCAG

F	Mouse beta-a-globin	94 Bases

ATGGTTGCACCTGACTGATGCTGAGAAGTCTGCTGTCTCTTGCCTGTGGGCA
AAGGTGAACCCCGATGAAGTTGGTGGTGAGGCCCTGGGCAGG

G	Rabbit beta-globin	90 Bases

ATGGTGCATCTGTCCAGTGAGGAGAAGTCTGCGGTCACTGCCCTGTGGGGC
AAGGTGAATGTGGAAGAAGTTGGTGGTGAGGCCCTGGGC

H	Rat beta-globin	92 Bases

ATGGTGCACCTAACTGATGCTGAGAAGGCTACTGTTAGTGGCCTGTGGGGA
AAGGTGAACCCTGATAATGTTGGCGCTGAGGCCCTGGGCAG

When two sequences are to be compared qualitatively, the easiest way to see whether there are potential regions of similarity is probably by a graphical display called dot matrix plots (Gibbs and McIntyre, 1970, and States and Boguski, 1991). A dot matrix plot program called *Dotter* is available at http://www.cgb.ki.se/cgb/groups/sonnhammer/Dotter.html. Simple as it is, the dot matrix plot is still a popular tool for researchers to visually inspect the similarity between two sequences, and most sequence analysis packages will have one or more programs to produce these plots. In a dot matrix plot, one sequence is plotted on each axis, and a dot is drawn where the two sequences "match". The general rule for dot matrix plots is to examine the characters one by one, starting from the first character in the sequence on the vertical axis, and place a dot at locations in the row in the other sequence where the same character is found. Any region of similar sequence is revealed by a diagonal row of dots. Isolated dots represent random matches that are probably not related to any significant alignment.

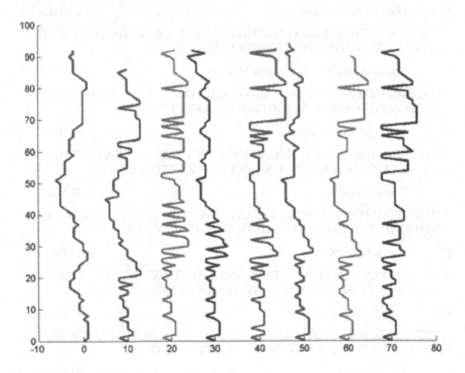

Fig. 4.5. The AC DB-Curve of the DNA sequences of the first exons of beta-globin genes for eight different species shown in Table 4.3

For a DNA sequence with only four alphabets, the above rule would put dots in about 25% of the possible places and fill the plot so that any real matches become impossible to see. Detection of matching regions may be improved by filtering out random matches in the dot matrix plot. Instead of comparing single characters, a window is used to compare a group of characters in both sequences (Maizel and Lenk, 1981). A dot is drawn in the plot if a certain minimal number of matches occur in the window. Figure 4.4 shows an example of a dot plot (produced with *Dotter*), comparing the alpha chain of human hemoglobin to the beta chain of human hemoglobin with a window length of 31. Matches and mismatches were assigned similarity values of +5 and -4, respectively, and the gray values of the dots scale with the similarity of two windows. One can clearly discern a diagonal trace along the entire length of the two sequences.

For relatively short sequences, sequence comparison can also be done visually by sequence visualization techniques. One such 2D visualization technique is the DB-Curve (Dual-Base Curve) (Wu et al., 2003a). In DB-curve DNA sequence visualization, two out of the four bases are considered at a time. The two bases are assigned +45° and −45° vectors, respectively, whereas the remaining bases are assigned +90° vectors. Starting at the origin, a DNA sequence can be mapped to a 2D curve by a cumulative plot of the bases in the sequence using the assigned vectors. Figure 4.5 shows the AC DB-Curve of the DNA sequences of the first exons of beta-globin genes for the eight different species shown in Table 4.3. Similarities and differences in the sequences can be readily observed from the plots.

Gene Prediction

Gene prediction has been an area of active research in bioinformatics (Mathe et al., 2002). Gene prediction requires the integration of many different signals such as promoter regions, translation start and stop codons, reading frame periodicities, polyadenylation (polyA) signals, and, for eukaryotes, intron splicing signals, base compositional bias between codon positions for exons and introns, and various coding statistics. Many of these signals and statistics are related to each other, and are often complementary in the sense that some may be weak when others are strong. Therefore, a combination of these signals is often employed in most existing gene prediction algorithms.

In prokaryotes, gene finding is made simpler by the fact that coding regions are not interrupted by intervening sequences such as introns. Still, for short open reading frames, it is highly nontrivial to distinguish between sequences that represent true genes and those that do not. A eukaryotic gene typically consists of exons interrupted by non-coding regions, such as introns or intergenic regions. Prediction of a eukaryotic gene is therefore a much more difficult problem.

In general, three approaches of gene prediction can be distinguished: similarity-based, content-based, and site-based. Similarity-based methods make use of already determined sequences by a comparison of sequence data. Content-based methods determine the overall properties of a sequence in terms of the various coding statistics. Site-based methods determine transcription factor binding sites, polyA signals, start and stop codons, splice junctions, and other specific subsequences or sequence patterns.

Since it is reasonable to assume that similar sequences would have similar biological and functional roles, the availability of a vast number of sequences in various databases means that similar sequences with the genes annotated in them could be used to annotate new uncharacterized sequences. Thus, a first step in gene finding would be to perform a database search using search tool like BLAST. The probable gene candidates obtained from the search could then be subjected to more sophisticated analysis, either algorithmic or experimental, to further validate the findings. The use of available site knowledge from already annotated sequences often results in substantial reduction in effort.

A sequence can also be analyzed for regions of high coding potential by an examination of various coding statistics. Such an approach has the advantage that no similar sequence is needed, as the information to predict the protein coding genes in the sequence is mined from the sequence itself. Of course, the sensitivity and accuracy of the prediction depends on the statistics used. Finding powerful coding statistics is still an area of active research in bioinformatics.

A coding statistic describes the likelihood that a DNA sequence is coding for a protein. Many such statistics have been proposed by various researchers. Some of these coding statistics are codon usage bias, base compositional bias between codon positions, and periodicity in base occurrence. Several excellent reviews of such statistics and algorithms are available (Fickett and Tung, 1992; Fickett, 1996; Burset and Guigo, 1996; and Guigo, 1999). The coding statistics can be furher divided into two classes (Guigo, 1999): model dependent and model independent. Model dependent statistics require a representative sample of coding DNA from the species under consideration to estimate the parameters of the model. For example, the codon usage table for *homo sapiens* (see Table 4.4 below) shows the relative frequency of usage of each codon in human coding regions versus the relative frequency of each codon among synonymous codons. Significant, non-random differences in codon usage frequency have been observed in the table. Thus, regions in which codons are used with frequencies similar to the typical species codon frequencies are likely to code for protein (Staden and McLachlan, 1982, and Staden, 1990). The bias in codon usage could also be used to identify the correct reading frame for an uncharacterized sequence.

Recognition of coding regions or ORFs in the human genome based on coding statistics is a difficult problem due to the short exon length, where the average length of exons of the vertebrate gene is only 137 bp (Hawkins, 1988). While good recognition rates can be achieved in the recognition of coding and non-coding regions in the yeast genome (Zhang and Wang, 2000), the strengths of the statistical features alone are generally not sufficient to identify human exons due to their limited average length. The use of splicing signals, such as stop codons, together with the coding statistics results in better prediction power (Thanaraj, 2000).

Table 4.4. The relative frequency of codon usage in *homo sapiens* (from http://www.kazusa.or.jp/codon/, where the statistics are computed from the Gen-Bank Release 139 database).

Amino acid	Codon	Freq per 1000	Fraction
Gly	GGG	16.49	0.25
Gly	GGA	16.41	0.25
Gly	GGT	10.81	0.16
Gly	GGC	22.52	0.34
Glu	GAG	39.99	0.58
Glu	GAA	29.04	0.42
Asp	GAT	22.03	0.46
Asp	GAC	25.52	0.54
Val	GTG	28.53	0.47
Val	GTA	7.06	0.12
Val	GTT	10.97	0.18
Val	GTC	14.60	0.24
Ala	GCG	7.53	0.11
Ala	GCA	16.04	0.23
Ala	GCT	18.62	0.26
Ala	GCC	28.27	0.40
Arg	AGG	11.69	0.21
Arg	AGA	11.72	0.21
Ser	AGT	12.11	0.15
Ser	AGC	19.47	0.24
Lys	AAG	32.18	0.57
Lys	AAA	24.04	0.43
Asn	AAT	16.74	0.47
Asn	AAC	19.18	0.53
Met	ATG	22.19	1.00
Ile	ATA	7.26	0.16
Ile	ATT	15.78	0.36
Ile	ATC	21.02	0.48
Thr	ACG	6.15	0.12
Thr	ACA	14.96	0.28

Thr	ACT	13.01	0.24
Thr	ACC	19.08	0.36
Trp	TGG	13.03	1.00
End	TGA	1.23	0.49
Cys	TGT	10.27	0.45
Cys	TGC	12.47	0.55
End	TAG	0.57	0.23
End	TAA	0.69	0.28
Tyr	TAT	12.09	0.44
Tyr	TAC	15.38	0.56
Leu	TTG	12.77	0.13
Leu	TTA	7.45	0.07
Phe	TTT	17.15	0.46
Phe	TTC	20.34	0.54
Ser	TCG	4.47	0.06
Ser	TCA	12.05	0.15
Ser	TCT	14.93	0.19
Ser	TCC	17.62	0.22
Arg	CGG	11.63	0.21
Arg	CGA	6.26	0.11
Arg	CGT	4.63	0.08
Arg	CGC	10.63	0.19
Gln	CAG	34.43	0.74
Gln	CAA	12.06	0.26
His	CAT	10.67	0.42
His	CAC	15.03	0.58
Leu	CTG	40.07	0.40
Leu	CTA	7.04	0.07
Leu	CTT	13.01	0.13
Leu	CTC	19.62	0.20
Pro	CCG	7.04	0.11
Pro	CCA	16.90	0.28
Pro	CCT	17.45	0.28
Pro	CCC	20.03	0.33

Not all types of coding statistics are equally powerful for any one species. Choosing the coding statistics that have the most discriminating power would lead to better recognition results. We have recently performed a study of several coding statistics for the recognition of human, yeast and C. elegans coding and non-coding sequences (Liew et al., 2004). The statistics we considered are listed below:

1. Two ATG triplet features
   Note that the ATG triplet that is involved in the initiation of translation is called start codon.
   - Let the total number of the triplet ATGs contained in all three frames in a sequence be denoted by n. The number of frames containing the triplet ATG in a sequence is denoted by K, i.e., $K = 0, 1, 2, 3$. The ATG triplet statistic is defined by $f_1 = (1 + K^2) \times n$.
   - $f_2 = N_{ATG}$, where N_{ATG} is the number of triplet ATGs in the sequence.
2. Two stop codon features
   The number of triplets TAA, TAG, and TGA occurring in each frame of the sequence is counted.
   - As with f_1, the stop codon feature is defined by $f_3 = (1 + K^2) \times n$. This feature has been used by Wang et al. (2002).
   - $f_4 = \max(N_{TAA}, N_{TAG}, N_{TGA})$.
3. Three asymmetric features of distribution of nucleotides at the three triplet positions
   - The Position Asymmetry (PA) of the sequence (Guigo, 1999)
     Let $f(b, r)$ be the relative frequency of nucleotide b at triplet position r. Let $f(b) = \sum_{r=1}^{3} (f(b, r))/3$ be the average frequency of nucleotide b at the three triplet positions, and define the asymmetry in the distribution of nucleotide b as the variance of this frequency, i.e., $asym(b) = \sum_{i=1}^{3} (f(b, i) - f(b))^2$; the PA of the sequence is defined as $f_5 = PA = asym(A) + asym(C) + asym(G) + asym(T)$.
   - One Purine feature
     It is well known that the predominant bases at the first codon position in the reading frame are purines and this fact is independent of species, whereas bases in non-coding regions tend to be randomly distributed. The occurrence frequencies of purines in the three reading frames are denoted by $(a_i + g_i)$, $i = 1, 2, 3$, and the purine feature is defined as $f_6 = \max_i (a_i + g_i)$, $i = 1, 2, 3$.
   - One Pyrimidine feature

It is well known that the predominant bases at the third codon position in the reading frame are pyrimidines and this fact is independent of species. The occurrence frequencies of pyrimidines in the three frames are denoted by $(c_i + t_i)$, $i = 1, 2, 3$. The pyrimidine feature is defined by $f_7 = \max_i (c_i + t_i)$, $i = 1, 2, 3$.

4. Nine Z-Curve features (Zhang and Zhang, 1994)

The Z-Curve features are based on the differences of single nucleotide frequencies at the three codon positions between the protein coding ORFs and the non-coding ones. The frequencies of bases A, C, G, and T occurring in an ORF or a fragment of DNA sequence with bases at positions 1, 4, 7, ...; 2, 5, 8,...; and 3, 6, 9, ... are denoted by a_1, c_1, g_1, and t_1; a_2, c_2, g_2, and t_2; and a_3, c_3, g_3, and t_3, respectively. They are actually the frequencies of bases at the first, second, and third codon positions. Let x_1, y_1, z_1; and x_2, y_2, z_2; x_3, y_3, z_3 be given by

$$\begin{cases} x_i = (a_i + g_i) - (c_i + t_i) \\ y_i = (a_i + c_i) - (g_i + t_i), & i = 1, 2, 3 \\ z_i = (a_i + t_i) - (g_i + c_i) \end{cases} \tag{4.1}$$

Then the nine Z-Curve features, f_8 to f_{16}, are defined by

$$\begin{cases} f_8 = x_1, f_9 = y_1, f_{10} = z_1 \\ f_{11} = x_2, f_{12} = y_2, f_{13} = z_2 \\ f_{14} = x_3, f_{15} = y_3, f_{16} = z_3 \end{cases} \tag{4.2}$$

5. Three Simple Z-Curve (SZ) features (Wu et al., 2002)

The SZ features, f_{17} to f_{19}, are defined by

$$\begin{cases} f_{17} = \max_i [(a_i + g_i) - (c_i + t_i)] \\ f_{18} = \max_i [(a_i + c_i) - (g_i + t_i)], & i = 1, 2, 3 \\ f_{19} = \max_i [(a_i + t_i) - (g_i + c_i)] \end{cases} \tag{4.3}$$

6. Three periodic correlations features between nucleotide positions (Fickett, 1982, and Guigo, 1999)

- Periodic Asymmetry Index (PAI)

  Given a sequence, the following three distinct probabilities can be considered (Konopka, 1994):

  - the probability P_{in} of finding pairs of the same nucleotide at distances $k = 3, 6, 9, ...$,

- the probability P_{out}^1 of finding pairs of the same nucleotide at distances $k = 1, 4, 7,...$, and

- the probability P_{out}^2 of finding pairs of the same nucleotide at distances $k = 2, 5, 8,....$

Note that nucleotide pairs at distances of $k = 3, 6, 9, ...$ nucleotides are at the same codon position, whereas nucleotide pairs at other distances are not. Because of the 3-base periodic pattern, P_{in} will be larger than the other two probabilities in coding regions, while in non-coding regions the three probabilities will be similar. The tendency to cluster homogeneous dinucleotides in a 3-base periodic pattern can be measured by the Periodic Asymmetry Index

$$f_{20} = PAI = \frac{\max\left(P_{in}, P_{out}^1, P_{out}^2\right)}{\min\left(P_{in}, P_{out}^1, P_{out}^2\right)} \tag{4.4}$$

- Average Mutual Information (AMI) (Grosse et al., 2000)

It is well known that a coding sequence exhibits a 3-base periodicity due to non-uniform codon usage, and this periodicity shows up as the correlation between nucleotide i and nucleotide j at a distance of k nucleotides (Li W., 1997). For each distance k, sixteen different individual correlations can be calculated. A measure that summarizes all individual correlations at a given distance k is the mutual information function,

$$I(k) = \sum_{i,j \in \{A,C,G,T\}} P_{ij}(k) \log_2 \left(\frac{P_{ij}(k)}{P_i P_j}\right) \tag{4.5}$$

The mutual information $I(k)$ quantifies the amount of information that can be obtained from one nucleotide about another nucleotide at a distance k. For a coding sequence, $I(k)$ has larger values for $k = 3, 6, 9, ...$, and the 3-base periodic pattern in coding sequences is obvious. Thus, in coding DNA, $I(k)$ oscillates between two values, while in non-coding DNA, $I(k)$ is rather flat. Herzel and Grosse (1995) called the two values between which $I(k)$ oscillates in coding DNA the in-frame mutual information I_{in} at distances $k = 3, 6, 9,...$, and the out-of-frame mutual information I_{out} at $k = 4, 5, 7, 8,...$ In order to reduce the pairs of numbers I_{in} and I_{out} to a single quantity, they compute the Average Mutual Information (AMI) as (Grosse et al., 2000)

$$f_{21} = AMI = \frac{I_{in} + 2I_{out}}{3} \tag{4.6}$$

- Fourier Spectrum feature

  Periodic correlations in DNA sequences can also be examined by means of Fourier analysis (Tiwari et al., 1997). DNA coding regions reveal the characteristic 3-base periodicity, which shows up as a distinct peak at the frequency index $k = N/3$, where N is the length of the sequence. No such peak is apparent for non-coding sequences. The Fourier Spectrum feature f_{22} is defined as follows. Let $A_d(t)$, $C_d(t)$, $G_d(t)$, and $T_d(t)$ be the number of distinct pairs of nucleotide bases A, T, G, and C, respectively, in a DNA sequence separated by a distance t, where t ranges from 1 to N. Let $s(t) = A_d(t) + C_d(t) + G_d(t) + T_d(t)$. Let $S(k)$ be the Discrete Fourier Transform (DFT) of $s(t)$, i.e.,

$$S(k) = \sum_{t=0}^{N-1} s(t)e^{-j2\pi kt/N} \tag{4.7}$$

For 3-base periodicity, $S(k)$ should exhibit a strong peak at the frequency index $k = N/3$. Let $P(k) = |S(k)|^2$ be the power spectrum of $S(k)$, then the Fourier Spectrum feature f_{22} is defined as

$$f_{22} = \frac{P(k)}{\frac{1}{2w+1} \sum_{j=k-w}^{j=k+w} P(j)} \tag{4.8}$$

where $k = N/3$ and $2w+1$ is the window used to obtain the average power spectrum within the window.

Altogether, 22 statistical features are compared. Their discriminating power for coding and non-coding sequences is evaluated using the information-theoretic measure called mutual information, which essentially measures the information the feature gives us about the two class labels (i.e., coding vs non-coding). The mutual information of every feature has been computed in the 6,000 Yeast ORFs and 6,000 Yeast NoFeature sequences, 3,000 C. elegans coding sequences and 3,000 small non-coding RNAs, 1,500 Human exons and 1,500 introns, respectively. The results are presented in Table 4.5 and Fig. 4.6.

We see that, in general, the discriminating power of most of the statistical features, with the exception of PA, PAI, AMI, and the last SZ feature, is significantly lower for human than for yeast or C. elegans. For the recognition of human exons, it seems that statistics that measure the asymmetry in nucleotide distribution at the three codon positions (PA), and those that measure the periodic structure in the sequence (PAI and AMI) have better discriminating power than the other statistics (except the three SZ features). One can also observe that the three SZ features perform reasonably well for the recognition of human exons. In fact, the third SZ feature has the second largest discriminating power among all 22 features tested. The three SZ features also perform better than almost all Z Curve features for Human, although the two sets of features are quite closely related. This observation is less valid for the other two species.

Table 4.5. Comparison of mutual information of 22 statistical features for three different species.

		Human	Yeast	C.elegans
	f1 = ATG triplet feature 1	0.0378	0.2507	0.2912
	f2 = ATG triplet feature 2	0.0550	0.2748	0.3032
	f3 = Stop Codon feature 1	0.1000	0.1856	0.2152
	f4 = Stop Codon feature 2	0.0110	0.1665	0.1759
	f5 = Position Asymmetry (PA)	0.3073	0.1320	0.1066
	f6 = First Codon (Purines)	0.0629	0.2884	0.2308
	f7 = Third Codon (pyrimidines)	0.0546	0.2435	0.2857
Z	f8 = (a1+g1)-(c1+t1)	0.0451	0.5377	0.4459
	f9 = (a1+c1)-(g1+t1)	0.0417	0.1592	0.0662
	f10 = (a1+t1)-(c1+g1)	0.0826	0.0702	0.0565
	f11 = (a2+g2)-(c2+t2)	0.0862	0.1082	0.0999
	f12 = (a2+c2)-(g2+t2)	0.0839	0.3791	0.2127
	f13 = (a2+t2)-(c2+g2)	0.1111	0.1646	0.2736
	f14 = (a3+g3)-(c3+t3)	0.0388	0.1439	0.1252
	f15 = (a3+c3)-(g3+t3)	0.0215	0.1083	0.1133
	f16 = (a3+t3)-(c3+g3)	0.0683	0.1489	0.1034
SZ	$f17 = \max_i[(a_i + g_i)-(c_i + t_i)]$	0.1406	0.4270	0.2623
	$f18 = \max_i[(a_i + c_i)-(g_i + t_i)]$	0.0985	0.3188	0.2339
	$f19 = \max_i[(a_i + t_i)-(g_i + c_i)]$	0.2977	0.1813	0.2304
	f20 = PAI	0.1478	0.0308	0.0930
	f21 = AMI	0.1760	0.0020	0.0558
	f22 = FFT	0.1182	0.5155	0.4308

Another important observation is that features that do well on Yeast and C. elegans perform rather poorly on Human. The converse is generally true as well. We see that PA, which is the most discriminating feature among all 22 features for Human, has a fairly low discriminating value for both Yeast and C. elegans. The first SZ feature and the FFT feature are good for Yeast and C. elegans, and are also fairly good for human. These two features could potentially be useful for independent recognition of exons of species.

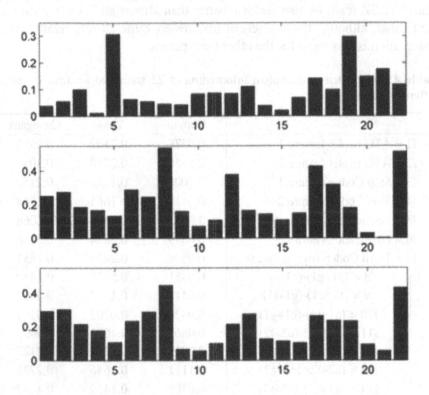

Fig. 4.6. The MI of 22 features for Human (top), Yeast (middle), and C.elegans (bottom)

From the above study, we see that certain statistical features are more species-dependent than others. Choosing the better features, and a good classification algorithm, would potentially give a better recognition rate. To illustrate, we perform classification experiments using the two most discriminating features for Human, i.e., set1 = (f_5, f_{19}), and the two most discriminating features for Yeast and C. elegans, i.e., set2 = (f_8, f_{22}) (see Fig. 4.6 for their MI values relative to other features). Using a simple K-Nearest-Neighbor (KNN) classifier, we obtain classification accuracy for

Human of 80.33% for set1, and only 63.16% for set2. For Yeast, the accuracy is 81.74% for set1 and 90.89% for set2, while for C. elegans, the accuracy is 80.28% for set1 and 89.83% for set2. In another experiment using just the three SZ features, the PA feature, and the first stop codon feature, we were able to obtain around 90~92% accuracy in the classification of short human exons and introns using the same KNN classifier, without compromising sensitivity and specificity (Wu et al., 2003b, and Liew et al., 2004).

Besides consideration of coding statistics, gene prediction could also involve identification of splice sites, promoter regions, transcription factors binding sites, and polyA sites (Mount, 2001). Many database and algorithms have been created for this purpose.

Although significant advances in gene prediction algorithms have been made, gene prediction in the complex genome of higher eukaryotes is still a difficult problem. Some of the latest gene prediction algorithms have used machine learning techniques such as neural networks, pattern recognition methods, and rule-based methods and probabilistic models such as Hidden Markov models to achieve better prediction results. Some examples of these algorithms are GRAIL (Uberbacher et al., 1996), GeneScan (Tiwari et al., 1997), Glimmer (Salzberg et al., 1998a), GeneMark.hmm (Lukashin and Borodovsky, 1998), MZEF (Zhang, 1997), GeneFinder (http://dot.imgen.bcm.tmc.edu:9331/gene-finder/gf.html), and MORGAN (Salzberg et al., 1998b).

It is clear that additional work is required to further improve the detection rates and to decrease the level of falsely predicted genes. Such improvements may come from the incorporation of new and better submodels of promoters or initial and terminal exons, as well as of other physical properties and signals present in the DNA, such as bendability or nucleosome positioning.

Phylogenetic Analysis

Analysis of multiple DNA sequences for phylogenetic study is an important area of sequence analysis. A phylogenetic analysis of a family of related DNA or protein sequences is a determination of how the family might have been derived during molecular evolution (Li W.H., 1997; Graur and Li, 2000; and Swofford et al., 1996). Phylogenetic analysis leads to the construction of an evolution tree. The evolutionary relationships among the sequences are depicted by placing the sequences the leaves on the tree in such a way that the branching relationship in the tree reflects the degree to which different sequences are related. Phylogenetic study performed on a gene family could also aid in the prediction of genes with equivalent or similar functions. It could also be used to track changes in the genome of a rapidly changing (i.e., by mutation) species, such as a virus.

Phylogenetic analysis is closely linked to sequence alignment. Three methods that are commonly used to derive the phylogenetic tree that best account for the observed variation in a group of sequences are: maximum parsimony method, distance method, and maximum likelihood method (Felsenstein, 1996). The choice of method depends on the results of the multiple sequence alignment performed on the set of sequences, and whether the assumptions underlying the method fit well with the data.

For parsimony analysis, the best results are obtained when the amount of variation among all pairs of sequences is similar and the amount of variation is small. It is not good for reconstructing ancient phylogenies. If variation among sequences is present (some sequences are more similar than others) and the amount of variation is intermediate, distance method can be used. In the distance method, the concept of genetic distance between two sequences needs to be defined appropriately, depending on the type of sequences in consideration, and on their structural properties. Algorithms are also available for converting sequence similarity scores into distance scores (Feng and Doolittle, 1996, Altschul and Gish, 1996). The genetic distances between sequences are then used to construct the phylogenetic tree. Maximum likelihood methods are particularly useful when the sequences are more variable. The method uses probability calculations based on an explicit evolutionary model, e.g., the F84 substitution model in the PHYLIP package (Felsenstein, 1993) and the TN93 substitution model (Tamura and Nei, 1993), to find a tree that best accounts for the variation in the sequence.

Phylogenetic analysis programs are widely available. Two main ones are PHYLIP (available at http://evolution.genetics.washington.edu/phylip.html) and PAUP (available at http://www.lms.si.edu/PAUP/). Both packages provide the three main methods for phylogenetic analysis described above, as well as many types of evolutionary models for sequence variation.

4.4 Protein Data Analysis

4.4.1 Protein and Amino Acid Sequence

Protein synthesis constitutes the final stage of information flow within a cell, where the genetic code in the coding regions of a DNA sequence is translated into biomolecular end products that perform specific cellular and biological functions. Proteomics, the study of proteins and their interactions, is emerging as an important area of bioscience. An understanding of proteins and their functions would lead to new approaches for the diagnosis and treatment of diseases, for the discovery of new drugs, and for disease control.

Proteins are composed of linear, unbranched chains of amino acids (from an alphabet of 20 amino acids), linked together by peptide bonds. Amino acids, the basic building blocks of proteins, have a general structure, as shown in Fig. 4.7 The general structure consists of two functional groups (amino group, NH_2, and carboxyl group, COOH), an H atom, and a distinctive side group R, all bound to a carbon center called the alpha-carbon. The differences between the 20 amino acids are in the nature of the R groups. These vary considerably in their chemical and physical properties. It is the chemistry of the R groups that determine the many interactions that stabilize the structure of protein and enable its biological function. Special roles are played by glycine (G), which has only a hydrogen atom as its side group, and therefore has greater local flexibility in structures, and cysteine (C), which can react with another cysteine to form a cross-link (disulphide bond) that can stabilize the protein structure. The amino acids are linked together by peptide bonds to form a polypeptide chain. The peptide bond results from a condensation reaction involving the amino and carboxylic acid moieties on two amino acids (see Fig. 4.8). The peptide bond is very stable and has unusual conformational properties.

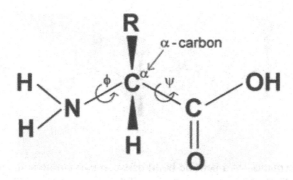

Fig. 4.7. General structure of amino acid

Proteins are complex organic molecules that perform their functions through interactions with other molecules at the molecular level. A full understanding of the molecular functions of proteins therefore requires information about their 3D structures at the molecular level. Protein structures are hierarchical (Branden and Tooze, 1999). The *primary structure* of protein refers to the sequence of amino acids that make up the protein. The *secondary structure* refers to the local folding pattern of the polypeptide chain. The *tertiary structure* describes how the secondary structure elements are arranged to form the overall 3D folding pattern. The tertiary structure is held together by hydrogen, ionic, and disulphide bonds between amino acids. It is this unique structure that gives a protein is specific function. Examples of proteins with tertiary structure include enzymes. The *quaternary structure* describes the interaction of two or more globular or tertiary structures and other groups such as metal ions or cofactors that make up the functional protein. The quaternary structure is held together by ionic, hydrogen, and disulfide bonds between amino acids. An example of a protein with a quaternary structure is hemoglobin.

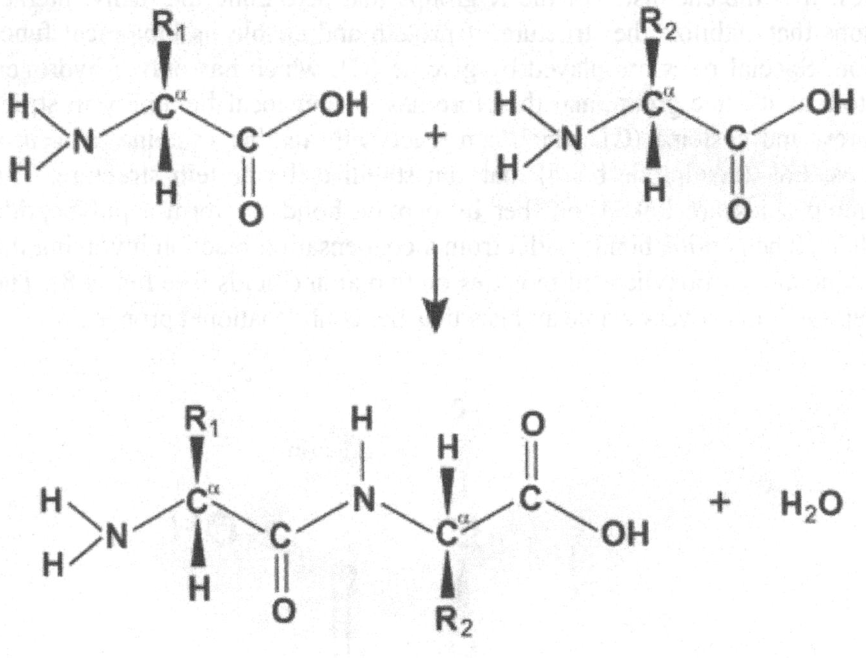

Fig. 4.8. The formation of a peptide bond between two amino acids to form a peptide chain. The N-Cα-N sequence is repeated throughout the protein and forms the backbone of the 3D structure

The secondary structure of proteins is predominantly stabilized by hydrogen bonds and is generally classified into four types: α-helix, β-sheet, loop, and random coil. The α-helix is the most common form of secondary structure in proteins. The helix has 3.6 amino acid residues per turn, and is stabilized by hydrogen bonding between the backbone carbonyl oxygen of one residue and the backbone NH of the fourth residue along the helix. Certain amino acids have a distinct preference for α-helices. Alanine (A), glutamic acid (E), leucine (L), and methionine (M) are good helix formers, whereas praline (P), glycine (G), tyrosine (Y), and serine (S) are helix-breaking residues. This preference forms the basis for computer prediction of the general locations of α-helices in a new protein sequence.

The second most common element of secondary structure in proteins is the β-sheet. A β-sheet is formed from several individual β-strands that are distant from each other along the primary protein sequence (see Figure. 4.9). β-strands are usually five to 10 residues long, and are in fully extended conformation. The individual strands are aligned next to each other in such a way that carbonyl oxygens are hydrogen-bonded with neighboring NH groups. Two types of connection topology are seen in β-sheets. The most stable is the antiparallel β-sheet. In antiparallel sheets, the β-strands are connected sequentially. Parallel β-sheets are less stable due to the hydrogen bonds not being optimally aligned, and are formed from segments of a peptide backbone distantly connected by other types of secondary structures. It is more difficult to predict the location of β-sheets than of α-helices.

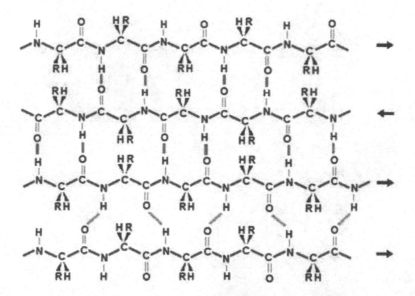

Fig. 4.9. Hydrogen bond patterns in beta sheets. Here, a four-stranded beta sheet, which contains three antiparallel and one parallel strand, is drawn schematically. Hydrogen bonds are indicated with red lines (antiparallel strands) and green lines (parallel strands) connecting the hydrogen and receptor oxygen

96   W.-C. Liew et al.

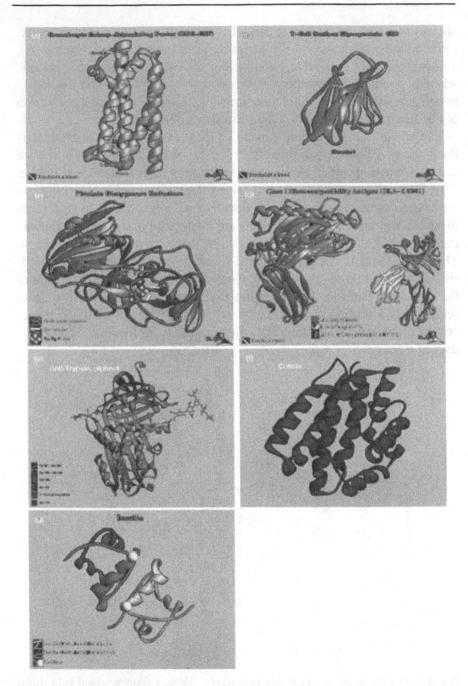

Fig. 4.10. Seven protein classes as defined in SCOP. Images are taken from http://scop.mrc-lmb.cam.ac.uk/scop/

Loops are regions of a protein chain that connect α-helices and β-strands or sheets to each other. In general, the helices and sheets form the stable hydrophobic core of the protein, and the connecting loops are to be found on the surface of the structure. Loops are rich in polar and charged amino acids, and are frequently a component of binding sites and enzyme active sites. Because amino acids in loops are not constrained by space and environment, unlike amino acids in the core region, and because they do not have an effect on the arrangement of secondary structures in the core, more substitutions, insertions, and deletions may occur. Thus, in a sequence alignment, the presence of these features may be an indication of a loop.

Random coil is the term used for segments of polypeptide chains that do not form regular secondary structures. Such conformations are not really random: they are the result of a balance of interactions between amino acid side chains and the solvent and interactions between sidechains. The predominant hydrogen-bonding pattern in random coils is between polypeptide and water; concerted hydrogen bonding networks are absent.

Depending on the type of secondary structures present, the tertiary structure of a protein is classified into seven classes in the SCOP database (structural classification of proteins, http://scop.mrclmb.cam.ac.uk /scop/):

1. All α proteins (Fig. 4.10a)
2. All β proteins (Fig. 4.10b)
3. Alpha and beta proteins (α / β) (Fig. 4.10c)
   Mainly parallel β-sheets with intervening α-helices
4. Alpha and beta proteins (α +b) (Fig. 4.10d)
   Mainly segregated α-helices and antiparallel β-sheet
5. Multi-domain proteins (α and β) (Fig. 4.10e)
   Folds consisting of two or more domains belonging to different classes
6. Membrane and cell surface proteins and peptides (Fig. 4.10f)
   Exclude proteins in the immune system
7. Small proteins (Fig. 4.10g)
   Usually dominated by metal ligand, heme, and/or disulfide bridges

Some of the internet resources on protein structure classification, modeling, and databases are listed below:

• http://www.biochem.ucl.ac.uk/bsm/cath/class.html
  The CATH database is a hierarchical domain classification of protein structures in the Brookhaven protein databank (Orengo et al., 1997, and Pearl et al., 2000). The four major levels in the hierarchy are class, architecture, topology (fold family), and homologous superfamily.
• http://scop.mrc-lmb.cam.ac.uk/scop/

The SCOP (Structural Classification of Proteins) database aims to provide a detailed and comprehensive description of the structural and evolutionary relationships between all proteins whose structure is known, including all entries in the Protein Data Bank (Murzin et al., 1995; Lo Conte et al., 2002; and Andreeva et al., 2004). The SCOP classification of proteins has been constructed manually by visual inspection and comparison of structures. Proteins are classified to reflect both structural and evolutionary relatedness. The principal levels of hierarchy in SCOP are family, superfamily, and fold.

- http://www.expasy.org/swissmod/SWISS-MODEL.html
  SWISS-Model is a fully automated protein structure homologymodeling server (Schwede et al., 2003). A variety of methods are used in Swiss-Model.

- http://www.rcsb.org/pdb/
  Protein Data Bank (PDB) (Berman et al., 2000) is a repository of 3D protein structure data determined from X-ray or nuclear magnetic resonance (NMR). The 3D coordinates of each atom in the protein molecule is deposited as a PDB entry. PDB files can be retrieved and displayed with a molecular viewer such as Rasmol (available at http://www.bernstein-plus-sons.com/software/rasmol/) or Swiss-PdbViewer (available at http://us.expasy.org/spdbv/).

- http://www2.ebi.ac.uk/dali/
  The DALI (Distance ALIgnment tool) server is a network service for comparing protein structures in 3D. A user submits the coordinates of a query protein structure and DALI compares them against those in the PDB.

- http://www2.ebi.ac.uk/dali/fssp/fssp.html
  The FSSP (Fold classification based on Structure-Structure alignment of Proteins) database is based on an exhaustive all-against-all 3D structure comparison of protein structures currently in the PDB using the DALI program (Sander, 1996a). The classification and alignments are automatically maintained and continuously updated using the DALI search engine.

- http://www.compbio.dundee.ac.uk/3Dee/
  3Dee contains structural domain definitions for all protein chains in the PDB that have 20 or more residues and are not theoretical models (Siddiqui et al., 2001). The domains have been clustered by both sequence and structural similarity.

- http://www.sander.ebi.ac.uk/dssp/
  The DSSP (Database of Secondary Structure in Proteins) database is a database of secondary structure assignments for all protein entries in the

Protein Data Bank (PDB). The DSSP program was designed by Wolf-gang Kabsch and Chris Sander (Kabsch and Sander, 1983) to standard-ize secondary structure assignment. The DSSP program defines secon-dary structure, geometrical features, and solvent exposure of proteins given the 3D atomic coordinates in Protein Data Bank format. The pro-gram does not predict protein structure.

Before a protein can be studied, it has to be identified. There are two main approaches for protein identification (Figeys, 2002): (i) identification by 2D gel electrophoresis, which separates proteins by both size and over-all electrical charge, and (ii) identification by mass spectrometry, where the exact mass of each peptide fragment cleaved by using a selective pro-tease, for example, the enzyme trypsin, can be determined. Knowledge of the exact mass of each of the protein fragments serves as a "fingerprint," and allows the identification of the protein's gene and, thus, its amino acid sequence.

As proteins are amino acid sequences, and the amino acid composition is dictated by the genetic code in a DNA sequence, proteins can also be de-rived, in principle, directly from DNA sequence data. The determination of proteins by direct translation from DNA sequences is an attractive ap-proach in view of the large amount of nucleotide sequences available to-day. However, the existence of introns in a (eukaryotes) gene and the oc-currence of alternative splicings make the prediction of protein from a nucleotide sequence a difficult task.

4.4.2 Protein Data Analysis

Protein Sequence Comparison

Proteins can be compared in terms of sequence similarity or structural similarity. There is one important difference between sequence and struc-tural similarity. Significant sequence similarity is usually an important in-dicator of an evolutionary relationship between sequences. In contrast, sig-nificant structural similarity is common, even among proteins that do not share any sequence similarity or evolutionary relationship.

The similarity between two protein sequences can be assessed by se-quence comparison. In protein sequence alignment, the problem of degen-eracy in the genetic code (where multiple DNA triplets may code for the same amino acid) does not occur. In addition, it is much less likely that two proteins will have the same letter (amino acid), by chance alone, at any position, since protein sequences are written with a 20-letter alphabet (see Table 4.1 in Subsection 4.2.1). Many of the sequence alignment and comparison tools that are used for DNA sequence comparison can also be used for protein sequences. In protein sequence alignment, the amino acid sequence of a protein is aligned to another amino acid sequence, with possible insertions (i.e., gaps) and deletions, such that the distance between the two sequences is minimized or the similarity score is maximized.

To align and assess the similarity of two protein sequences, the varying degrees of similarity between amino acids needs to be taken into account. The varying degrees of similarity reflect the different likelihoods of one amino acid being substituted for another during the course of molecular evolution. Quantification of the similarity between amino acids is by means of scoring matrices. The 20 by 20 matrices, relating each amino acid to every amino acid, fall into the PAM, Percent or Point Accepted Mutation (Dayhoff et al., 1978; Schwartz and Dayhoff, 1978; and Jones et al., 1992b), and BLOSUM, BLOcks SUbstitution Matrix (Henikoff and Henikoff, 1992, 1994) classes.

PAM is a unit introduced by Dayhoff et al. to quantify the amount of evolutionary change in a protein sequence. One PAM unit is the amount of evolution which will change, on average, 1% of amino acids in a protein sequence. A PAM(x) substitution matrix is a lookup table in which scores for each amino acid substitution have been calculated based on the frequency of that substitution in closely related proteins, i.e., global alignments of protein sequences that are at least 85% identical, that have experienced a certain amount x of evolutionary divergence. Other PAM matrices are extrapolated from PAM1 by matrix multiplication.

The BLOSUM matrix is constructed from blocks of sequences derived from the Blocks database (http://www.blocks.fhcrc.org/). The Blocks database contains multiply aligned ungapped segments or blocks that correspond to the most highly conserved regions of proteins. BLOSUM is constructed from these blocks by examining the substitution frequencies of each amino acid pair. The matrix number in a BLOSUM matrix, e.g., as in BLOSUM 62, means that the matrix is derived from blocks containing (≥62%) identities in ungapped sequence alignment. Unlike with PAM, at least that many BLOSUM matrices are based on observed alignments and are not extrapolated from comparisons of closely related proteins. In general, BLOSUM performs better than PAM. BLOSUM 62 is the default matrix for the standard protein BLAST program.

Alignment tools for protein sequences are very similar to those for nucleotide sequences. Some popular alignment tools are: (i) the BLAST family (http://www.ncbi.nlm.nih.gov/BLAST/), i.e., *blastp*, phi-*blast*, *psi-blast*, (ii) FASTA (http://www.ebi.ac.uk/fasta33/#), and (iii) ClustalW (for multiple sequence alignment, http://www.ebi.ac.uk/clustalw/).

Protein Structure Comparison

The 3D structure of a protein can be determined by X-ray crystallography or nuclear magnetic resonance (NMR) spectroscopy (Branden and Tooze, 1999). The procedure for X-ray crystallography requires the protein to first be in the form of crystals. A narrow beam of X-rays is then directed at the protein crystal, where the atoms in the protein molecules scatter the incoming X-rays. These scattered waves either reinforce or cancel one another, producing a complex diffraction pattern. The position and intensity of each spot in the diffraction pattern contain information about the position of the atoms in the protein crystal that can be deciphered by a computer. By combining this information with the known amino acid sequence of the protein, an atomic model of the protein's structure can be generated. In NMR spectroscopy, a solution of pure protein is placed in a strong magnetic field and then bombarded with radio waves of different frequencies. The hydrogen nuclei in the protein would generate an NMR signal that can be used to determine the distances between the amino acids and between different parts of the protein. The NMR spectrum, together with the known amino acid sequence, would allow us to compute the 3D structure of the protein.

As more and more protein structures have been determined and deposited in various protein structure databases, the prediction of protein structure by computer algorithms is becoming more feasible. When proteins of unknown structure are similar to a protein of known structure at the sequence level, the 3D structure of the proteins can be predicted. The stronger the similarity and identity, the more similar are the 3D folds and other structural features of the proteins. However, it should be noted that proteins with no apparent sequence similarity could also have very similar structure, and that the 3D structure of protein is much more highly conserved than the amino acid sequence (Mizuguchi and Blundell, 2000, Shapiro and Harris, 2000). By tracking their structural similarities, very distant evolutionary relationships between proteins may be inferred.

Several methods have been proposed to compare protein structures and measure the degree of structural similarity between them. These methods are based either on alignment of intra- and inter-molecular atomic distances (e.g., DALI) or on alignment of secondary structure elements (e.g., VAST). In the latter case, two proteins are compared based on the types and arrangements of their α-helices and β-strands, as well as on the ways in which these elements are connected. Because there are relatively few secondary structural elements in proteins, vectors giving their lengths, relative positions, and directions may provide a fast and reliable way to align structures.

The well known program DALI (Distance ALIgnment tool) is based on the alignment of 2D distance matrices, which represent all intra-molecular Cα-Cα distances of a protein structure (Holm and Sander, 1993, and Holm and Sander, 1996a). For a given pair of structures, DALI attempts to compute the optimal arrangement of similar contact patterns from their respective distance matrices. Each distance matrix is first split into hexapeptide fragments, and all pairs of similar fragments from the two structures are stored in a pair list. The final alignment is computed by assembling pairs of overlapping fragments from the pair list. The scoring function for an alignment of two structures is based on the intra-molecular distances. DALI has been used to perform an exhaustive all-against-all 3D structure comparison of protein structures currently in the Protein Data Bank (PDB) to create the FSSP database (Holm and Sander, 1996b; http://www2. ebi.ac.uk/dali/fssp/fssp.html) and the classification and alignments in FSSP are automatically maintained and continuously updated using DALI.

The program VAST (Vector Alignment Search Tool) is based on aligning secondary structure elements (Madej et al., 1995, and Grindley et al., 1993). In VAST, all pairs of secondary structure elements (one from each structure) that have the same type are represented as nodes of a graph. Two nodes are connected by an edge if the distance and angle between the corresponding pairs of secondary structure elements from the two proteins are within some threshold. The graph therefore represents correspondences between pairs of secondary structure elements that have the same type, relative orientation, and connectivity. This correspondence graph is then searched to find the maximal subgraph such that every node in the subgraph is connected to every other node in the subgraph and is not contained in any larger subgraph with this property. This finds the initial secondary structure alignment. VAST then extends this initial alignment to a residue level alignment using a Gibbs sampling technique. VAST only reports alignments that yield a P-value less than 0.05. A P-value of 0.05 indicates that *VAST* expects to find an alignment with the same degree of similarity by chance in 5% of all pair-wise comparisons. VAST has been used to compare all known PDB domains to each other. The results of this computation are included in NCBI's Molecular Modeling Database at http://www.ncbi.nlm.nih.gov/Structure/VAST/vast.html.

Protein Structure Prediction

Comparative Modeling

The structure of a new protein could be predicted based on the presence of certain patterns or motifs, such as specific amino acid patterns or profiles that are known to have specific structures. This type of prediction is also called *comparative modeling*, and is useful when there is a clear sequence relationship between the target structure and one or more known structures. To facilitate such motif-based protein structure prediction, known proteins are being analyzed computationally to discover the motif-structure relationship in several motif-based protein family databases. The PROSITE database (http://us.expasy.org/prosite/) (Sigrist et al., 2002) is an annotated collection of motif descriptors dedicated to the identification of protein families and domains. The motif descriptors used in PROSITE are either patterns or profiles that are derived from multiple sequence alignments of homologous sequences. Patterns, which are typically around 10 to 20 amino acids in length, arise because specific residues or regions thought or proved to be important to the biological function of a group of proteins are conserved in both structure and sequence during evolution. Patterns are qualitative motif descriptors; they either do or do not match. In contrast, profiles are quantitative motifs providing numerical weights for each possible match and mismatch between a sequence residue and a profile position. Profiles characterize protein domains over their entire length, not just over their most conserved parts. A mismatch at a highly conserved position can still be accepted provided the rest of the sequence displays a sufficiently high level of similarity. The generalized profiles used in PROSITE allow the detection of even poorly conserved domains or families.

Several other motif-based protein family databases are: Pfam (Protein families database of alignments and HMMs, at http://www.sanger.ac.uk /Software/Pfam/ (Sonnhammer et al., 1998), BLOCKS, at http://blocks. fhcrc.org/ (Henikoff et al., 2000), and eMOTIF, at http://dna.stanford.edu /emotif (Huang and Brutlag, 2001). Pfam is a collection of protein families and domains, based on multiple protein alignments and profile-HMMs of these families. BLOCKS is a collection of multiply aligned ungapped segments that correspond to the most highly conserved regions of proteins. eMOTIF is a collection of protein sequence motifs representing conserved biochemical properties and biological functions derived from the BLOCKS and PRINTS, at http://www.bioinf.man.ac.uk/dbbrowser/ PRINTS/ (Attwood, 2002), databases.

Ab Initio Structure Prediction

The function of a protein is directly related to the 3D shape, i.e., the folding, of the molecule, and the 3D shape is directly determined by the sequence of amino acids in the molecule. Thus, the primary structure, i.e., the sequence of amino acids, ultimately determines the fold (3D structure) and function of a protein. A major goal in bioinformatics and structural molecular biology is to understand the relationship between the amino acid sequence and the 3D structure in protein, and to predict the fold based on the amino acid sequence alone. This type of structure prediction directly from the amino acid sequence is called ab initio structure prediction. The protein folding problem is often described as the most significant problem remaining in structural molecular biology, and to solve the protein folding problem is to break the second half of the genetic code. Solving the protein folding problem is the key to rapid progress in the fields of protein engineering and rational drug design.

However, protein fold prediction from an amino acid sequence is still a distant goal, and most current algorithms aim at predicting only the secondary structures, such as α-helices, β-strands, and loops/coils. The prediction of the secondary structure is an essential intermediate step on the way to predicting the full 3D structure of a protein. If the secondary structure of a protein is known, it is possible to derive a comparatively small number of possible tertiary (3D) structures using knowledge about the ways that the secondary structural elements pack.

The assumption on which all secondary structure prediction methods are based is that there is a correlation between the amino acid sequence and the secondary structure, and that a given short stretch of sequence may be more likely to form one type of secondary structure than another. Some of the major computational methods of secondary structure prediction are: (1) statistical feature-based method, (2) nearest neighbor method, and (3) neural network-model method.

In the statistical feature-based method of secondary structure prediction, the frequency of occurrence of each of the 20 amino acids in different secondary structures is used to create a scoring matrix. The method is based on the observation that certain amino acids have preference for certain secondary structures. For example, it was found that amino acids Ala (A), Glu (G), Leu (L), and Met (M) are strong predictors of α-helices, but that Pro (P) and Gly (G) are predictors of a break in a helix (Chou and Fasman, 1978). To predict a secondary structure, a sequence is scanned using a sliding window for the occurrence of amino acids that have a high probability for one type of structure, as measured by the scoring matrices. In the Garnier, Osguthorpe, and Robson (GOR) method (Garnier et al., 1978, 1996), a window of 17 residues is used for the prediction of the structural conformation of the central amino acid in the window. The GOR method estimates the joint probabilities of secondary structure S and amino acid a from sequences in structural databases, and uses these probabilities to estimate the information difference between the hypotheses that residual a is in structure S and residual a is not in structure S. Besides considering the influence of each amino acid in the window independently, a recent version of GOR (GOR IV, http://abs.cit.nih.gov/gor/) also considers the influence of pairwise combinations of amino acids in the flanking region, or of a flanking amino acid and the center amino acid when predicting the structural conformation of the center amino acid. GOR IV is reported to have a mean accuracy of Q3 = 64.4% for a three state prediction (Q3 is the percentage of residues correctly predicted for all three structures; α-helix, β-strand, and coil).

Nearest-neighbor method of secondary structure prediction predicts the secondary structural conformation of an amino acid in the query sequence by identifying training sequences of known structures that are homologous to the query sequence (Yi and Lander, 1993). The nearest-neighbor method requires the availability of a set of training sequences with known structures but with minimal sequence similarity to each other, and a scoring scheme for measuring similarity between sequence segments. A large list of short sequence fragments is then generated by sliding a window of length n (e.g., $n = 17$) along each training sequence, and the secondary structure of the center amino acid in the window is recorded. For structure prediction, a window of the same size is applied to the query sequence and the amino acid in the window is compared to each of the sequence fragments. The k (e.g., $k = 50$) bestmatching fragments are identified and the frequencies of the known secondary structures of the center amino acids in each of the matching fragments are used to predict the secondary structure of the center amino acid in the query window. Outputs from several nearest-neighbor predictors (i.e., with different parameters for n and k, and balanced or unbalanced prediction) could be combined using a simple majority vote rule or a more sophisticated machine learning algorithm such as neural network to improve the prediction accuracy. Finally, a set of filtering rules could be applied to exclude unrealistic predictions such as unusually short α-helices and β-strands.

The program NNSSP at http://searchlauncher.bcm.tmc.edu/pssprediction/Help/nnssp.html (Salamov and Solovyev, 1995, 1997) is a nearest-neighbor based secondary structure prediction algorithm. NNSSP uses a scoring system that combines an amino acid sequence similarity matrix with the local structural environment scoring method of Bowie et al. (1991), and takes into consideration the N- and C-terminal positions of α-helices, β-strands, and β-turns as distinctive types of secondary structures. Using multiple sequence alignments and a simple jury decision procedure, and by excluding the subset of most dissimilar sequences from the training database, an overall three-state accuracy (Q3) of 72.2% was reported (Salamov and Solovyev, 1995). Further improvement in NNSSP prediction accuracy (up to 73.5%) was achieved by using non-intersecting local sequence alignments of the query sequence with sequences having known 3D structures (Salamov and Solovyev, 1997). Another method that also uses nearest-neighbor prediction is the program called PREDATOR (Frishman and Argos, 1996, 1997).

The neural network-based method uses an artificial neural network which simulates the neural system in the brain for structure prediction. The general architecture for a neural network model consists of three layers of processing units or nodes – the input layer, the hidden layer, and the output layer (Lippmann, 1987). The main class of neural network relevant to protein secondary structure prediction is the *feed-forward network*, or multi-layer perceptron (MLP). In a feed-forward network, signals are sent from the nodes in the input layer to the nodes in the hidden layer and from the nodes in the hidden layer to the nodes in the output layer through links between units. The links may amplify or attenuate the signals by a weighting factor associated with each link. Except for the input layer nodes, the net input to each node is the sum of the weighted outputs of the nodes in the prior layer. Each node in the hidden and output layers is activated and produces an output signal in accordance with the inputs to the node, the activation function of the node (typically a sigmoidal function), and the bias of the node. The outputs of the input layer nodes may be taken to be equal to the inputs, or to be normalized within a range, i.e., -1 to +1. Figure 4.11 shows the typical architecture of a three-layer feed-forward network.

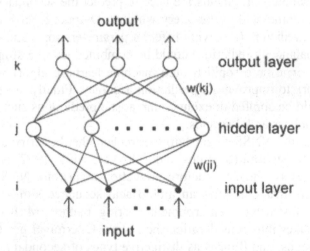

Fig. 4.11. A three-layer feed-forward neural network

Neural networks generalize by extracting the underlying physicochemical principles from the training sequence data. Training the network is the process of adjusting the weights w associated with each link. Initially, the weights are assigned random values. A sliding window of 13-17 amino acid residues is positioned along a training sequence and the predicted output is compared to the known structure of the center amino acid residue. Errors in the predictions are used for adjusting the weights using the back-propagation algorithm (Rumelhart et al., 1986). The back-propagation algorithm uses a gradient search technique to minimize a cost function equal to the mean square difference between the desired and the actual network outputs. Training by back-propagation is stopped when the errors cannot be reduced further.

The PHDsec is a neural network-based secondary structure prediction algorithm (Rost and Sander, 1993, 1994, and Rost 1996) (http://www. embl-heidelberg.de/predictprotein/). PHDsec predictions have three main features: (1) improved accuracy by using evolutionary information contained in multiple sequence alignments as input to the neural networks, (2) improved β-strand prediction accuracy through a balanced training procedure, and (3) more accurate prediction of secondary structure segments by using a multi-level system. The first level in PHDsec is a three-layer feed-forward neural network. Input to this first level sequence-to-structure network consists of two contributions: one from the local sequence, i.e., taken from a window of 13 adjacent residues, and another from the global sequence statistics. Output of the first level network is the 1D structural state of the residue at the center of the input window, i.e., α-helix (H), β-strand (E), and loop (L). The second level is a three-layer feed-forward structure-to-structure network. The output for the second level network is identical to the first level. The second level network introduces a correlation between adjacent residues with the effect that the predicted secondary structure segments have length distributions similar to the observed distributions. The third level consists of an arithmetic average over independently trained networks (jury decision). The final level is a simple filter that affects only drastic, unrealistic predictions (e.g., HEH to HHH; EHE to EEE; and LHL to LLL). PHDsec is reported to have a prediction accuracy of Q3 > 72%.

PSIPRED (Jones, 1999, and McGuffin et al., 2000) (http://bioinf. cs.ucl.ac.uk/psipred/) is another neural network-based secondary structure prediction algorithm that was reported to have very high prediction accuracy, with a Q3 score of 76.5% to 78.3%. PSIPRED incorporates two simple feed-forward neural networks that perform analysis on the iterated profile (position-specific scoring matrix) obtained from PSI-BLAST, and Position Specific Iterated - BLAST (Altschul et al., 1997). The high sensitivity and accuracy of the PSI-BLAST alignments was thought to be a major contributing factor to the high prediction rate of the PSIPRED method.

Hidden Markov Models (HMM) have also been applied in protein structure prediction. In one example of this approach, the models are trained on patterns of α-helix, β-strand, tight turns, and loops in specific structural classes, which then may be used to provide the most probable secondary structure and structural class of a protein (Stultz et al., 1993, 1997, and Hubbard and Park 1995; http://bmerc-www.bu.edu/psa/index.html).

A center that is focused on the prediction of protein structure is the *Protein Structure Prediction Center* (http://predictioncenter.llnl.gov/Center-.html), supported by the National Institutes of Health, National Library of Medicine, and the U.S. Department of Energy, Office of Biological and Environmental Research. It is a part of the Biology and Biotechnology Research Program at the Lawrence Livermore National Laboratory. The center's goal is to advance the methods of protein structure prediction from sequences and to provide the means for objective testing of prediction methods via the process of blind prediction. Since 1994, the center has organized a biannual CASP (Critical Assessment of techniques for protein Structure Prediction) event that aims to promote an objective evaluation of prediction methods on a continuing basis. The series of CASP experiments (from CASP1 in 1994 to CASP5 in 2002) attempts to establish the current state-of-the-art in protein structure prediction to identify what progress has been made and to highlight where future effort may be most productively focused.

Threading

More and more emphasis has been placed on tertiary structure prediction in the later CASP experiments, indicating that techniques for tertiary structure prediction are making substantial headway. Since the ways that protein can fold appear to be limited, there is considerable optimism that methods will eventually be found to predict the fold of any protein, given just its amino acid sequence. One popular and quite successful method for tertiary structure prediction is threading (Lemer et al., 1995; Lathrop et al., 1998; Mirny and Shakhnovich, 1998; Thiele et al., 1999; Panchenko et al., 2000; and Mirny et al., 2000).

In threading, a new sequence is mounted on a series of known folds (a sequence-structure alignment) from homologous sequences with the goal of finding a fold that provides the best score (lowest energy). Two commonly used techniques for deciding whether a given protein sequence is compatible with a known fold are the environmental template (or structural profile) method (Bowie et al., 1996; Johnson et al., 1996; and Panchenko et al., 2000) and the contact potential method (Jones et al., 1992a; Bryant and Lawrence, 1993; and Panchenko et al., 2000).

In the environmental template method, the environment, e.g., the secondary structure of the buried status, the polarity, the types of nearby side chains, and the hydrophobicity, of each amino acid in each known structural core is determined. The frequencies of different amino acids within multiple alignments in different environments are then counted and used to create structural 3D profiles. Dynamic programming is used to align a sequence to a string of descriptors that describe the 3D environment of the target structure, and the new sequence is predicted to have a fold similar to that of the target core if a significantly high score is obtained. In the contact potential method, the number of and closeness between amino acids in the core are analyzed, and each structural core is represented as a 2D contact matrix. The query sequence is evaluated for amino acid interactions that will correspond to those in the core and that will contribute to the stability of the protein. The most energetically stable conformations are assumed to be the most likely 3D structures.

References

Alberts, B., Bray, D., Lewis, J., Raff, M., Roberts, K. and Watson, J.D., (1989) Molecular Biology of the Cell. Garland Publishing, New York and London.

Altschul, S.F., Gish, W., Miller, W., Myers E.W. and Lipman, D.J., (1990) Basic local alignment search tool. J. Mol. Bio. 215: 403-410.

Altschul, S.F. and Gish, G., (1996) Local alignment statistics. Methods Enzymol. (Series title: Computer methods for macromolecular sequence analysis) 266: 460-480.

Altschul, S.F., Madden, T.L., Schaffer, A.A., Zhang, J., Zhang, Z., Miller, W. and Lipman, D.J., (1997) Gapped BLAST and PSI-BLAST: a new generation of protein database search programs. Nucl. Acids Res. 25: 3389-3402.

Andreeva, A., Howorth, D., Brenner, S.E., Hubbard, T.J.P., Chothia, C., and Murzin, A.G. (2004). SCOP database in 2004: refinements integrate structure and sequence family data. Nucl. Acid Res. 32:D226-D229.

Attwood, T.K. (2002) The PRINTS database: a resource for identification of protein families.

Ball, C.A., Sherlock, G., Parkinson, H., Rocca-Sera, P., Brooksbank, C., Causton, H.C., Cavalieri, D., Gaasterland, T., Hingamp, P., Holstege, F., Ringwald, M., Spellman, P., Stoeckert, C.J.Jr, Stewart, J.E., Taylor, R., Brazma, A. and Quackenbush, J. (2002) An open letter to the scientific journals. Published in Science 298(5593):539 and Bioinformatics 18(11):1409.

Benson, D.A., Karsch-Mizrachi, I., Lipman, D.J., Ostell, J. and Wheeler, D.L. (2003) GenBank. Nucl. Acids. Res. 31: 23-27.

Bowie, J.U., Luthy, R. and Eisenberg, D. (1991) A method to identify protein sequences that fold into a known three-dimensional structure. Science **253**: 164–170.

Bowie, J.U., Zhang, K., Wilmanns, M. and Eisenberg D (1996) Three-dimensional profiles for measuring compatibility of amino acid sequence with three-dimensional structure. Methods Enzymol. (Series title: Computer methods for macromolecular sequence analysis) **266**: 598-616.

Branden, C. and Tooze, J. (1999) Introduction to Protein Structure. 2nd Ed., Garland Science Publishing, New York

Brazma, A., Hingamp, P., Quackenbush, J., Sherlock, G., Spellman, P., Stoeckert, C, Aach J, Ansorge, W., Ball, C.A., Causton, H.C., Gaasterland, T., Glenisson, P., Holstege, F.C.P., Kim, I.F., Markowitz, V., Matese, J.C., Parkinson H., Robinson, A., Sarkans, U., Schulze-Kremer, S., Stewart, J., Taylor, R., Vilo, J. and Vingron, M. (2001) Minimum information about a microarray experiment (MIAME)—toward standards for microarray data. Nature Genetics **29**: 365 - 371

Bryant, S.H. and Lawrence, C.E. (1993) An empirical energy function for threading protein sequence through the fold motif. Proteins Struct. Funct. Genet. **16**: 92-112.

Burset, M. and Guigo, R. (1996) Evaluation of Gene Structure Prediction Programs. Genomics **34**: 353-367

Chou, P.Y. and Fasman, G.D. (1978) Prediction of the secondary structure of proteins from their amino acid sequence. Adv. Enzymol. Relat. Areas Mol. Biol. **47**: 45-147.

Dayhoff, M.O., Schwartz, R.M. and Orcutt BC (1978) A model of evolutionary change in proteins. Atlas of Protein Science and Structure, vol. 5, supplement 3, National Biomedical Research Foundation, Washington, DC, pp. 345-351

Dovichi, N.J. and Zhang, J.Z. (2001) DNA sequencing by capillary array electrophoresis. Methods Mol. Bio. **167**: 225-239.

Eddy, S.R. (1998) Profile Hidden Markov models. Bioinformatics **14**: 755-763.

Felsenstein, J. (1993) PHYLIP 3.5 (phylogeny inference package). Department of Genetics, University of Washington, Seattle.

Felsenstein, J. (1996) Inferring phylogeny from protein sequences by parsimony, distance and likelihood methods. Methods Enzymol. (Series title: Computer methods for macromolecular sequence analysis) **266**: 418-427.

Feng, D.F. and Doolittle, R.F. (1996) Progressive alignment of amino acid sequences and construction of phylogenetic trees from them. Methods Enzymol. (Series title: Computer methods for macromolecular sequence analysis) **266**: 368-382.

Fickett, J.W. (1982) Recognition of protein coding regions in DNA sequences. Nucl. Acids Res. **10**: 5303-5318.

Fickett, J.W. (1996) Finding genes by computer: the state of the art. Trends Genet. **12**: 316–320.

Fickett, J.W. and Tung, C.S. (1992). Assessment of protein coding measures. Nucl. Acids Res. **20**: 6641-6450.

Frishman, D. and Argos, P. (1996) Incorporation of long-distance interactions into a secondary structure prediction algorithm. Protein Engineering **9**: 133-142.

Frishman D and Argos, P. (1997) 75% accuracy in protein secondary structure prediction. Proteins **27**: 329-335.

Galperin, M.Y. (2004) The Molecular Biology Database Collection: 2004 update. Nucl. Acids Res. **32**: D3-D22.

Garnier, J., Osguthorpe, D.J. and Robson, B. (1978) Analysis of the accuracy and implications of simple methods for predicting the secondary structure of globular proteins. J. Mol. Biol. **120**: 97-120.

Garnier, J., Gilbrat, J.F. and Robson, B. (1996) GOR method for predicting protein secondary structure from amino acid sequence. Methods Enzymol. (Series title: Computer methods for macromolecular sequence analysis) **266**: 540-553.

Geer, R.C. and Sayers, E.W. (2003) Entrez: Making use of its power. Briefings in Bioinformatics 4:1779-184

Gibbs, A.J., McIntyre, G.A. (1970) The diagram, a method for comparing sequences. Its use with amino acid and nucleotide sequences. Eur. J. Biochem. **16**: 1-11.

Graur, D., Li, W.H. (2000) Fundamentals of molecular evolution. (2nd ed.) Sinauer Associates, Sunderland, Massachusetts.

Grosse, I., Buldyrev, S.V., Stanley, H.E., Holste, D. and Herzel, H. (2000) Average mutual information of coding and noncoding DNA. Pacific Symposium on Biocomputing **5**:611-620.

Guigo, R. (1999) DNA Composition, Codon Usage and Exon Prediction. In: Genetic Databases, (ed. M.J. Bishop), chap.4, pp. 53-80, Academic Press.

Henikoff, S., Henikoff, J.G. (1992) Amino acid substitution matrices from protein blocks. Proc. Natl. Acad. Sci. USA **89**: 10915-10919.

Henikoff, S. and Henikoff, J.G. (1994) Protein family classification based on searching a database of blocks. Genomics **19**:97-107.

Henikoff, J.G., Greene, E.A., Pietrokovski, S. and Henikoff S (2000) Increased coverage of protein families with the blocks database servers. Nucl. Acids Res. **28**:228-230.

Herzel, H. and Grosse, I. (1995) Measuring correlations in symbol sequences. Physica A **216**: 518-542.

Hawkins, J.D. (1988) A survey on intron and exon lengths. Nucl. Acids Res. **16**: 9893-9908.

Helt, G.A., Lewis, S., Loraine, A.E. and Rubin, G.M. (1998) BioViews: Java-based tools for genomic data visualization. Genome Res. **8**: 291-305.

Hoersch, S., Leroy, C., Brown, N.P., Andrade, M.A., and Sander, C. (2000) The GeneQuiz Web server: protein functional analysis through the Web. Trends in Biochem. Sci. **25**: 33-35.

Holm, L. and Sander, C. (1993) Protein structure comparison by alignment of distance matrices. J. Mol. Biol. **233**: 23-138,

Holm, L. and Sander, C. (1996a) Mapping the protein universe. Science **273**:595-602.

Holm, L. and Sander, C. (1996b) The FSSP database: fold classification based on structure-structure alignment of proteins. Nucl. Acids Res. **24**: 206-209

Hughey, R. and Krogh, A. (1996) Hidden Markov models for sequence analysis: Extension and the analysis of the basic method. Comput. Appl. Biosci. **12**: 95-107.

Huang, J.Y. and Brutlag, D.L. (2001). The eMOTIF database. Nucl. Acids Res. **29**:202-204.

Johnson, M.S., May, A.C. and Ridionov, M.A., Overington JP (1996) Discrimination of common protein folds: Application of protein structure to sequence/structure comparisons. Methods Enzymol. (Series title: Computer methods for macromolecular sequence analysis) **266**: 575-598.

Jones, D.T. (1999) Protein secondary structure prediction based on position-specific scoring matrices. J. Mol. Biol. **292**: 195-202.

Jones, D.T., Taylor, W.R. and Thornton, J.M. (1992a) A new approach to protein fold recognition. Nature **358**: 86-89.

Jones, D.T., Taylor, W.R. and Thornton, J.M. (1992b) The rapid generation of mutation data matrices from protein sequences. Comp. Appl. Biosci. **8**: 275-282.

Kabsch, W. and Sander, C. (1983) Dictionary of protein secondary structure: pattern recognition of hydrogen-bonded and geometrical features. Biopolymers **22**: 2577-2637.

Kim, J., Pramanik. S. and Chung, M.J. (1994). Multiple sequence alignment by simulated annealing. Comput. Appl. Biosci. **10**: 419-426.

Konopka, A.K. (1994) Structure and Methods: VI. Human Genome Initiative and DNA Recombination, chapter Towards Mapping Functional Domains in Indiscriminantly Sequenced Nucleic Acids: A Computational Approach. Adenine Press, Guilderland, New York.

Kulikova, T., Aldebert, P., Althorpe, N., Baker, W., Bates, K. and Browne, P., van den Broek A, Cochrane G, Duggan K, Eberhardt R, Faruque N, Garcia-Pastor M, Harte N, Kanz C, Leinonen R, Lin Q, Lombard V, Lopez R, Mancuso R, McHale M, Nardone F, Silventoinen V, Stochr P, Stoesser G, Tuli MA, Tzouvara K, Vaughan R, Wu D and Zhu W, Apweiler R (2004) The EMBL Nucleotide Sequence Database. Nucl. Acids Res. **32**: D27–D30.

Lathrop, R.H., Rogers R.G. Jr., Bienkowska J., Bryant B.K.M, Buturovic L.J., Gaitatzes C., Nambudripad R., White J.V., and Smith T.F. (1998). Analysis and algorithms for protein sequence-structure alignment. *Computational methods in molecular biology.* S. Salzberg, D. Searls, and S. Kasif Eds. Elsevier Press. Amsterdam, Chapter 12, pp. 227-283.

Lathrop, R.H., Rogers, R.G. Jr., Bienkowska, J., Bryant, B.K.M., Buturovic, L.J., Gaitatzes, C., Nambudripad, R., White, J.V., Smith, T.F. (1988) Analysis and algorithms for protein sequence-structure alignment. New Compr. Biochem. (Series title: Computational methods in molecular biology) **32**: 337-355.

Lemer, C.M., Rooman, M.J. and Wodak, S.J. (1995) Protein structure prediction by threading methods: evaluation of current techniques. Proteins **23**(3):337-55.

Li, W. (1997) The study of correlation structures of DNA sequences: a critical review. Computer and Chemistry **21**:257-271.

Li, W.H. (1997) Molecular evolution. Sinauer Associates, Sunderland, Massachusetts.

Liew, A.W.C., Wu, Y., Yan, H. and Yang, M. (2004) A Study on the Effective Statistical Coding Features for Coding/Non-coding DNA Sequence Classification for Yeast, C. elegans and Human. Submitted.

Lippmann, R.P. (1987) An introduction to computing with neural nets. IEEE ASSP Magazine. 4(2): 4-22.

Lo Conte, L., Brenner, S.E., Hubbard, T.J.P., Chothia, C. and Murzin, A. (2002) SCOP database in 2002: refinements accommodate structural genomics. Nucl. Acid Res. 30: 264-267.

Lukashin, A.V., Borodovsky, M. (1998) GeneMark.hmm: new solutions for gene finding. Nucl. Acids Res. 26: 1107-1115.

Madej, T., Gibrat, J.F. and Bryant, S.H. (1995) Threading a database of protein cores. Proteins, 23: 356-369.

Markel, S. and Leon, D. (2003) Sequence Analysis in a nutshell: a guide to common tools and databases. O'Reilly and Associates, Inc., USA

Martz, E. (2003) 3D molecular visualization with Protein Explorer. In: Introduction to Bioinformatics: A Theoretical and Practical Approach, (S.A. Krawetz, D.D. Womble eds.), Humana Press, Totowa, New Jersey

Maizel, J.V. Jr. and Lenk, R.P. (1981) Enhanced Graphic Matrix Analysis of Nucleic Acid and Protein Sequences. Proc. Natl. Acad. Sci. USA. 78; 7665-7669

Mathe, C., Sagot, M.F., Schiex, T. and Rouze, P. (2002) Current methods of gene prediction, their strengths and weakness – survey and summary. Nucl. Acids Res. 30: 4103-4117

McGuffin, L.J., Bryson, K. and Jones D.T. (2000) The PSIPRED protein structure prediction server. Bioinformatics 16: 404-405.

Mirny, L.A. and Shakhnovich, E.I. (1998) Protein structure prediction by threading -Why it works and why it does not. J. Mol. Biol. 283(2):507-526.

Mirny, L.A., Finkelstein, A.V. and Shakhnovich, E.I. (2000) Statistical significance of protein structure prediction by threading. Proc. Natl. Acad. Sci. USA. 97(18): 9978–9983.

Miyazaki, S., Sugawara, H., Gojobori, T. and Tateno, Y. (2003) DNA Data Bank of Japan (DDBJ) in XML. Nucl. Acids. Res. 31: 13-16.

Miyazaki, S., Sugawara, H., Ikeo, K., Gojobori, T. and Tateno, Y. (2004). DDBJ in the stream of various biological data. Nucl. Acids. Res. 32: D31-D34.

Mizuguchi, K., Blundell, T.L. (2000) Analysis of conservation and substitutions of secondary structure elements within protein superfamilies. Bioinformatics 16: 1111-1119.

Mount, D.W. (2001) Bioinformatics – Sequence and Genome Analysis. Cold Spring Harbor Laboratory Press, New York.

Murzin, A.G., Brenner, S.E., Hubbard, T. and Chothia, C. (1995) SCOP: a structural classification of proteins database for the investigation of sequences and structures. J. Mol. Biol. 247: 536-540.

Needleman, S.B. and Wunsch, C.D. (1970) A general method applicable to the search for similarities in the amino acid sequence of two proteins. J. Mol. Bio. 48: 443-453.

Notredame, C. and Higgins, D.G. (1996) SAGA: Sequence alignment by genetic algorithm. Nucl. Acids Res. **24**: 1515-1524.

Orengo, C.A., Michie, A.D., Jones S., Jones D.T., Swindells M.B., and Thornton J.M. (1997). CATH- A Hierarchic Classification of Protein Domain Structures. Structure **5**(8):1093-1108.

Panchenko, A.R., Marchler-Bauer, A., Bryant, S.H. (2000) Combination of threading potentials and sequence profiles improves fold recognition. J. Mol. Biol. **296**(5):1319-1331.

Pearl, F.M.G., Lee, D., Bray, J.E,, Sillitoe, I., Todd A.E. and Harrison A.P., Thornton J.M., and Orengo C.A. (2000). Assigning genomic sequences to CATH. Nucl. Acids Res. **28**(1): 277-282.Andrade MA, Brown NP, Leroy C, Hoersch S, de Daruvar A, Reich C, Franchini A, Tamames J, Valencia A, Ouzounis C, Sander C (1999) Automated genome sequence analysis and annotation. Bioinformatics **15**: 391-412.

Pearson, W.R. (1990) Rapid and sensitive comparison with FASTP and FASTA. Methods Enzymol. (Series tile: Molecular evolution: computer analysis of protein and nucleic acid sequences) **183**: 63-98.

Pearson, W.R. and Lipman, D.J. (1988) Improved tools for biological sequence comparison. Proc. Natl. Acad. Sci. U.S.A. **85**:2444-8.

Rost, B. (1996) PHD: predicting one-dimensional protein structure by profile based neural networks. Methods Enzymol. (Series title: Computer methods for macromolecular sequence analysis) **266**: 525-539.

Rost, B. and Sander, C. (1993) Prediction of protein secondary structure at better than 70% accuracy. J. Mol. Biol. **232**: 584-599.

Rost, B. and Sander, C. (1994) Combining evolutionary information and neural networks to predict protein secondary structure. Proteins **19**: 55-77.

Rumelhart, D.E., Hinton, G.E. and Williams, R.J. (1986) Learning internal representations by error propagation. Parallel Distributed Processing: Explorations in the Microstructure of Cognition. Vol. 1: Foundations. D.E. Rumelhart and J.L. McClelland Eds. MIT Press, pp 318-362.

Salamov, A.A. and Solovyev, V.V. (1995) Prediction of protein secondary structure by combining nearest-neighbor algorithms and multiply sequence alignments. J. Mol. Biol. **247**: 11-15.

Salamov, A.A. and Solovyev, V.V. (1997) Protein secondary structure prediction using local alignments. J. Mol. Biol. **268**: 31-36.

Salzberg, S.L., Delcher, A.L., Kasif, S. and White, O. (1998a) Microbial gene identification using interpolated Markov models. Nucl. Acids Res. **26**: 544-548.

Salzberg, S.L., Delcher, A.L., Fasman, K.H. and Henderson, J. (1998b) A decision tree system for finding genes in DNA. J. of Comp. Biol. **5**: 667-680.

Sanger, F., Nicklen, S. and Coulson, A.R. (1977) DNA sequencing with chain terminating inhibitors. Proc. Natl. Acad. Sci. USA. **74**: 5463-5467.

Schwartz, R.M. and Dayhoff, M.O. (1978) Matrices for detecting distant relationships. Atlas of Protein Science and Structure, vol. 5, supplement 3, National Biomedical Research Foundation, Washington, DC, pp 353-358.

Serov, V.N. and Spirov, A.V., Samsonova MG (1998) Graphical interface to the genetic network database GeNet. Bioinformatics **14**: 546-547.

Shapiro, L. and Harris, T. (2000) Finding function through structural genomics. Current Opinion in Biotechnology **11**: 31-35.

Siddiqui, A.S., Dengler, U. and Barton, G.J. (2001) 3Dee: A database of protein structural domains. Bioinformatics **17**: 200-201.

Sigrist, C.J., Cerutti, L., Hulo, N., Gattiker, A., Falquet, L., Pagni, M., Bairoch, A., Bucher, P.. (2002) PROSITE: a documented database using patterns and profiles as motif descriptors.

Smith, T.F. and Waterman, M.S. (1981a) Identification of common molecular subsequences. J. Mol. Bio. **147**: 195-197.

Smith, T.F. and Waterman, M.S. (1981b). Comparison of biosequences. Adv. Appl. Math. **2**: 482-489.

Sonnhammer, E.L.L., Eddy, S.R., Birney, E., Bateman, A. and Durbin, R. (1998) Pfam: multiple sequence alignments and HMM-profiles of protein domains. Nucl. Acids Res. **26**:320-322.

Staden, R. (1990) Finding protein coding regions in genomic sequences. Methods Enzymol. (Series title: Molecular evolution : computer analysis of protein and nucleic acid sequences) **183**: 163-80.

Staden R, McLachlan AD (1982) Codon preference and its use in identifying protein

States, D.J., Boguski, M.S. (1991) Similarity and homology. In: Sequence Analysis Primer, (ed. M. Gribskov and J. Devereux), pp. 92-124, Stockton Press, New York.

Swofford, D.L., Olsen, G.J., Waddell, P.J., Hillis, D.M. (1996) Phylogenetic inference. In Molecular Systematics 2nd ed., (ed. D.M. Hillis et al.), chap. 5, pp 407-514, Sinauer Associates, Sunderland, Massachusetts.

Tamura, K. and Nei, M. (1993) Estimation of the number of nucleotide substitutions in the control region of mitochandrail DNA in humans and chimpanzees. Mol. Bio. Evol. **10**: 512-526.

Tateno, Y., Imanishi, T., Miyazaki, S., Fukami-Kobayashi, K. and Saitou, N., Sugawara H, Gojobori T (2002) DNA Data Bank of Japan (DDBJ) for genome scale research in life science. Nucl. Acids. Res. **30**: 27-30.

Thanaraj, T.A. (2000) Positional characterisation of false positives from computational prediction of human splice sites. Nucl. Acids Res. **28**: 744-754.

Thiele, R., Zimmer, R. and Lengauer, T. (1999) Protein threading by recursive dynamic programming. J. Mol. Biol. **290**(3):757-779.

Thompson, J.D., Higgins, D.G. and Gibson, T.J. (1994) CLUSTAL W: Improving the sensitivity of progressive multiple sequence alignment through sequence weighting, position-specific gap penalties and weight matrix choice. Nucl. Acids Res. **22**: 4673-4680.

Thompson, J.D., Gibson, T.J., Plewniak, F., Jeanmougin, F. and Higgins, D.G. (1997) The CLUSTAL X windows interface: Flexible strategies for multiple sequence alignment aided by quality analysis tools. Nucl. Acids Res. **25**: 4876-4882.

Tiwari, S., Ramachandran, S., Bhattacharya, A., Bhattacharya, S., Ramaswamy, R. (1997) Prediction of probable genes by fourier analysis of genomic sequences. Computer Applications in the Biosciences **13**: 263-270.

Uberbacher, E.C., Xu, Y. and Mural, R.J. (1996) Discovering and understanding genes in human DNA sequence using GRAIL. Methods Enzymol. (Series title: Computer methods for macromolecular sequence analysis) **266**: 259-281.

Vilo, J., Kapushesky, M., Kemmeren, P., Sarkans, U. and Brazma, A. (2003) Expression Profiler. In: The analysis of gene expression data: methods and software (Parmigiani G; Garrett E; Irizarry R; Zeger S L, eds.), Springer, NY.

Wang Y., Zhang C.T., and Dong P. (2002). Recognizing shorter coding regions of human genes based on the statistics of stop codons. Biopolymers **63**(3): 207-216.

Williams, G. (1999) Nucleic acid and protein sequence databases. In: Genetic Databases, (ed. M.J. Bishop), chap.2, pp. 11-37, Academic Press.

Wu, S., Liew, A.W.C. and Yan, H. (2003) Cluster Analysis of Gene Expression Data Based on Self-Splitting and Merging Competitive Learning. To appear in IEEE Transactions on Information Technology in Biomedicine.

Wu, Y., Liew, A.W.C., Yan, H. and Yang, M. (2003a) DB-Curve: A Novel 2D Method of DNA Sequence Visualization and Representation. Chem. Phys. Lett. **367**: 170-176.

Wu, Y., Liew, A.W.C., Yan, H. and Yang, M. (2003b) Classification of short human exons and introns based on statistical features. Phys. Rev. E. 67(6): Art. No. 061916.

Zhang, M.Q. (1997) Identification of protein coding regions in the human genome by quadratic discriminant analysis. Proc. Natl. Acad. Sci. USA. 94: 565-568.

Zhang, C.T., Wang, J. (2000) Recognition of protein coding genes in the Yeast genome at better than 95% accuracy based on the Z curve. Nucl. Acids Res. **28**: 2804-2814.

Zhang, R. and Zhang, C.T. (1994). Z Curves, an Intuitive Tool for Visualizing and Analyzing DNA sequences. Journal Biomolecular Structure Dynamics 11:767-782.

5 Machine Learning in Bioinformatics

Supawan Prompramote[1], Yan Chen[1] and Yi-Ping Phoebe Chen[1,2]

[1] School of Information Technology
Faculty of Science and Technology
Deakin University, 221 Burwood Highway, VIC3125, Australia
[2] ARC Centre in Bioinformatics

5.1 Introduction

Given the complexity and gigantic volume of biological data, the traditional computer science techniques and algorithms fail to solve complex biological problems of the real world. However, there are modern computational approaches called machine learning that can address the limitations of the traditional techniques. Machine learning is an adaptive process that enables computers to learn from experience, learn by example, and learn by analogy. Learning capabilities are essential for automatically improving the performance of a computational system over time on the basis of previous results. A basic learning model typically consists of the following four components:

- learning element, responsible for improving its performance,
- performance element, which decides the choice of actions to be taken,
- critical element, which tells learning element how the algorithm performs, and
- problem generator, responsible for suggesting actions that could lead to new or informative experiences (Adeli, 1995; Finlay and Dix 1996;

Kuonen, 2003; Narayanan et al., 2002; Negnevitsky, 2002; Nilsson, 1996; Baldi and Brunak, 2001; and Westhead et al., 2002).

Machine learning typically can be divided into three phases, as follows:

1. analysis of a training set of examples and generation of a set of rules from training set,
2. verification of the rules by human experts or automatic knowledge based components and
3. use of the validated rules in responding to some new testing datasets (Finlay and Dix 1996).

There are a number of reasons why machine learning approaches are widely used in practice, especially in bioinformatics (Narayanan et al., 2002; Nilsson, 1996; Baldi and Brunak, 2001; and Westhead et al., 2002)

- Traditionally, a human being builds such an expert system by collecting knowledge from specific experts. The experts can always explain what factors they use to assess a situation; however, it is often difficult for the experts to say what rules they use, for example, for disease analysis and control. This problem can be resolved by machine learning mechanisms. Machine learning can extract the description of the hidden situation in terms of those factors and then fire rules that match the expert's behavior.
- Systems often produce results different from the desired ones. This may be caused by unknown properties or functions of inputs during the design of systems. This situation always occurs in the biological world because of the complexities and mysteries of life sciences. However, with its capability of dynamic improvement, machine learning can cope with this problem.
- In molecular biology research, new data and concepts are generated every day, and those new data and concepts update or replace the old ones. Machine learning can be easily adapted to a changing environment. This benefits system designers, as they do not need to redesign systems whenever the environment changes.
- Missing and noisy data is one characteristic of biological data. The conventional computer techniques fail to handle this. Machine learning techniques are able to deal with missing and noisy data.
- With advances in biotechnology, huge volumes of biological data are generated. In addition, it is possible that important hidden relationships and correlations exist in the data. Machine learning methods are de-

signed to handle very large data sets, and can be used to extract such relationships.

Table 5.1. The existing research on bioinformatics that has applied machine learning techniques.

Research Area	Application	Reference
Sequence alignment	BLAST	http://www.ncbi.nlm.nih.gov/BLAST/
	FASTA	http://www.ebi.ac.uk/fasta33/
Multiple sequence alignment	ClustalW	http://www.ebi.ac.uk/clustalw/
	MultAlin	http://prodes.toulouse.inra.fr/multalin/multalin.html
	DiAlign	http://www.genomatix.de/cgi-bin/dialign/dialign.pl
Gene finding	Genscan	http://genes.mit.edu/GENSCAN.html
	GenomeScan	http://genes.mit.edu/genomescan/
	GeneMark	http://www.ebi.ac.uk/genemark/
Protein domain analysis and identification	Pfam	http://www.sanger.ac.uk/Software/Pfam/
	BLOCKS	http://www.blocks.fhcrc.org/
	ProDom	http://prodes.toulouse.inra.fr/prodom/current/html/ home.php
Pattern identification	Gibbs Sampler	http://bayesweb.wadsworth.org/gibbs/gibbs.html
	AlignACE	http://atlas.med.harvard.edu/cgi-bin/alignace.pl
	MEME	http://meme.sdsc.edu/meme/website/intro.html
Protein folding prediction	PredictProtein	http://www.embl-heidelberg.de/predictprotein/ predictprotein.html
	SwissModle	http://www.expasy.org/swissmod/ SWISS-MODEL.html

- There are some biological problems in which experts can specify only input/output pairs, but not the relationships between inputs and outputs, such as the prediction of protein structure and structural and functional sequences. This limitation can be addressed by machine learning methods. They are able to adjust their internal structure to produce approximate results for the given problems.

Machine learning mechanisms form the basis of adaptive systems. In bioinformatics research, a number of machine learning approaches are applied to discover new meaningful knowledge from the biological databases, to analyze and predict diseases, to group similar genetic elements, and to find relationships or associations in biological data. Examples of machine learning approaches in bioinformatics research are shown in Table 5.1.

In this chapter, the most popular of machine learning approaches, namely, artificial neural networks, genetic algorithms, and fuzzy expert systems, are elaborated. The basic background, definition, and models of each method are presented. Further, a survey of tools for using the learning techniques used in bioinformatics is included.

5.2 Artificial Neural Network

The process of learning is a complex phenomenon. Many puzzling questions arise from of it. How can one recognize the faces of others? How can one identify complex patterns from the faces? How does one discriminate images and backgrounds? How does one learn a shortcut to go to his or her university? In order to answer these questions, one needs to know how the brain works.

The human brain has been studied since the late Middle Ages; however, its detailed structure began to be unraveled only in the nineteenth century. Neuronists claim that the brain is a collection of about 10 billion densely interconnected cellular units called neurons. The structure of a neuron and its network is shown in Fig. 5.1.

Each neuron consists of a cell body called soma, a number of root-like extensions connected to a thousand adjacent neurons called dendrites, and a single transmission line extending out from the soma called axon. The two specialized extensions of a soma are responsible for carrying information from/to a cell body. Dendrites bring information to a cell body and axons take information away from a cell body. The connection between two neurons, in particular, between an axon terminal and another neuron, is called synapse.

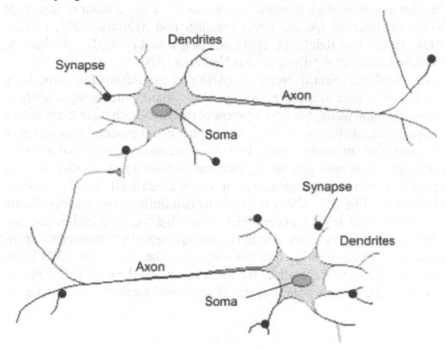

Fig. 5.1. Biological neural network (Adapted from: http://ffden2.phys.uaf.edu/-212_fall2003.web.dir/Keith_Palchikoff/Intro_page.html)

Each neuron uses biochemical reactions to receive processes and transmit information. Neurons communicate with each other through an electrochemical process. This means that chemicals create an electrical signal. When a neuron does not send a signal, it is in a resting state. The inside of the neuron has a negative electric potential. When a neuron sends a signal, it causes a change in the electrical potential of the cell body. The change occurs due to the release of chemical substances from the synaptic cell, called neurotransmitter. When the potential exceeds a certain threshold, an action potential occurs. Consequently, the neuron will fire the electrical signal down the axon. The occurrence of action potential can be increased or decreased by changing the constitution of various neurotransmitters.

An essential characteristic of biological neural networks is plasticity, an ability of the brain to reorganize with learning, based on experience or sensory stimulation. Scientists believe that there are two types of modifications that form the basis of learning in the brain, namely, 1) a change in the internal structure of the synapses and 2) an increase in the number of synapses between neurons.

The natural and power of a biological neural network, in particular, the potential of learning process, motivated computer scientists to design and develop a new network platform that worked in a way similar to that of the biological neurons (Adeli, 1995; Freeman and Skapura, 1991; Haykin, 1994; Müller and Reinhardt, 1990; and Negnevitsky, 2002). This leads to the introduction of Artificial Neural Networks (ANNs).

An Artificial Neural Network (ANN) is an information processing model that is able to capture and represent complex input-output relationships. The motivation the development of the ANN technique came from a desire for an intelligent artificial system that could process information in the same way the human brain. Its novel structure is represented as multiple layers of simple processing elements, operating in parallel to solve specific problems. An architecture of a typical artificial neural network is illustrated in Fig. 5.2. ANNs resemble human brain in two respects: learning process and storing experiential knowledge. An artificial neural network learns and classifies a problem through repeated adjustments of the connecting weights between the elements. In other words, an ANN learns from examples and generalizes the learning beyond the examples supplied. For instance, human beings learn to recognize faces from examples of faces.

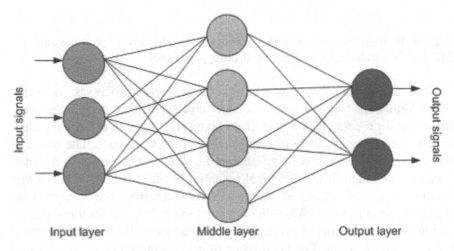

Fig. 5.2. Schematic representation of a generic ANN

Each element (analogous to a neuron) in the network is connected to its neighbors with weights (analogous to synapses) that represent the strengths of the connections. Typically, a single processing element receives a number of inputs (analogous to dendrites) through its connection, combines them, performs a (non-)linear operation on the result, and then produces the final result (analogous to an axon). The input can be information from external environments or outputs of other neurons. The output can be either a final solution to the problem or an input to other neurons. Figure 5.3 illustrates a neuron model, and Table 5.2 shows that the artificial neural network concepts are similar to those of the biological brain.

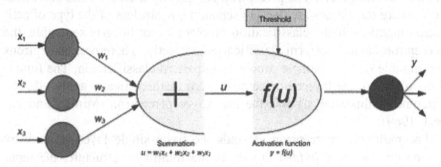

Fig. 5.3. A neuron model

The neuron determines its output on the basis of the weighted sum of the inputs, a threshold value (θ), and an activation function. An activation function of a neuron can be any mathematical function. In practice, four functions are commonly used. They are step function, sign function, sigmoid function, and linear function. If one chooses a sign function as an activation function and the net input is less than θ, the neuron output is 1; otherwise, it is -1.

Table 5.2. An analogy between the biological and artificial neural networks and the functions of their components

Function of each component	Biological neural networks	Artificial neural networks
Accept Inputs	Dendrite	Input
Process the inputs	Soma	Neuron
Turn the processed inputs into outputs	Axon	Output
Involve learning process	Synapse	Weight

To build an artificial network, one must decide which network architecture and learning algorithm should be used. Network architecture tells how the neurons are used, and how they are connected in a network. The aim of the learning function is to modify the weights of the inputs to achieve the desired outputs.

Based on the arrangement of the internal nodes in the network layer, the neural network architecture can be classified into different types, namely, perceptron, feedforward networks, and feedback networks. The simplest type of neural network is a perceptron (Rosenblatt, 1958). It consists of a single layer wherein weights are trained to produce a correct output when presented with inputs. The perceptron is typically used for class classification, where the classes are linearly separable, regardless of the type of activation function. If the classification problem is not linearly separable, the perceptron cannot perform classification correctly. Therefore, perceptrons are suitable only for simple problems in pattern classification. The limitations of the single layered perceptron were mathematically analyzed. The outcome of this analysis was the multilayer perceptron (Minsky and Papert, 1969).

The multilayer perceptron expands the basic single layer network by having one or more *hidden layers*. In the multilayer structure, the input layer accepts information from the external environment and passes the information to all units in the first hidden layer. The outputs from the first hidden layer are redistributed to the next hidden layer, and so on. The output layer accepts output from the last hidden layer and generates the final output of the entire network.

A feedforward network is a network of neurons that have signals traveling from input layer to output layer only. In contrast, feedback networks allow signals traveling in both directions (from input layer to output layer and vice versa). A type of feedback network is a recurrent neural network.

One important function of the human brain is to collect down and recall the memories. This is done with short and long term memories. The human memory is associative, that is, people recognize an input pattern by comparing it with patterns stored in their memories. If the input pattern is noisy, the associative memory returns the closest stored pattern. In other words, if a corrupted image is given to a network, the network will automatically reconstruct a perfect image. A *recurrent neural network*, a variation of the multilayer perceptron, is able to emulate the associative characteristics. It is a modification to the multilayer neural networks, trained with the backpropagation algorithm; that is, a recurrent neural network has feedback loops from its outputs to its inputs. As in backpropagation learning, the feedbacks are used to adjust the weights of inputs. Then the output is computed again. The algorithm is repeatedly iterated until output becomes convergent.

Learning in neural networks can be divided into two types: supervised and unsupervised learning. In supervised learning, an artificial neural network is trained by an external teacher who presents inputs, weights, and desired outputs to a network. Weights are randomly initialized to the inputs of the network to compute the actual outputs. The actual outputs are compared to the desired outputs. The weights are then adjusted by the network to produce actual outputs that are close to the desired outputs. The input weights are continuously modified until acceptable actual outputs are achieved. In contrast, unsupervised learning, also known as self-supervised learning, does not require an external teacher. During the training phase, a neural network receives a number of inputs, discovers regularities in the inputs, and learns how to organize itself.

With remarkable abilities such as nonlinearity, adaptive learning, self organization, real-time operation, very large-scale integrated implementation, and fault tolerance via redundant information coding, neural networks are able to solve complex problems that human and other computer techniques cannot do. For example, neural networks outperform the decision tree approach on the same data. However, neural networks have some limitations. For instance, complex neural network models lack explanations to interpret the decisions of each node in the network as rules; as testing and verification. This problem comes from adaptive learning capability, in which a network learns how to solve problem by itself, and its operations cannot therefore be interpreted.

The neural network is one of several machine learning approaches that have been successfully applied to solving a wide variety of bioinformatics problems. In sequence analysis, ANNs have been applied or integrated with other methods or systems. For example, a knowledge-based neural network system was applied to analyzing DNA sequence (Fu, 1999). An artificial neural network was trained to predict the sequence of the human TP53 tumor suppressor gene based on a p53 GeneChip (Spicker et al., 2002). A multilayered feed-forward ANN was developed as a tool to predict a mycobacterial promoter sequence in a nucleotide sequence (Kalate et al., 2003).

There are two popular gene finder tools that accommodated ANNs. GRAIL (Uberbacher and Mural, 1991) is the first gene finder program, which was designed to identify genes, exons, and various features in DNA sequences. It uses a neural network that combines a series of coding prediction algorithms to recognize coding potential in fixed length windows without looking for additional features. Figure 5.4 shows a snapshot of the GRAIL tool screen.

Another gene finder system is GeneParser (Synder and Stormo, 1993, 1997). It was designed to identify and determine the fine structure of protein genes in genomic DNA sequences. It comprises two variations of a single layer network, namely, 1) one fully connected and one partially connected with an activation bias added to some inputs, and 2) a partially connected two-layer network. Dynamic programming has been used as the learning algorithm to train the system for protein sequencing.

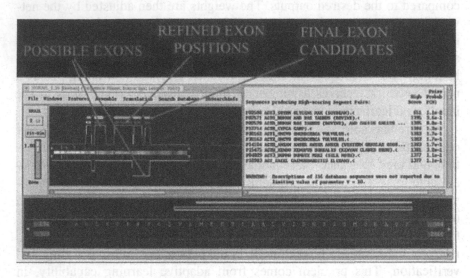

Fig. 5.4. GRAIL gene finding tool (Source from: Presentation slides appeared in Bioinformatics Forum, Thailand. 2002)

ANN has been widely used in protein structural and functional prediction. The prediction of protein secondary structure using neural networks was formerly carried out in 1988 (Bohr et al., 1990, and Qian and Sejnowski, 1988). However, this has requirements of training several neural networks and of adding an extra layer. Much work has been done to improve the effective methods (Baldi, 2000; Fairchild et al., 1995; Riis and Krogh, 1996; and Rost and Sander, 1993). Most of the recent methods use ensembles of neural networks.

ANN has also been used to carry out expression analysis. An artificial neural system for gene classification called GenCANS was developed to analyze and manage a large volume of molecular sequencing data from the Human Genome Project (Wu, 1993, 1996; and Wu et al., 1992). Gen-CANS is based on a three-layered feed-forward backpropagation network. GenCANS was initially designed to classify unknown sequences into known classes. There are two extensive works of GenCANS – GenCANS-RDP (Wu and Shivakumar, 1994) and GenCANS-PIR (Wu, 1995). Gen-CANS-RDP is the RNA classification system which groups a number of small subunit ribosomal RNAs together based on RDP (Ribosomal Database Project) phylogenetic classes. GenCANS-PIR is the protein classification system which currently classifies protein sequences into more than 3,300 PIR (Protein Identification Resource) superfamilies.

Unsupervised learning neural networks can be generally categorized into the following types:

- self-organizing map (SOM) (Golub, 1999; Tamayo et al., 1999; Toronen et al., 1999),
- self-organizing tree (SOTA) (Herrero et al., 2001), and
- adaptive resonance theory (ART) (Azuaje, 2003, and Tomida et al., 2001).

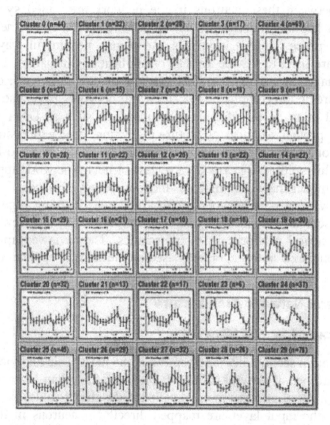

Fig. 5.5. The 828 genes of yeast cell cycle were grouped into 30 clusters (source: Tamayo et al., 1999)

They have been used to analyze gene expression data. ART was used to show that unsupervised learning neural network tools outperform for the analysis and visualization of gene expression profiles. Figure 5.5 shows an example result of applying SOM to analyze gene expression data.

5.3 Neural Network Architectures and Applications

Neural networks are parallel and distributed information processing systems that are inspired by and derived from biological learning systems such as the human brain. The architecture of neural networks consists of a network of nonlinear information processing elements that are normally arranged in layers and executed in parallel. This layered arrangement is referred to as the topology of a neural network. The nonlinear information processing elements in the network are called neurons, and the interconnections between these neurons in the network are called synapses or weights. A learning algorithm must be used to train a neural network so that it can process information in a useful and meaningful way. Neural networks are used in a wide variety of applications in pattern classification, language processing, complex systems modeling, control, optimization, and prediction (Lippman, 1987). Neural networks have also been actively used in many bioinformatics applications such as DNA sequence prediction, protein secondary structure prediction, gene expression profile classification, and analysis of gene expression patterns (Wu and McLarty, 2000). In this section, we provide a review of neural network applications in bioinformatics that accommodates the most recent advances.

A review of neural network architectures and learning algorithms is briefly presented in the next section. This is followed by a review of applications of neural networks in bioinformatics. The reviewed applications are then compared and categorized based on the areas of application.

5.3.1 Neural Network Architecture

Feed-Forward Neural Networks

As discussed in section 5.2, a perceptron is the most basic and the simplest feed-forward neural network model. It consists of an input layer and a single output layer of processing units called nodes. Input values presented to neurons in the input layer are mapped directly to neurons in the output layer. There are no intermediate processing steps. Each input is associated with a weight to reflect the significance of the input to the output. Given a set of training patterns that consist of exemplar "input" and "desired output" pairs, the perceptron is trained by feeding the input patterns to it and minimizing the error between its outputs and the desired outputs. Since the perceptron performs a direct mapping of input to output, it is a linear classifier, because only its weights define a hyperplane that divides input space into regions of pattern classes. The perceptron, therefore is, incapable of performing tasks that require nonlinear mappings between input and output.

For more complicated problems, a linear hyperplane is not good enough as a separator. A nonlinear surface that separates the classes is used instead. This can be achieved by the multi-layer perceptron (MLP), or the feed-forward network that consists of three layers of nodes, or neurons. Besides having an input layer and output layer, MLP has one (or several) hidden layer(s) in the middle. All artificial neural networks have a similar structure or topology, as shown in Fig. 5.6.

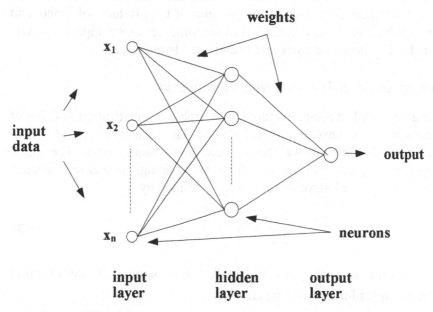

Fig. 5.6. The architecture of a multi-layer perceptron

Input data is a long continuous-valued vector that contains n elements, $x = (x_1, x_2,...,x_n)$. The n elements can be considered as the lengths of the inputs, and are determined by the problem specification. Each hidden neuron ($i = 1, 2,...,m$) stores an exemplar training sample faithfully as its weight vector $w = (w_{i,1}, w_{i,2},...,w_{i,n})$. A hidden neuron i is computed from the inputs

$$h_i = F(\sum_n w_{i,n} x_n)$$

(5.1)

where x_n denotes the nth input and $w_{i,n}$ denotes the weights between the input and hidden layers.

The hidden neurons are then used as inputs for the output y

$$y_i = G(\sum_n v_{i,n} h_n) \qquad (5.2)$$

where $v_{i,n}$ denotes the weights between the hidden and output layers. The activation function F or G is a sigmoid or logistic function which is usually differentiable and contributes to stability in neural network learning (Narayanan et al., 2003a).

Despite the simplicity of neural network, the summation functions can be more complex than just the simple sum of the products of inputs and their weights. The specific algorithm to combine neural inputs is determined by the chosen network architecture and hypothesis.

Training of Feed-Forward Neural Networks

Once a network has been structured for a problem specification, training of the network is the next step to be followed. The training of the network is nothing but finding the weights to minimize possible error. The initial weights are allocated randomly. Then, the training, or learning, begins. The commonly used algorithm for error is defined by

$$E = \frac{1}{2}\sqrt{\sum_i (t_i - O_i)^2} \qquad (5.3)$$

where t_i is the target output and O_i is the actual output. The steps used to find the weights for minimizing error are:

- choose the initial weights randomly for a sample input values,
- compare the actual output value with the target output value,
- calculate the error, and
- modify the weights so that the actual output is closer to the target output next time, with smaller error.

This process is repeated for all samples in the dataset and results, and then repeated until the output error for all the samples achieves an acceptable low value, which indicates the end point of the training. Once the training is finished, testing can be done using the rest of the data set, not used during the training phase, to test the trained neural network. If the testing is not satisfactory, further modification of the weights has to be done. Otherwise, the output value of the tested data is preserved for any decision making.

5.3.2 Neural Network Learning Algorithms

There are many different types of neural networks. Based on the type of learning, they can be categorized into supervised and unsupervised neural networks.

Supervised Learning Neural Networks

Most neural networks are trained with supervised training algorithms. This means that the desired output must be provided for each input used in the training. In other words, both the inputs and the outputs are already known. In supervised training, a network processes the inputs and compares its actual outputs against the expected outputs. Errors are then propagated back through the network, and the weights that control the network are changed. This process is repeated until the errors are minimized. This means that the same dataset is processed many times while the weights between the layers of the network are being refined during the training of the network. Figure 5.7 demonstrate the architecture for a supervised neural network that includes three layers, namely, input layer, output layer and, a hidden layer in the middle.

Support vector machines (SVMs) are considered supervised computer learning methods. Since the support vector machine (SVM) is well known as a training algorithm for learning classification from data, SVMs, as one of the major supervised neural networks, are widely used for the applications of classification and pattern recognition problems in bioinformatics (Vapnik, 1995, and Cristianini and Shawe-Taylor, 2000).

The theory of SVMs can be applied to the clustering of yeast microarray expression data. When the misclassification rates of SVMs are compared with those of other machine learning approaches, SVMs are found to be the best performing methods (Brown et al., 2000). In addition to their use for evaluating microarray expression data, SVMs have been shown to perform well in multiple areas of biological analysis, including detecting remote protein homologies (Jaakkola, 1999) and recognizing translation initiation sites. SVMs can also be used to analyze expression data (Furey et al., 2000). Gene expression data is usually high dimensional data that constitutes a serious problem in several machine learning methods. Dimensionality reduction can be used, but it leads often to information loss and performance degradation. Fortunately, SVMs can overcome this problem as they can generalize high dimensional data well (Valentini, 2002).

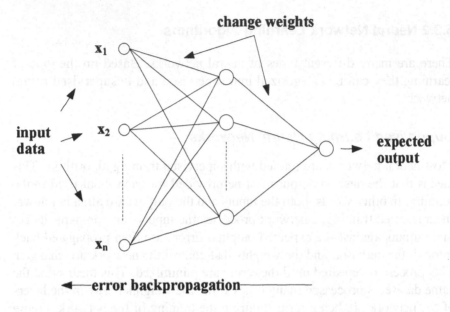

Fig. 5.7. A sample structure of supervised neural network

Unsupervised Learning Neural Networks

The learning algorithm used in unsupervised neural networks is an unsupervised learning algorithm. In unsupervised training, the network is provided only with inputs, while the expected output is unknown. The neural network must itself choose features to group the input data without being trained (Agatonovic-Kustrin and Beresford, 2000). Once an unsupervised neural network has been trained, it must be tested to show that the network really represents the data; the data is expected to be well represented in clusters.

A self-organizing network known as self-organizing map (SOM), or Kohonen network, is the most common algorithm used in unsupervised neural networks (Kohonen, 1982). It is different from the supervised learning described earlier. The neighborhood of a neuron is used to find and group the data that has the similarity. The grouped neurons are arranged in a matrix pattern called a map. Every input neuron is connected to other neurons in this map. Finally, these neurons form the output of the neural network, as shown Fig. 5.8.

The SOM consists of an input layer and a competitive output layer. The output layer is normally organized into a two-dimensional grid of fully connected neurons, as illustrated in Fig. 5.8. The input vectors are fed into input layer and mapped with competitive neurons in the output layer. The competition learning algorithm in the output layer ensures that similar input vectors are mapped with competitive neurons that are closer to each other in the grid than dissimilar ones. In SOM, input vectors in high dimensional space are, therefore, projected on to two-dimensional output space based on their spatial similarities. Similar input patterns are clustered into one small region in the grid of the output layer.

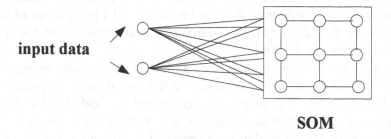

SOM

Fig. 5.8. Self-organizing map (adapted from Narayanan et al., 2003a)

The SOM is widely used as a data mining and visualization method in bioinformatics. It is a more robust and accurate method for the clustering of large amounts of noisy data than hierarchical clustering methods are for analyzing the gene expression data. In the analysis of the Stanford yeast gene expression dataset using SOMs, the best performance of gene expression analysis was the result of combining clustering and visualization methods (Torkkola et al., 2001). SOMs, can be used to reduce the amount of data through clustering, and to construct a nonlinear projection of the data onto a low dimensional display simultaneously. Therefore, SOMs can be used to combine aspects of gene analysis, namely, clustering and visualization.

Nevertheless, this approach presents several problems (Fritzke, 1994). They are as follows:

- As the SOM is a topology-preserving neural network, the number of clusters is randomly fixed from the beginning. Therefore, the clustering obtained is not proportionate.
- The lack of a tree structure makes it impossible to detect higher order relationships between clusters.

The hierarchical clustering and the SOM can be combined to surmount the problems faced by these methods in analysing the gene expression profiles and the gene expression data from DNA array experiments (Herrero et al., 2001, and Dopazo and Carazo, 1997).

The advantages of SOTA are as follows:

- the clustering obtained is proportional to the heterogeneity of the data
- the binary topology produces a nested structure in which nodes at each level are averages of the items below them.

An alternative way to avoid the problems is to use Fuzzy Kohonen Neural Networks that combines a Kohonen network and a fuzzy c-means algorithm to keep the advantages and overcome the shortcomings of both techniques (Granzow et al., 2001).

The advantages of the SOM can be attributed to its ability to map high dimensional data onto more comprehensible lower dimensional space and to its fast execution. It is potentially very useful for dealing with high dimensionality and large-scale databases to extract information from gene expression data. However, the effectiveness of its combining with database queries warrants further investigation. SOM also has limitations, namely, 1) no convergence guarantee and 2) the nondeterministic results that depend on learning rates.

5.3.3 Neural Network Applications in Bioinformatics

Neural networks have been widely used in biology since the early 1980s (Brusic and Zeleznikow, 1999). They can be used to

- predict the translation initiation sites in DNA sequences (Stormo et al., 1982).
- explain the theory of neural networks using applications in biology (Baldi and Brunak, 1998).
- predict immunologically interesting peptides by) combining an evolutionary algorithm (Brusic et al. 1998a)
- study human TAP transporter (Brusic et al., 1998b).
- carry out pattern classification and signal processing successfully in bioinformatics; in fact, a large number of applications of neural network can be found in this area
- perform protein sequence classification; neural networks are applied to protein sequence classification by extracting features from protein data

and using them in combination with the Bayesian neural network (BNN) (Wu et al., 1993, 1995, 1997, 2000).

- predict protein secondary structure prediction (Qian and Sejnowski, 1988).
- analyze the gene expression patterns as an alternative to hierarchical clusters (Toronen, Kolehmainen, et al., 1999; Wang, Ma, et al., 2000; Bicciato, Pandin, et al., 2001; and Torkkola, Gardner, et al., 2001); gene expression can even be analyzed using a single layer neural network (Narayanan, Keedwell, et al., 2003b).

In summary, a neural network is presented with a pattern on its input nodes, and the network produces an output pattern based on its learning algorithm during the training phase. Once trained, the neural network can be applied to classify new input patterns. This makes neural networks suitable for the analysis of gene expression patterns, prediction of protein structure, and other related processes in bioinformatics..

5.4 Genetic Algorithm

The genetic algorithm is an artificial system based on biological evolutionary mechanisms (Holland, 1975). A modern biological evolutionary theory came into existence by incorporating genetics and population biology theory into the classical evolution theory of Charles Darwin (Darwin, 1859). It can be defined as the inheritable changes, via genetic materials in a population of chromosomes, from one generation to the next generation. The main goal of evolution is to produce a population of chromosomes with increasing fitness. The fitness is a quantitative measure of the success of a chromosome in survival and reproduction. The main processes of natural evolution are reproduction of some chromosomes within a population, mutation in the DNA sequence within a gene or chromosome of an organism to create a new character not found in the parental type, and competition and fitness selection to limit expanding populations of different species in finite space.

The recombination (or crossover) first occurs during reproduction, resulting in the combination of genes from parents to form a new chromosome. The new chromosome, which consists of genes or blocks of DNA, can be mutated. The mutation can be caused, for example, by errors in copying genes from parents. These errors change the gene's position (or locus) in the chromosome, and this change is called genetic variation. But one might question which parents should be chosen to form a new chromosome. Naturally, parental chromosomes are selected to produce new chromosome according to the fitness of the genotypes. A chromosome with higher fitness has a higher chance than other chromosomes of being selected to reproduce. Natural evolution is a gradual, continuous, and never ending process.

The biological evolutionary theory inspired computer scientists to develop an intelligent system that is capable of imitating the principles of natural evolution.

An automatic mechanism to adapt and learn is desirable for producing good solutions. This is the starting point of a genetic algorithm.

The genetic algorithm is a search algorithm that operates on pieces of information. It is similar to a natural evolutionary process that operates on the information stored in genes. In the genetic algorithm, chromosomes are represented as binary strings; these strings are modified in the same way that populations of chromosomes evolve in nature. The population of strings improves its fitness over interactions, and after a number of generations the population finally evolves to the best solution for a given problem. In each generation, all strings are evaluated by a fitness function for their performance. Based on these evaluations, a new population of strings, with well adapted effectiveness, is formed by using genetic operators such as selection, crossover, and mutation.

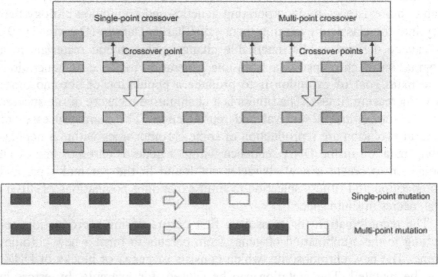

Fig. 5.9. The illustration showing how crossover and mutation operators work

The selection operator selects the as many survival chromosomes as possible from a given population based on their fitness values. The aim of the selection is to increase the occurrence of fitter chromosomes in the population over subsequent generations. There exist a wide number of selection techniques (Forrest, 1985; Goldberg and Deb, 1991; and Grefenstette and Baker, 1989); however, a detailed discussion on the selection techniques is beyond the scope of this book. Further reading can be found in any genetic algorithm book.

The crossover operator breaks and then swaps some parts of two parental chromosomes. The mutation operator represents a mechanism through which a randomly chosen gene (or several genes) is (are) changed to some other gene. The mutation introduces diversity to the population and guarantees that the population is not trapped at a local maximum. Figure 5.9 shows a typical case of crossover and mutation operators.

As mentioned before, the genetic algorithm simulates the process of natural evolution. Analogies between the two can be found in Table 5.3.

Table 5.3. A comparison of the genetic algorithm and the natural evolutionary mechanism

Natural evolution	Genetic algorithm
Environment	Given problem
Chromosome	Binary string
Fitness of phenotype (probability of survival)	Fitness function
Locus	A position on the string
Selection, recombination, crossover, and mutation	Genetic operators
A population of chromosomes that suits to the environment	The optimal solutions to a given problem

The genetic algorithm is a simple computational model compared to the natural mechanism; however, complex and interesting structures have been developed using genetic algorithms. Most genetic algorithms consist of the following steps (Coley, 1999; Ghanea-Hercock, 2003; and Goldberg, 1989):

Step 1 (a) Encode the problem variables as a chromosome, representing a fixed-length binary string.
(b) Choose a population size, N.

(c) Define a fitness function to measure the probability that a chromosome will be selected as a parent chromosome to further generate new chromosomes.

Step 2   Randomly generate a population of chromosomes of size, N.

Step 3   Test each chromosome in the population with the fitness function.

Step 4   Perform the following sub-steps until termination condition such as specified best fitness values, is satisfied.

(a) Select a pair of chromosomes from the population with the higher fitness value as parent chromosomes for reproduction.

(b) Apply the genetic operators to selected parent chromosomes to create a pair of offspring chromosomes.

(c) Allow the offspring chromosomes and their parents to form the new population.

(d) Replace the current chromosome population with the new population.

(e) Calculate the fitness value of each chromosome of the new population.

Step 5   Output the optimal solutions to a given problem as the fittest chromosomes.

Genetic algorithms have a number of advantages.

- A genetic algorithm is a parallel search, that is, in each generation several solutions are checked at once. It generates optimized and robust solutions via powerful operators; for example, bad solutions are filtered out by selection, and local optimal solutions can be avoided by mutation.
- A genetic algorithm can provide good solutions even if very little information about the problem is provided. As a result, genetic algorithms are widely used in classification and optimization.

However there are limitations with the genetic algorithm.

- Encoding a given problem in a suitable representation (for example, bit string) is difficult and often changes the nature of the problem being investigated. Natural evolution does not always produce a good solution. Nor does a genetic algorithm. It frequently converges to a local optimum.
- A genetic algorithm involves several parameters, such as representation, population size, and fitness function. In practice, it is difficult to define

or create these parameters due to the lack of guidelines for choosing them.

It is expected that new developments in genetic algorithms may overcome the limitations.

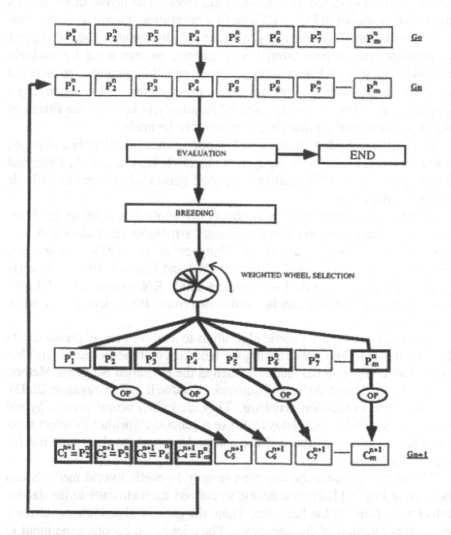

Fig. 5.10. The layout of the SAGA algorithm (Notredame and Higgins, 1996)

The genetic algorithm has been successfully applied for solving many practical problems in many disciplines, in particular, in bioinformatics. Genetic algorithms have been used to solve multiple sequence alignment problems. One well known approach is SAGA (Ohno-Machado et al., 2002). SAGA randomly creates an initial population of alignments and evolves them in a quasi-evolutionary manner. Through each generation, the fitness of the population is gradually improved. The authors show that SAGA outperforms the most common solution of the multiple alignment problem that uses progressive approach (Barton and Sternberg, 1987; Feng and Doolitle, 1987; and Thompson et al., 1994). The layout of the SAGA algorithm is shown in Fig. 5.10. The first generation initially creates a random population (G_0) consisting of a set of alignments. The subsequent generations are derived from better parents, as measured by multiple alignment quality. When creating children, genetic operators are involved in selecting the better parents, in mixing the contents, and in modifying a single parent. These steps are repeated iteratively to increase the fitness of the population until no more improvement can be made.

In addition to SAGA, there are a few approaches (Chellapilla and Fogel, 1999; Isokawa et al., 1996; Nguyen et al., 2002; Wayama et al., 1995; and Zhang and Wong, 1997) that have applied genetic algorithms to multiple sequence alignment.

Genetic algorithms have been commonly applied to a set of RNA sequences to find common RNA secondary structures (Benedetti and Morosetti, 1995; Chen et al., 2000; Gultyaev et al., 1995; Shapiro and Navetta, 1994; Shapiro et al., 2001; and Wu and Shapiro, 1999). The early proposed methods can deal only with a single RNA sequence, while the latest improved methods can be used to determine RNA structures in RNA sequences.

The trend to use pure genetic algorithms to analyze gene expression data has diminished. The new techniques tend to combine genetic algorithm with other computational methods, such as the K-nearest Neighbor Method (Li et al., 2001) and the neural network (Keedwell and Narayanan, 2003), to solve gene expression problems. They are called neural-genetic hybrid methods. Keedwell and Narayanan use a genetic algorithm to select a set of genes for classification and use a neural network to determine the fitness of the genes.

The steps that are to be followed in neural-genetic hybrid methods can be seen in Fig. 5.11. Preprocessing, to convert each attribute in the dataset into binary field, is the first step. Then, the genetic algorithm initializes a random population of chromosomes. The population becomes the input to the neural network. The network is trained till the desired output (minimum error) is produced. The error from each chromosome acts as a fitness function to determine mutation, crossover, and selection for the next generation of chromosomes. The generation creation process is iterated until the maximum number of generations is satisfied, that is, until the correct classification of genes is finally discovered.

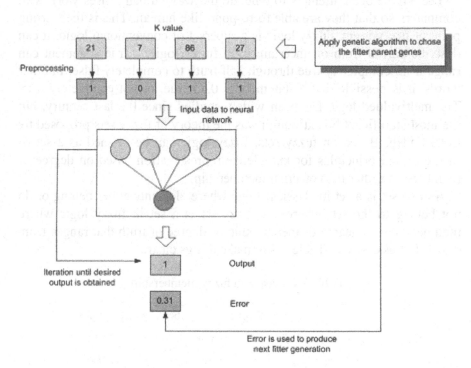

Fig. 5.11. The visual layout of neural-genetic algorithm (adapted from Keedwell and Narayanan, 2003)

5.5 Fuzzy System

A fuzzy system is an expert system that uses a collection of fuzzy membership functions and rules, instead of Boolean logic, to reason about data. It provides a rich meaningful addition to classical logic. The basic concepts of a fuzzy system include fuzzy logic and fuzzy set theory. In order to understand a fuzzy expert system, related terminologies and theories are first explained.

A characteristic of human mind is its ability to reason about vague and ambiguous terms. For example, today may feel hot because the temperature is more than 33°C. If the temperature tomorrow is 31°C, human senses can immediately interpret it as moderately hot. However, a computer with conventional logic cannot replicate that statement. The reason is that in conventional logic a statement is either true or false, and not multi-valued or partially true or false.

There have been attempts to emulate the way human senses work with computers so that they are able to respond like human. This is the starting point of fuzzy logic. Fuzzy logic is a superset of conventional logic. It can describe partial truth or uncertainty. In fuzzy logic, a true statement can range from completely true through half truth to completely false. In other words, it is possible that a statement is 0.75 true, or not completely true. The multivalued logic has been widely studied since the last century, but the most significant breakthrough was the theory of fuzzy sets proposed by Lotfi Zadeh. Based on fuzzy sets, fuzzy logic can be defined as a set of mathematical principles for knowledge representation based on degree of membership rather than on crisp membership.

A crisp set is a set in classical logic where elements either belong or do not belong to the set, whereas a fuzzy set is a set in fuzzy logic where members have a degree of membership or degree of truth that ranges from 0 to 1. Let us consider Table 5.4 to make things clear.

Table 5.4. Crisp and fuzzy membership

Day	Temperature, °C	Degree of membership of "Hot day"	
		Crisp	Fuzzy
1	5	0.0	0.0
2	10	0.0	0.0
3	25	0.0	0.1
4	27	0.0	0.3
5	29	0.0	0.5
6	30	0.0	0.8
7	33	1.0	1.0
8	35	1.0	1.0
9	40	1.0	1.0

In crisp set theory, days 1 through 9 fall into only two groups (hot and not hot), depending on their temperatures (°C). If the temperature is less than 33°C, the day is considered not hot. Unlike crisp set theory, fuzzy set theory classifies its members (days) by regarding the degree of truth (hotness). Therefore, there are more than two groups of days. It is a cold day if the temperature is less than or equal 10°C and it is hot day if the temperature is equal to or more than 33°C. For example, days 1 and 2 are hot with

0 degree of truth; days 3 through 6 are hot with 0.10, 0.30, 0.50, and 0.80 degrees of through respectively; and days 7 through 9 are considered hot day with 1 degree of truth. The question is how to find the degree of membership.

In classical set theory, the degree of membership can be calculated by a characteristic function. For example, the crisp set "Hot day" can be defined as

$$f_{Hot\ day}(temperature)=\begin{cases}1 & if\ temperature \geq 33 \\ 0 & otherwise\end{cases} \tag{5.4}$$

The function $f_{Hot\ day}(temperature)$ maps each temperature value onto 0 or 1. In a fuzzy set, the mapping function, called membership function, maps each temperature value onto the real interval [0, 1]. In the "Hot day" case, the membership function can be defined as

$$\mu_{Hotday}(temperature)=\begin{cases}1 & if\ temperature \geq 33 \\ 0 & if\ temperature \leq 10 \\ between\ 0\ and\ 1 & if\ 10 < temperature < 33\end{cases} \tag{5.5}$$

In a manner similar to that of producing crisp and fuzzy sets of "Hot day", crisp and fuzzy sets of "Fine day" and "Cold day", and their degrees of membership, can be obtained as shown in Table 5.5.

Table 5.5. Crisp and fuzzy set temperatures, with members Cold, Fine, and Hot

| Day | Temperature °C | Degree of membership | | | | | |
| | | Crisp | | | Fuzzy | | |
		Cold	Fine	Hot	Cold	Fine	Hot
1	5	1.0	0.0	0.0	1.0	0.0	0.0
2	10	1.0	0.0	0.0	1.0	0.0	0.0
3	25	0.0	1.0	0.0	0.8	0.8	0.1
4	27	0.0	1.0	0.0	0.5	1.0	0.3
5	29	0.0	1.0	0.0	0.3	1.0	0.5
6	30	0.0	1.0	0.0	0.1	0.8	0.8
7	33	0.0	0.0	1.0	0.0	0.0	1.0
8	35	0.0	0.0	1.0	0.0	0.0	1.0
9	40	0.0	0.0	1.0	0.0	0.0	1.0

The characteristic and membership functions that describe how to translate from temperature in value to temperature in words, and vice versa, are shown in Fig. 5.12.

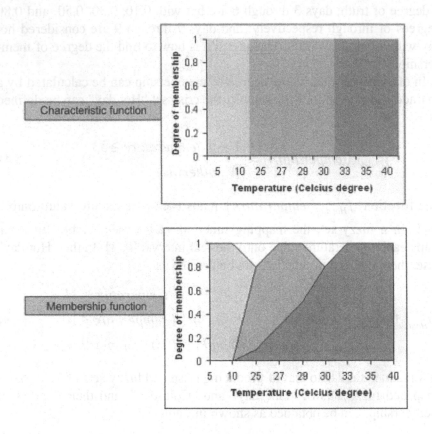

Fig. 5.12. Characteristic and membership functions of Cold, Fine, and Hot day

Another important concept of fuzzy set theory is the linguistic variable. It is used to construct the fuzzy rules. For example, "Temperature" is called a linguistic variable, and "hot", "fine", and "cold" are called linguistic values. A simple fuzzy rule can be represented in the following way:

$$\text{IF} \quad x \text{ is A} \quad \text{THEN} \quad y \text{ is B} \tag{5.6}$$

where x and y represent linguistic variables and A and B are linguistic values. One can use operations, including EQUAL, COMPLEMENT (NOT), CONTAINMENT, UNION (OR), and INTERSECTION (AND), to construct a more complex fuzzy rule such as:

$$\text{IF (x is A) AND (y is B) AND (…) OR NOT (…) THEN } z \text{ is Z}$$

$$\tag{5.7}$$

$$\text{IF } x \text{ is A THEN (y is B) AND (…) AND } z \text{ is Z}$$

where x, y, and z are variables and A, B, and Z are values. The IF part of the rule is called the rule antecedent and the THEN part of the rule is called the rule consequent. If the antecedent part is true with a degree of membership, then consequent part is also true with the same degree. The outputs of fuzzy sets are aggregated into a single. Then the single output is transformed to a single output number. Many researchers have proposed techniques (Mamdani and Assilian, 1975) that facilitate the whole process from the beginning to the end. The most significant technique is fuzzy inference. Fuzzy inference is a tool used to evaluate a knowledge base. It takes a given input and fires an output by using the theory of fuzzy sets. Generally, it consists of four steps: fuzzification of the input variables, rule evaluation, aggregation of the rule outputs, and defuzzification, as shown in Fig. 5.13.

The development of the fuzzy expert system (FES) is an iterative process. A typical process involves the following four steps:

- determine problem input and output variables and their ranges,
- define fuzzy sets and construct fuzzy rules,
- perform fuzzy inference process, and
- evaluate and tune the system.

The basic structure of a fuzzy system can be seen in Fig. 5.14. It consists of four basic components: a fuzzifier, an inference engine, a defuzzifier, and a knowledge base. More details of these components are beyond the scope of this chapter; however, they can be found in general artificial intelligence or soft computing books (Kruse et al., 1994).

Fuzzy systems have been successfully applied to several areas in practice. In bioinformatics, fuzzy systems play an important role for building knowledge-based systems. Most systems involve fuzzy logic-based and fuzzy rule-based models. They can control and analyze processes and diagnose and make decisions in biomedical sciences (Adriaenssens et al., 2004; Boegl et al., 2004; Saritas et al., 2003; Sarkar and Leong, 2003; Schneider et al., 2003; Seker et al., 2003; and Virant-Klun and Virant, 1999).

A fuzzy expert system for the diagnosis of prostate cancer (Saritas et al., 2003), has been explained in detail. The authors use prostate-specific antigen (PSA), age, and prostate volume (PV) as input parameters, and prostate cancer risk as output. The input values are converted to the linguistic variables, with degree of truth. This conversion is done by the membership function. Then, 80 rules are formed. The output of each rule has a degree of truth, obtained from fuzzy operation (MIN and MAX). Finally, the fuzzy outputs are converted into real output values. Figure 5.15 shows the overview of the FES system and its components.

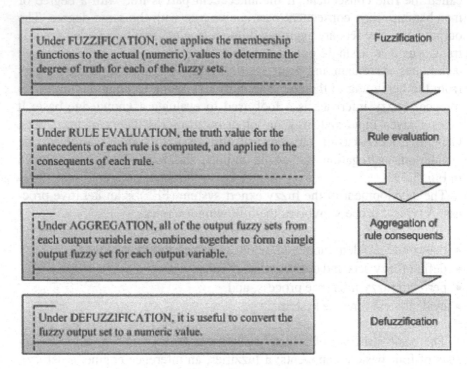

Fig. 5.13. The general steps of fuzzy inference

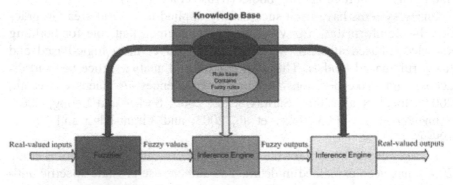

Fig. 5.14. The basic components of fuzzy expert system

In addition, fuzzy logic has been recently applied to analyze (Woolf and Wang, 2000) and to classify (Ohno-Machado et al., 2002) gene expression data. The fuzzy logic-based classifier gives results similar to those of other classifiers, but are much simpler and easier to interpret (Ohno-Machado et al., 2002). Fuzzy logic accounts for noisy data from a large number of biological patterns.

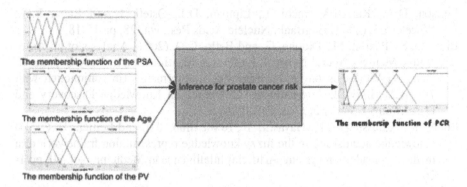

Fig. 5.15. The structure of the fuzzy expert system (FES) for diagnosis of prostate cancer (adapted from Saritas et al., 2003)

References

Adeli, H. (1995) Machine learning : neural networks, genetic algorithms, and fuzzy systems. New York: Wiley.

Adriaenssens, V., Baetsb, B.D., Goethalsa, P.L.M. and Pauwa, N.D. (2004) Fuzzy rule-based models for decision support in ecosystem management. Science of The Total Environment, vol. 319, pp 1-12.

Agatonovic-Kustrin, S., Beresford, R. (2000). Basic concepts of artificial neural network (ANN) modeling and its application in pharmaceutical research. Journal of Pharmaceutical and Biomedical Analysis 22(5): 717-727.

Azuaje, F. (2003) A computational evolutionary approach to evolving game strategy and cooperation. IEEE Transactions on Systems, Man, and Cybernetics, Part B, vol. 33, pp 498-503.

Baldi, P. and Brunak, S. (2001) "Bioinformatics The Machine Learning Approach", The MIT Press.

Baldi, P., Brunak, S., Frasconi, P., Pollastri, G. and Soda, G. (2000) Bidirectional IOHMMs and Recurrent Neural Networks for Protein Secondary Structure Prediction. In: Protein Sequence Analysis in the Genomic Era, R. Casadio and L. Masotti, Eds. CLUEB, Bologna, Italy.

Baldi, P. and Brunak, S. (1998) Bioinformatics: the Machine Learning Approach. MIT Press.

Barton, G.J. and Sternberg, M.J.E. (1987) A strategy for the rapid multiple alignment of protein sequences: Confidence levels from tertiary structure comparisons. Journal of Molecular Biology, vol. 198, pp 327-337.

Baxevanis, A.D., Ouellette, B.F.F. (2001) Bioinformatics : a practical guide to the analysis of genes and proteins, 2nd ed ed. New York: Wiley-Interscience.

Benedetti, G. and Morosetti, S. (1995) A genetic algorithm to search for optimal and suboptimal RNA secondary structures. Biophysical Chemistry, vol. 55, pp 253-259.

Benson, D.A., Karsch-Mizrachi, I., Lipman, D.J., Ostell, J. and Rapp, B.A., Wheeler DL (2002) GenBank. Nucleic Acids Res., vol. 28, pp 15-18.

Bicciato, S., Pandin, M., Didone, G. and Bello, C.D. (2001) Analysis of an Associative Memory Neural Network for Pattern Identification in Gene Expression Data. 1st Workshop on Data Mining in Bioinformatics (in conjunction with 7th ACM SIGKDD International Conference on Knowledge Discovery and Data Mining), San Francisco, CA, USA.

Boegl, K., Adlassnig, K.P., Hayashi, Y., Rothenfluh, T.E. and Leitich, H. (2004) Knowledge acquisition in the fuzzy knowledge representation framework of a medical consultation system. Artificial Intelligence in Medicine, vol. 30, pp 1-26.

Bohr, H., Bohr, J., Brunak, S., Cotteril, R.M., Fredholm, H., Lautrup, B. and Peterson, S.B. (1990) A novel approach to prediction of the 3-dimensional structures of protein backbones by neural networks. FEBS Letters, vol. 261, pp 43-46.

Brown, M.P.S., Grundy, W,N., et al. (2000) Knowledge-based analysis of microarray gene expression data by using support vector machines. Proceedings of the National Academy of Sciences 97(1): 262-267

Brusic, V., Rudy, G., Honeyman, M., Hammer, J. and Harrison, L. (1998a) Prediction of MHC class-II binding peptides using an evolutionary algorithm and artificial neural network. Bioinformatics 14, 121-130.

Brusic, V., Van Endert, P., Zeleznikow, J., Daniel, S., Hammer, J. and Petrovsky, N. (1998b) A Neural Network Model Approach to the Study of Human TAP Transporter. Silico biology 1, 0010.

Brusic, V. and Zeleznikow, J. (1999) Knowledge discovery and data mining in biological databases. The Knowledge Engineering Review 14, 257-277.

Chellapilla, K. and Fogel, G.B. (1999) Multiple sequence alignment using evolutionary programming. Congress on Evolutionary Computation, pp 445-452.

Chen, J-H., Le, S-Y. and Maizel, J.V. (2000) Prediction of common secondary structures of RNAs: a genetic algorithm approach. Nucleic Acids Res., vol. 28, pp 991-999.

Coley, D.A. (1999) An introduction to genetic algorithms for scientists and engineers. Singapore: World Scientific.

Cristianini, N. and Shawe-Taylor, J. (2000) An Introduction to Support Vector Machines (and other kernel-based learning methods), Cambridge University Press.

Darwin, C. (1859) On the Origin of Species by means of natural selection: John Murray, London.

Dopazo J and Carazo JM (1997) Phylogenetic reconstruction using a growing neural work that adopts the topology of a phylogenetic tree. Journal of Moleculer Evolution 44: 226-233.

Fairchild, S., Pachter, R. and Perrin, R. (1995) Protein Structure Analysis and Prediction. The Mathematica Journal, vol. 5.

Feng, D.F. and Doolitle, R.F. (1987) Progressive sequence alignment as a prerequisite to correct phylogenetic trees. Journal of Molecular Evolution, vol. 25, pp 351-360.

Finlay, J. and Dix, A. (1996) Introduction to artificial intelligence: Taylor and Francis.

Forrest, S. (1985) Documentation for prisonner dilemna and norms programs that use the genetic algorithm. University of Michigan, Technical report.

Freeman, J.A. and Skapura, D.M. (1991) Neural networks : algorithms, applications, and programming techniques. Reading, Mass: Addison-Wesley.

Fritzke, B (1994) Growing cell structures--a self -organizing network for unsupervised and supervised learning. Neural Networks 7: 1141-1160.

Fu, L. (1999) Knowledge Discovery Based on Neural Networks. Communications of the ACM (CACM), vol. 42, pp 47-50.

Furey, T.S., Cristianini, N., et al. (2000) Support vector machine classification and validation of cancer tissue samples using microarray expression data. Bioinformatics 16(10): 906-914.

Ghanea-Hercock, R. (2003) Applied evolutionary algorithms in Java. New York: Springer.

Goldberg, D.E. (1989) Genetic algorithms in search, optimization, and machine learning: Addison-Wesley Pub. Co.

Goldberg, D.E., Deb, K. (1991) A comparison of selection schemes used in genetic algorithms. In: Foundations of Genetic Algorithms, G. J. E. Rawlins, Edn. pp 69-93.

Golub, T.R. (1999) Molecular classification of cancer: class discovery and class prediction by gene expression monitoring. Science, vol. 286, pp 531-537.

Granzow, M., Berrar, D., et al. (2001) Tumour classification by gene expression profiling: comparison and validation of five clustering methods. ACM SIGBIO Newsletter 21(1): 16 – 22.

Grefenstette, J.J., Baker, J.E. (1989) How genetic algorithms work: A critical look at implicit parallelism. Presented at Proc. 3rd Intl. Conf. Genetic Algorithms, San Mateo, CA.

Gultyaev, A.P., Batenburg, F.H.D., Pleij, C.W.A. (1995) The Computer Simulation of RNA Folding Pathways using a Genetic Algorithm. Journal of Molecular Biology, vol. 250, pp 37-51.

Han, J. and Kamber, M. (2001) Data mining : concepts and techniques. San Francisco, Calif.: Morgan Kaufmann Publishers.

Haykin, S. (1994) Neural networks : a comprehensive foundation. Upper Saddle River, N.J.: Prentice Hall.

Herrero, J., Valencia, A. and Dopazo, J. (2001) A hierarchical unsupervised growing neural network for clustering gene expression patterns. Bioinformatics, vol. 17, pp 126-136.

Herrero, J., Valencia, A., et al. (2001) A hierarchical unsupervised growing neural network for clustering gene expression patterns. Bioinformatics 17(2): 126-136.

Holland, J.H. (1975) Adaptation in Natural and Artificial Systems: University of Michigan Press, Ann Arbor.

Isokawa, M., Wayama, M. and Shimizu, T. (1996) Multiple sequence alignment using a genetic algorithm. Genome Informatics, vol. 7, pp 176-177.

Jaakkola, T., Diekhans, M., et al. (1999) Using the Fisher kernel method to detect remote protein homologies. 7th International Conference on Intelligent Systems for Molecular Biology, Menlo Park, CA.

Jagota, A. (2000) Data analysis and classification for bioinformatics. California: Bay Press.

Kalate, R.N., Tambe, S.S., Kulkarni, B.D. (2003) Artificial neural networks for prediction of mycobacterial promoter sequences. Comput Biol Chem, vol. 27, pp 555-564.

Kandel, A. (1992) Fuzzy expert systems. Boca Raton, FL: CRC Press.

Keedwell, E.C., Narayanan, A. (2003) Genetic algorithms for gene expression analysis. Presented at Applications of Evolutionary Computation: Proceedings of the 1st European Workshop on Evolutionary Bioinformatics (EvoBIO 2003).

Kohonen, T. (1982) Self-organized formation of topologically correct feature maps. Biological Cybernetics 43: 59-69.

Kohonen, T. (1990) The self-organizing map. Proceedings of IEEE 78(9): 1464-1480.

Kruse, R., Gebhardt, J., Palm, R. (1994) Foundations of fuzzy systems. Chichester, West Sussex, England; New York: Wiley & Sons.

Kruse, R., Gebhardt, J., Palm, R. (1994) Fuzzy systems in computer science. Braunschweig: Vieweg.

Kuonen, D. (2003) Challenges in Bioinformatics for Statistical Data Miners. Bulletin of the Swiss Statistical Society, vol. 46, pp 10-17.

Li, L., Weinberg, C.R., Darden, T.A. and Pedersen, L.G. (2001) Gene selection for sample classification based on gene expression data: study of sensitivity to choice of parameters of the GA/KNN method. Bioinformatics, vol. 17, pp 1131-1142.

Lippman, R.P. (1987) An introduction to computing with neural nets. IEEE Acoustics, Speech, and Signal Processing Magazine 4(2): 4-22.

Mamdani, E.H. and Assilian, S. (1975) An Experiment in Linguistic Synthesis with a Fuzzy Logic Controller. International Journal of Man-Machine Studies, vol. 7, pp 1-13.

Minsky, M. and Papert, S. (1969) Perceptrons: MIT Press, Cambridge.

Müller, B. and Reinhardt, J. (1990) Neural networks: an introduction. Berlin; New York: Springer-Verlag.

Narayanan, A., Keedwell, E., et al. (2003a) Artificial Intelligence Techniques for Bioinformatics. Applied Bioinformatics 1(4): 191-222.

Narayanan, A., Keedwell, E., et al. (2003b) Single-Layer Artificial Neural Networks for Expression Analysis. Special Issue on Bioinformatics of Neurocomputing.

Gene Narayanan, A., Keedwell, E.C. and Olsson, B. (2002) Artificial intelligence techniques for bioinformatics. Applied Bioinformatics, vol. 1, pp 191-222.

Negnevitsky, M. (2002) Artificial Intelligence: A Guide to Intelligent Systems. New York: Addison Wesley.

Ng, S-K. and Wong, L. (2004) Accomplishments and Challenges in Bioinformatics. In: IT pro, pp 12-18.

Nguyen, H.D., Yoshihara, I., Yamamori, K. and Yasunage, M. (2002) A Parallel Hybrid Genetic Algorithm for Multiple Protein Sequence Alignment. Presented at Proceedings of the 2002 Congress on Evolutionary Computation CEC2002, Piscataway, NJ.

Nilsson, N.J. (1996) Introduction to Machine learning.

Notredame, C. and Higgins, D.G. (1996) SAGA: Sequence alignment by genetic algorithm. Nucleic Acids Res., vol. 24, pp 1515-1524.

Ohno-Machado, L. and Vinterbo, S., Weber, G. (2002) Classification of gene expression data using fuzzy logic. Journal of Intelligent and Fuzzy Systems, vol. 12, pp 19-24.

Qian, N. and Sejnowski, T.J. (1988) Predicting the secondary structure of globular proteins using neural network models. Journal of Molecular Biology 202: 865-884.

Qian, N. and Sejnowski, T.J. (1988) Predicting the secondary structure of globular proteins using neural network models. Journal of Molecular Biology, vol. 202, pp 865-884.

Riis, S.K. and Krogh, A. (1996) Improving prediction of protein secondary structure using structured neural networks and multiple sequence alignments. J Comput Biol., vol. 3, pp 163-183.

Rosenblatt, F. (1958) The perceptron: a probabilistic model for information storage and organization in the brain. Psychological Review, vol. 65, pp 386-408.

Rost, B. and Sander, C. (1993) Prediction of protein secondary structure at better than 70% accuracy. Journal of Molecular Biology, vol. 232, pp 584-599.

Saritas, I., Allahverdi, N. and Sert, I.U. (2003) A fuzzy expert system design for diagnosis of prostate cancer. Presented at International Conference on Computer Systems and Technologies, Sofia, Bulgaria.

Sarkar, M. and Leong, T-Y. (2003) Characterization of medical time series using fuzzy similarity-based fractal dimensions. Artificial Intelligence in Medicine, vol. 27, pp 201-222.

Schneider, J., Peltri, G., Bitterlich, N., Neu, K., Velcovsky, H.G., Morr, H., Katz, N. and Eigenbrodt, E. (2003) Fuzzy logic-based tumor marker profiles including a new marker tumor M2-PK improved sensitivity to the detection of progression in lung cancer patients. Anticancer Res., vol. 23, pp 899-906, 2003.

Seker, H., Odetayo, M.O., Petrovic, D. and Naguib, R.N.G. (2003) A fuzzy logic based-method for prognostic decision making in breast and prostate cancers. Information Technology in Biomedicine, IEEE Transactions, vol. 7, pp 114-122.

Shapiro, B.A. and Navetta, J. (1994) A massively parallel genetic algorithm for RNA secondary structure prediction. Journal of Supercomputing, vol. 8, pp 195-207.

Shapiro, B.A., Wu, JC., Bengali, D. and Potts, M.J. (2001) The massively parallel genetic algorithm for RNA folding: MIMD implementation and population variation. Bioinformatics, vol. 17, pp. 137-148.

Spicker, J.S., Wikman, F., Lu, M-L., Cordon-Cardo, C., Workman, C., Rntoft, T.F., Brunak, S. and Knudsen, S. (2002) Neural network predicts sequence of TP53 gene based on DNA chip. Bioinformatics, vol. 18, pp 1133-1134, 2002.

Stormo, G. D., Schneider, T. D., Gold, L. and Ehrenfeucht, A. (1982) Use of "Perceptron" algorithm to distinguish translatioanl initiation in E.coli. Nucleic Acids Research 10, 2997-3011.

Synder, E.E. and Stormo, G.D. (1993) Identification of coding regions in genomic DNA sequences: an application of dynamic programming and neural networks. Nucleic Acids Res., vol. 21, pp 607-613.

Synder, E.E. and Stormo, G.D. (1997) Identifying genes in genomic DNA sequences. In: DNA and Protein Sequence, M. J. Bishop and C. J. Rawlings, Edn. NewYork: Oxford University Press, pp 209-224.

Tamayo, P., Slonim, D., Mesirov, J., Zhu, Q., Kitareewan, S., Dmitrovsky, E., Lander, E.S. and Golub, T.R. (1999) Interpreting patterns of gene expression with self-organizing maps: methods and application to hematopoietic differentiation. Presented at Proc Natl Acad Sci, USA.

Thompson, J.D., Higgins, D.G. and Gibson, T.J. (1994) CLUSTAL W: Improving the sensitivity of progressive multiple sequence alignment through sequence weighting, position-specific gap penalties and weight matrix choice. Nucleic Acids Res., vol. 22, pp 4673-4680.

Tomida, S., Hanai, T., Honda, H. and Kobayashi, T. (2001) Gene Expression Analysis Using Fuzzy ART. Genome Informatics, vol. 12, pp 245-246.

Torkkola, K., Mike G.R., Kaysser-Kranich, T. and Ma, C. (2001) Self-organizing maps in mining gene expression data. Information Sciences 139, 79-96.

Toronen, P., Kolehmainen, M., Wong, C. and Castren, E. (1999) Analysis of gene expression data using self-organizing maps. In: FEBS Letters, vol. 451, pp 142-146.

Toronen, P., Kolehmainen, M., Wong, G. and Castrén, E. (1999) Analysis of gene expression data using self-organizing maps. Federation of European Biochemical Societies Letters 451, 142-146.

Uberbacher, E.C. and Mural, R.J. (1991) Locating Protein Coding Regions in Human DNA Sequences Using a Multiple Sensor-Neural Network Approach. Presented at Proc.Natl. Acad. Sci., USA.

Valentini, G. (2002). Gene expression data analysis of human lymphoma using support vector machines and output coding ensembles. Artificial Intelligence in Medicine 26(3): 281-304.

Vapnik, V. (1996) The nature of statistical learning theory, Springer.

Virant-Klun, I. and Virant, J. (1999) Fuzzy logic alternative for analysis in the biomedical sciences. Comput Biomed Res, vol. 32, pp 305-321.

Wang, J.T.L., Ma, Q., Shasha, D. and Wu, C.H. (2000) Application of neural networks to biological data mining: a case study in protein sequence classification. 6th ACM SIGKDD International Conference on Knowledge Discovery and Data Mining 20, 305 – 309.

Wayama, M., Takahashi, K., Shimizu, T. (1995) An approach to amino acid sequence alignment using a genetic algorithm. Genome Informatics, vol. 6, pp 122-123.

Westhead, D.R., Parish, J.H. and Twyman, R.M. (2002) "Bioinformatics", Instant Notes in Bioinformatics, BIOS Scientific Publishing.

Wong, L. (2000) Kleisli, a Funcitonal Query System. Journal of Functional Programming, vol. 10, pp 19-56.

Wong, L. (2002) Technologies for Integrating Biological Data. Briefings in Bioinformatics, vol. 3, pp 389-404, 2002.

Woolf, P.J. and Wang, Y. (2000) A fuzzy logic approach to analyzing gene expression data. Physiological Genomics, vol. 3, pp 9-15.

Wu, C. (1993) Classification Neural Networks For Rapid Sequence Annotation And Automated Database Organization. Computer & Chemistry, vol. 17, pp 219-227,.

Wu, C. (1996) Gene Classification Artificial Neural System. In: Methods In Enzymology: Computer Methods for Macromolecular Sequence Analysis, vol. 266, R. Doolittle, Ed, pp 71-88.

Wu, C., Berry M, Shivakumar S, McLarty J (1995) Neural Networks For Full-Scale Protein Sequence Classification: Sequence Encoding With Singular Value Decomposition. Machine Learning, vol. 21.

Wu, C. and Shivakumar, S. (1994) Back-Propagation And Counter-Propagation Neural Networks For Phylogenetic Classification Of Ribosomal RNA Sequences. Nucleic Acids Research, vol. 22, pp 4291-4299.

Wu, C., Whitson, G., McLarty, J., Ermongkonchai, A. and Chang, T. (1992) Protein Classification Artificial Neural System. Protein Science, vol. 1, pp 667-677.

Wu, C.H. (1997) Artificial neural networks for molecular sequence analysis. Computers and Chemistry 21(4): 237-256.

Wu, C.H., Berry, M.W., et al. (1993) Neural Networks for Molecular Sequence Classification. Proceeding of 1st ISMB.

Wu, C.H., Berry, M,W., et al. (1995) Neural Networks for Full-Scale Protein Sequence Classification: Sequence Encoding with Singular Value Decomposition. Machine Learning 21(1-2): 177-193.

Wu, C.H., McLarty, J.W. (2000) Neural Networks and Genome Informatics. Meth Comp Biol Biochem 1.

Wu, J.C. and Shapiro, B.A. (1999) A Boltzmann filter improves RNA folding pathway in a massively parallel genetic algorithm. Journal of Biomolecular Structure and Dynamics, vol. 17, pp 581-595.

Zhang, C. and Wong, A.K.C. (1997) A genetic algorithm for multiple molecular sequence alignment. Computer Application for Bioscience, vol. 13, pp 565-581.

6 Systems Biotechnology: a New Paradigm in Biotechnology Development

Sang Yup Lee[1,2], Soon Ho Hong[1], Dong Yup Lee[1,2], Tae Yong Kim[1]

[1] Metabolic and Biomolecular Engineering National Research Laboratory, Department of Chemical & Biomolecular Engineering and BioProcess Engineering Research Center, and
[2] Department of Biosystems and Bioinformatics Research Center, Korea Advanced Institute of Science and Technology 373-1 Guseong-dong, Yuseong-gu, Daejeon 305-701, Republic of Korea.
Mailing address: Metabolic and Biomolecular Engineering National Research Laboratory, Department of Chemical & Biomolecular Engineering and BioProcess Engineering Research Center, and Department of Biosystems and Bioinformatics Research Center, Korea Advanced Institute of Science and Technology 373-1 Guseong-dong, Yuseong-gu, Daejeon 305-701, Republic of Korea.

6.1 Introduction

Recent advances in high throughput biological research have accelerated the accumulation of a wide range of biological data and information at different levels ranging from DNA sequence to metabolic flux. This technology-driven discovery science is allowing not only the identification of individual components and molecules of a biological system, but also the characterization of their functions and interactions on a global scale (Lee, 2001; Ryu and Nam, 2000; and Williams, 1999). A vast amount of biologically relevant information on entire genome sequences, and proteome transcriptome and data of various living organisms being generated (Dongre et al., 2001; Fraser et al., 2000; Nelson et al., 2000; and Venter et al., 2001) await the development of new strategies for their integrated analysis. The individual components and molecules identified are insufficient alone to interpret the global behavior of the biological system.

As indicated elsewhere (Carlson and Doyle, 2002; Fukuda and Takagi, 2001; Hanahan and Winberg, 2000; Hartwell et al., 1999; Jordan et al., 2000; Karp, 2000; Somogyi et al., 1996; and Stelling et al., 2002), the biological system is complex: interactions between many simple and identical elements, as well as the selective and nonlinear communication of different multifunctional elements with others, lead to the complex and coherent behavior of the system. Moreover, even in a single cell, various types of biochemical processes are seamlessly integrated for generating mass and energy (metabolic), transmitting information (signaling), and regulating gene expression (gene regulatory) through complex networks and pathways of molecular interactions and reactions (Jeong et al., 2000). Thus, system-level approaches are indeed required to understand its organization in a global context, and to eventually discover a true knowledge map for deciphering the functions of a living system (Ideker et al., 2001; and Kitano, 2002a, 2002b); these approaches have collectively been referred to as "Systems Biology". While some formal frameworks have already been proposed (Kolpakov et al., 1998; and Rzhetsky et al., 2000), much remains to be done to design adequate models for representing, manipulating, and simulating the complex biological system (Alur et al., 2002; Endy and Brent, 2001; Leung et al., 2001; and Phair and Misteli, 2001). Consequently, an urgent need exists to investigate and integrate the relationships among all pathway information, protein interaction data, and biological process information for system-level understanding of the biological system.

This systems approach can be extended to the development of biotechnology, which we call "Systems Biotechnology". In other words, all the genomic, transcriptomic, proteomic, metabolomic, fluxomic, and other information and data available in public, and that generated in-house, are integrated at the system level for the development of complete a parts of bioprocesses. This poses a challenge that is reviewed in this chapter by presenting frameworks and methodologies.

6.2 Why Systems Biotechnology?

Biotechnology is considered one of the core technologies of the twenty-first century, considering its wide range of potential applications in the healthcare, pharmaceutical, chemical, food, and agricultural industries. As in other engineering disciplines, it is important to develop low cost and high yield biotechnological processes. To achive this goal, the development of improved strains by recombinant and other molecular biological methods and improvement of fermentation strategies have been subjects of significant research focus. However, efforts have not always been successful, due to unexpected changes in physiology and metabolism of host strains. Rational metabolic and cellular engineering approaches have been successfully taken in a number of cases to solve these problems, but they have been limited to the manipulation of only a handful (usually one or two) of enzymes and proteins. Development of high throughput experimental tools enabling thousands of analyses in parallel resulted in rapid accumulation of biological data, and provided a foundation for better understanding of biological processes. This means that biotechnology processes can be developed in rational and systematic ways (systems biotechnology), circumventing traditional "trial and error" approaches. Therefore, systems biotechnology will allow strain development based on a global understanding of metabolism and process development via upstream-to-downstream optimization, which will lead to the development of biotechnological processes with the high efficiencies. The essence of systems biotechnology resides in the integration of wet and dry experiments toward a goal of rational metabolic design, as shown in Fig. 6.1.

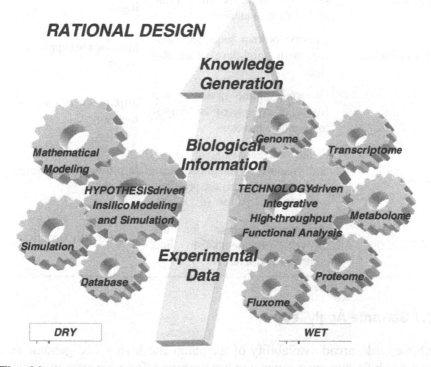

Fig. 6.1. Approaches in systems biotechnology. Various components of wet and dry experiments can be integrated to eventually allow rational metabolic design (shown in the figure) as well as upstream-to-downstream bioprocess optimization

6.3 Tools for Systems Biotechnology

With the advent of high throughput experimental tools such as the automatic genome sequencer, DNA microarray, 2-dimensional gel electrophoresis, and high performance gas chromatography mass spectrometry (GC/MS) and liquid chromatography mass spectrometry (LC/MS), multi-level data on DNA sequence and gene information of entire organisms (genomes), profiles of mRNA expression levels (transcriptomes), protein expression levels (proteomes), and metabolites (metabolomes), and intracellular flux distributions (fluxomes) are becoming available (Fig. 6.2).

Table 6.1. Genome sequence databases.

Database	Description	URL
GenBank	An annotated collection of all publicly available nucleotide and protein sequences	http://www.ncbi.nlm.nih.gov
SWISS-PROT	Curated protein sequence database with a high level of annotation	http://www.expasy.org/sport
GOLD	Genomes online database – a listing of completed and ongoing genome projects	http://www.genomesonline.org
KEGG	Kyoto encyclopedia of genes and genomes – integrated suite of databases on genes, proteins, and metabolic pathways	http://www.genome.ad.jp/kegg
BIOSILICO	Integrated database for the analysis of metabolism and compound structures	http://biosilico.kaist.ac.kr

6.3.1 Genome Analyses

With the widespread availability of the automatic high speed genome sequencer, whole genome sequencing has become affordable even in a small lab. Since the enormous volume of genomic information has been, is, and will be accumulated from genome sequencing projects, we are required to analyze the functions of predicted genes in a high throughput manner. A rapid automatic procedure for finding potential target genes is very attractive to all biotechnology-based industries, especially to many large pharmaceutical companies. However, the accuracy of functional annotations of genes in an entire genome is dependent on the applied annotation procedures. For example, there are significant differences between the novel genes predicted in the human genome by the International Human Genome Sequencing Consortium (HGSC) and Celera Genomics (Hogenesch et al., 2001). Due to limitations of the methods employed during the annotation procedure, genomic data is prone to errors (Devos and Valencia, 2001). Therefore, much improvement has to be made in bioinformatics analysis of genes and genomes in order to fully exploit the wealthy information in genome sequences. Furthermore, many of the results predicted by bioinformatics should be verified by wet experiments. Nonetheless, the genome sequence is a good starting point for analyzing the metabolism of an entire organism and for designing new strategies for biotechnological systems development. Several databases useful for genome analysis are listed in Table 6.1.

6.3.2 Transcriptome Analyses

Based on the availability of complete genome sequences and the development of DNA microarray technology, the study of gene expression of the model organisms on a genomic scale has become possible. Hence, an enormous amount of transcriptome data is being generated while data analysis is a bottleneck in transcriptome research (Berkum and Holstege, 2001). To overcome this problem, various strategies have been proposed. At present, clustering algorithms, which group genes showing similar patterns in expression profiles, are frequently employed to simplify analyses of large gene expression datasets (Eisen et al., 1998; and Sherlock, 2000).

DNA microarray technology has been intensively applied to medical studies since the physiological changes in normal and diseased cells and tissues can be deciphered by following drug targets (Hughes et al., 2000; and Marton et al., 1998). Differential or subtractive analyses of gene expression in drug-sensitive and drug-resistant cell lines or tumors have allowed the identification of genes that are potentially responsible for drug resistance, something that had not been recognized previously by traditional analytical approaches (Roberts, 2000; and Steele et al., 2003). Therefore, the mRNA expression profiles in various human cancers, including prostate, ovarian, lung, and breast cancers, had been extensively studied to find potential diagnostic markers and anticancer drug targets (Leerkes et al., 2002; Owens et al., 2002; Primiano et al., 2003; Robinson et al., 2003; and Waghray et al., 2001). Transcriptome profiling is increasingly used for understanding the effects of drugs and chemicals on cellular physiology. For example, the effect of cigarette smoking on gene expression in endothelial cells was also evaluated by DNA microarray, and the result indicated that a number of nicotine modulated genes encoding proteins involved in signal transduction and transcriptional regulation were identified (Zhang et al., 2001).

DNA microarray studies enable us to understand the global cellular physiologies and metabolisms of living organisms under various environmental disturbances. In this sense, transcriptome profiling of microorganisms is becoming popular for improving the performance in various biotechnology applications. For example, transcriptome profiling of *Bacillus subtilis*, widely used in bioindustry, was analyzed during glucose limiting and oxygen limiting conditions. The results suggested that several hundred genes involved in central metabolism, iron uptake, and stress response were differently regulated under these conditions, which provided insights on the complex regulatory network of *B. subtilis* (Ye et al., 2000; and Yoshida et al., 2001). The mRNA expression profiles of *Saccharomyces cerevisiae* at high salinity and high sugar conditions were also examined to decipher physiological changes under these conditions (Erasmus et al., 2003, and Yale and Bohnert, 2001).

As mentioned above, transcriptome analysis can enable identification of connections between regulatory circuits and metabolic pathways that have previously been unknown. This new information can be used to design metabolic and cellular engineering strategies for the improvement of biotechnological processes such as amino acid, organic acid, and recombinant protein production systems. Even though metabolic and cellular engineering at global level is the ultimate goal of systems biotechnology, we have only limited understanding of how to utilize the vast amounts of data. Under the circumstances, we should not be disappointed, as we can still rationally select local targets from the global scale data, as described below. For example, the transcriptome profiles of recombinant *Escherichia coli* producing human insulin-like growth factor I fusion proteins (IGF-Is) were analyzed (Choi et al., 2003). The transcriptome profiles indicated that the expression level of 529 genes were significantly affected by IGF-I overproduction, and among them over 200 genes were repressed during IGF-I production. Interestingly, the *prsA* and *glpF* genes encoding phosphoribosyl pyrophosphate synthase and glycerol transporter, respectively, were significantly down-regulated, which suggested a possible limitation of 5-phosphoribosyl-1-pyrophospahte, the precursor of nucleotides (purine, pyrimidine and incotinamide) and amino acids (histidine and tryptophan), and glycerol supply. When the *prsA* and *glpF* genes were coexpressed in recombinant *E. coli*, a more than two-fold increase of IGF-I concentration and IGF-I volumetric productivity could be achieved (Choi et al., 2003). It should be noted that these two genes would have not been the targets of metabolic engineering if a global analysis of gene expression was not carried out.

6.3.3 Proteome Analyses

Proteome profiling is another important tool for systems biotechnology, considering the fact that cellular behavior is more directly influenced by proteins rather than by mRNAs. Through proteome analysis, it is possible to monitor the presence of large numbers of proteins within a cell or tissue and to observe quantitatively how the protein levels change under different circumstances (Fig. 6.2). Proteome analysis has many applications in biotechnology, including the discovery of drug targets, development of diagnostic markers, monitoring of intracellular metabolism, and elucidating regulatory networks from proteins that undergo coordinated changes of expression.

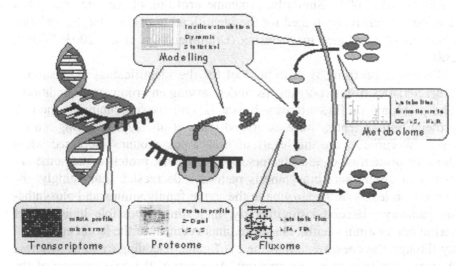

Fig. 6.2. Tools for Systems biotechnology

Therefore, proteome profiling has been applied to discover tumor markers for early detection and diagnosis, and to investigate drug resistance mechanisms in various human cancer cell lines (Poland et al., 2002; Verrills and Kavallaris, 2003; and Wu et al., 2002). Among the cancers, breast cancer is one of the most intensively studied, through proteomics. It was discovered that arylamine N-acetyltransferase-1 (NAT-1) was differentially expressed in normal and breast cancer tissues, indicating its importance in the metabolism of breast cancer cell lines. Besides its overexpression in cancer cell lines, it was reported that NAT-1 was also involved in the cytotoxic drug resistance mechanism of some cancer cell lines (Adam et al., 2003; and Stein and Zvelebil, 2002).

Proteome profiling of various human and animal pathogens has also been an important research topic. The resistance mechanism of *Helicobacter pylori* strains to metronidazole (MZT), revealed by proteome profiling, indicated that the expression levels of alkylhydroperoxide reductase (AHP) isozymes increased over two-fold suggesting its important role in MZT resistance (McAtee et al., 2001). Also, the mechanisms for regulating virulence factors in Bacillus cereus were investigated by proteome profiling (Gohar et al., 2002). The expression level of transcriptional activator PlcR was the highest at the stationary phase, under which most of the secreted enzymes were putative virulence-related enzymes. Based on this finding, the authors were able to significantly reduce or even abolish, the secretion of those virulence enzymes by knocking out the *plcR* gene, supporting the finding that PlcR is a key regulator of virulence in *B. cereus* (Gohar et al., 2002). Similarly, proteome profiling of parasite strains has also been intensively studied for the identification of drug targets and elucidations of resistance mechanisms (Drummelsmith et al., 2003; Seeber, 2003).

Proteome profiling is a useful tool for the identification of metabolic characteristics of microorganisms under varying environmental conditions. The proteome profiles of recombinant *E. coli* overproducing serine-rich protein, human leptin, were examined (Han et al., 2003). During human leptin overproduction, the levels of heat shock proteins increased while those of protein elongation factors, 30S ribosomal proteins, and some enzymes in amino acid biosynthesis pathways decreased. Interestingly, the expression levels of the enzyme in the serine family amino acid biosynthesis pathways decreased significantly, indicating a possible limitation of serine family amino acids. Therefore, improvement of the leptin productivity through the coexpression of the *cysK* gene, encoding cysteine synthase A, was examined as a new strategy. As a result, the coexpression of the *cysK* gene led to two- and four-fold increases of cell growth and leptin productivity, respectively (Han et al., 2003). In addition, it was further found that *cysK* coexpression could improve production of another serine-rich protein, interleukin-12 β chain, suggesting that this strategy may be useful for the production of other serine-rich proteins as well. This example demonstrates the power of global analysis, even though our current applications are limited to the engineering of local metabolic pathways.

6.3.4 Metabolome/Fluxome Analyses

Analysis of intracellular metabolome profiles is a powerful analytical tool allowing elucidation of intracellular metabolic conditions (Fig. 6.2). First, for the accumulation of metabolome data, various tools such as GC/MS, LC/MS, isotope ratio mass spectrometry (IRMS; Demmelmair et al., 1997) and gas chromatography/time of flight mass spectrometry (GC/TOFMS, Glassbrook et al., 2000) have been employed to quantify hundreds of metabolites. Then, intracellular flux distributions or fluxome data of living organisms can be estimated based on the time derivates of metabolite profiles (see below for the detail).

Since the flux distribution directly reflects metabolic conditions of a living organism, fluxome analysis is the most appropriate strategy for the estimation of metabolic characteristics such as metabolic responses caused by environmental and metabolic (genetic) disturbances. In one example, the metabolic response to toxic aromatic thiols such as thiophenol and 4-aminothiophenol was estimated. It was found that glycolysis, hexose monophosphate shunt, and methamoglobin formation were affected depending on the level of oxidative stress. Based on these results, it was revealed that thiol response mechanisms of human red blood cells are thiol exchange with glutathione and reduction of glutathione disulfide by the hexose monophosphate shunt (Amrolia et al., 1989). The effect of epinephrine on energy metabolism in human being was also evaluated by fluxome analysis (Matthews et al., 1990). Cancer is one of most important research areas in biotechnology, and fluxome analysis has been applied to understand metabolic characteristics of various cancer cell lines under various conditions. In pancreatic and colonic cancer cells, the glucose uptake rate and the lactic acid production rate increased (Li and Adrian, 1999).

Because fluxome analysis can provide information on intracellular flux distribution, it has been widely applied to the estimation of various microbial metabolite production systems. The variation of intracellular metabolic flux distribution during riboflavin production in *B. subtilis* was estimated (Dauner and Sauer, 2001, and Sauer et al., 1996). Also, the metabolic flux distributions in *S. cerevisiae* during overproduction of foreign protein were evaluated (Jin et al., 1997).

As the genome sequences of a number of organisms has become available, constructions of *in silico* metabolic network of living organisms, followed by *in silico* simulations have been carried out to predict metabolic characteristics under various conditions. Generally, the flux balance analysis (FBA) technique, which is based on the pseudo steady-state assumption or no intracellular accumulation of metabolites, is applied for the *in silico* simulation of a metabolic network. As an example, the effects of various single gene mutations on global metabolic characteristics were predicted through fluxome analysis using the *in silico* metabolic network of *E. coli*. It was predicted that 15 genes are essential for *E. coli* to grow from glucose under anaerobic conditions (Edwards and Palsson, 2000). Recently, metabolic characteristics of poly(3-hydroxybutyrate) producing *E. coli* were reported based on fluxome analysis of an *in silico E. coli* metabolic network; it was found that the Entner-Doudoroff (ED) pathway plays an important role in poly(3-hydroxybutyrate) production by supplying precursor metabolites of poly(3-hydroxybutyrate) in a particular *E. coli* strain examined. This prediction was verified by wet experiments employing mutant and engineered *E. coli* strains (Hong et al., 2003). It should be mentioned that current FBA is somewhat limited in its accuracy, as it is usually carried out by linear optimization (Edwards and Palsson, 2000, and Lee and Papoutsakis, 1999). Thus, improvement of mathematical analysis and application of more appropriate constraints are under investigation to make FBA a robust tool.

These days, GC/MS- and NMR-based flux analyses are becoming more popular, considering their advantages, such as high sensitivity and direct quantification of flux distributions. Recently, the responses of intracellular metabolism of *E. coli* to mutations in phosphoglucose isomerase and glucose-6-phosphate dehydrogenase were examined through a ^{13}C carbon substrate based fluxome analysis (Hua et al., 2003). Similarly, metabolic characteristics of industrial strain *Corynebacterium glutamicum*, which produces glutamate and lysine, were uncovered by a ^{13}C-labelling fluxome analysis (de Graaf et al., 2001; Sahm et al., 2000; and Wittmann and Heinzle, 2001).

6.4 Integrative Approaches

Due to the complexities of metabolic reactions and regulatory networks in living organisms, there is widespread belief that any of transcriptome, proteome, and fluxome data alone may provide incorrect information on cellular physiology and metabolism (Brent, 2000; Delneri et al., 2001; and Nielsen and Olsson, 2002). This perception arises from low correlations between levels of mRNA expression, protein expression, and flux distribution. Therefore, to understand the global cellular functions simultaneously at multiple controlling steps, combined analysis in an integrative manner is essential (Eymann et al., 2002; Phelps et al., 2002; Shimizu et al., 2002; and Yoshida et al., 2001).

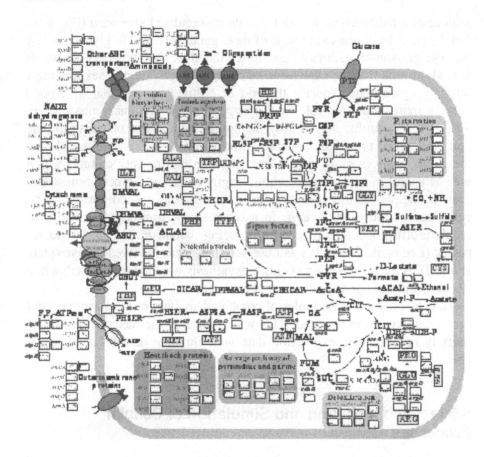

Fig. 6.3. AN integrated view of transcriptome and proteome profiles of E. coli during HCDC. The X axis denotes cell concentration (g DCW/L) and the Y axis denotes expression level in log2 scale for transcriptome (red) and in absolute value of volume % for proteome (blue). Gene names are colored red only when a transcription level is detected; otherwise, they are colored blue [reproduced from Yoon et al., 2002, with permission]

Recently, the integrated view of transcriptome and proteome profiles of *E. coli* during fed-batch fermentation by exponential feeding of nutrients, until cell density reached 74 g dry cell weight/L was reported (Yoon et al., 2002). A large-scale cultivation process employing high cell density culture techniques has usually been applied to produce biomaterials and biochemicals in large quantities (Lee, 1996). However, high cell density cultivation causes changes in physiology and metabolism of host strain and then often leads to reduced production yield in an unexpected way. The results of analyses indicated that the expression of genes of TCA cycle enzymes, NADH dehydrogenase and, ATPase was up-regulated during the exponential fed-batch period and was down-regulated afterward (Fig. 6.3). On the other hand, the expression of most genes involved in glycolysis and pentose phosphate pathway was up-regulated at the stationary phase. It was also found that the expression of phosphate starvation genes was most strongly up-regulated toward the end of cultivation, and that σ^E ($rpoE$) plays a more important role than σ^S ($rpoS$) at the stationary phase (Lee, 1996). These results, obtained by the combined analysis of transcriptome and proteome, provided valuable information about physiological and metabolic changes of $E.$ $coli$ during the high cell density culture, which will be useful in designing metabolic engineering and fermentation strategies for the production of recombinant proteins and metabolites by a high cell density culture of $E.$ $coli$. In another study, transcriptome and proteome profiles of a threonine overproducing mutant $E.$ $coli$ strain was reported (Lee et al., 2003). It was observed that genes involved in glyoxylate shunt, TCA cycle, and amino acids biosynthesis were overexpressed, while ribosomal protein genes were down-regulated.

To date, only a few examples of combined analysis of transcriptome and proteome have been reported. This will change as the methods for meaningfully linking these expression data with fluxome data becomes available.

6.5 In Silico Modeling and Simulation of Cellular Processes

As an alternative to *in vivo/in vitro* experiments for generating new knowledge in systems biotechnology, *in silico* modeling and simulation of cellular processes render it possible to predict the behavior of cells and organisms in response to genetic and environmental changes. Such *in silico* experiments, as pre-steps of real process development, can help biochemical engineers determine which genes or pathways should be manipulated to achieve improved properties for the cell. In spite of their benefits to biotechnology development, they cannot be truly implemented until a logical approach is developed for circumventing the combinatorial complexities involved in identifying biochemical or metabolic pathways in modeling intracellular metabolism.

Several approaches for quantitative *in silico* simulation of metabolic systems have been developed not only to understand the metabolic status, but also to design the metabolic engineering strategies; they include structural or topological pathway analysis (Schuster et al., 2000, and Simpson et al., 1999), flux-based model approaches such as metabolic flux analysis

(MFA), metabolic control analysis (MCA), and kinetics-based modeling for dynamic simulation (Table 6.2).

Table 6.2. Comparison of dynamic and static modeling methods.

	Model required	Requirements		
Topological pathway analysis	Stoichiometric model	Stoichiometric reactions Mass conservation	Elementary modes Extreme pathways Independent pathways	Network structure
Metabolic flux analysis	Stoichiometric model	Flux measurements (LC*, GC/MS*, NMR*)	Gross error detection Flux distribution	Flux distribution
Metabolic control analysis	Stationary Mechanistic model		Rate controlling steps Metabolite pool controlling steps	Pathway regulation MCA* coefficients
Dynamic simulation	Kinetic model	Enzyme kinetics (kinetic parameters) ODE* or DAE* solver	Dynamic behavior	System dynamics

*Abbreviations: LC, liquid chromatograph; GC/MS, gas chromatograph/mass spectrometer; NMR, nuclear magnetic resonance; MCA, metabolic control analysis; ODE, ordinary differential equation; DAE, differential algebraic equation.

6.5.1 Statistical Modeling

Among the available approaches for rational analysis of metabolic pathways, MFA is the most widely adopted one: it requires the least amount of information to quantify and analyze the metabolic system. Basically, under the pseudo steady-state assumption, MFA starts by constructing a stoichiometric model based on genome and metabolic information. In such a model, the relationships among all metabolites (intermediates) and reactions are balanced in terms of stoichiometry. Flux distribution is then calculated by matrix operations in the case of determined or overdetermined systems. If the resultant balanced reaction model is underdetermined in calculating the flux distribution due to insufficient measurements or constraints, the unknown fluxes within the metabolic reaction network are evaluated by means of FBA based on linear programming (LP), subject to the constraints pertaining to mass conservation, reaction thermodynamics, and enzymatic reaction capacity, as described elsewhere (Edwards and Palsson, 2000, and Lee and Papoutsakis, 1999). It should be noted that although FBA has been well established theoretically and experimentally, several issues still remain to be overcome. The problems are due to the availability of limited experimental observations and nonunique LP algorithms, resulting in different optimal solutions. In particular, multiple solutions may arise where different flux patterns occur for the same external conditions (Table 6.2).

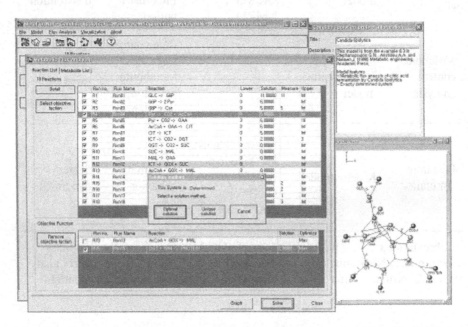

Fig. 6.4. Screen shot of the flux analysis part of MetaFluxNet. Flux distributions can be interactively determined and dynamically visualized via a user-friendly interface

A number of computer programs have been developed for analytical and computational implementations. An effort for establishing the steady-state simulation program was initiated by LabVIEW (Regan and Gregory, 1995). Since then, appreciable progress has been made through the devel-

opment of a number of programs. They include FBA (http://gcrg.ucsd.
edu/downloads/index.html), FluxAnalyzer (Klamt et al., 2003), Fluxmap
(http://www.biotecnol.com), INSILICO discovery (http://www.insilico-
biotechnology.com/products_en.html), and Metabologica (http://www-
.metabologica.com). Recently, MetaFluxNet, which is a stand-alone program package for the management of metabolic reaction information and
quantitative flux analysis, was developed (Lee et al., 2003). It allows users
to interpret and examine metabolic behavior in response to genetic and/or
environmental modifications (Fig. 6.4). As a result, quantitative *in silico*
simulations of metabolic pathways can be carried out to understand the
metabolic status and to design the metabolic engineering strategies. The
main features of the program include a well developed model construction
environment, a user-friendly interface for MFA, comparative MFA of
strains having different genotypes under various environmental conditions,
and automated pathway layout creation. The usefulness and functionality
of the program are demonstrated by applying it to the simulation of metabolic pathways in *E. coli* (Lee et al., 2003).

6.5.2 Dynamic Modeling

Considering the time variable nature of metabolism and the regulation
mechanism, various quantitative methodologies such as MCA (Fell, 1997),
biochemical systems analysis (Voit, 2000), and node flexibility analysis
(Stephanopoulos and Vallino, 1991) were developed to simulate intracellular metabolism. In addition, such regulatory aspects of metabolic networks
were also investigated in-depth in connection with the optimization of their
architectures (Hatzimanikatis et al., 1999). MCA is a statistical modeling
technique that can be used to understand the control of metabolic pathways
and pathway regulations. It has become the most widely used tool to gain a
quantitative understanding of metabolic networks. MCA allows us to understand how metabolic fluxes are controlled by certain enzyme activities
and metabolite concentrations. The major result of MCA is that the control
of a complex metabolic network is usually distributed over many enzymatic steps in a given pathway. This means that there is little chance that a
single genetic modification will result in a large alteration of the flux distribution (Table 6.2).

When a steady state is not assumed, and the profile of each reaction rate
is determined with time changes, intensive mathematical computing power
is needed to solve ordinary differential equations (ODEs). Dynamic simulations can be done using ODE solvers, but the amount of calculation re-

quired becomes easily unmanageable as the number of reactions in a metabolic network increases (Wiechert, 2002).

A number of computer programs have been developed for dynamic simulation and calculation of MCA coefficients – MetaModel (Cornish-Bowden and Hofmeyr, 1991), SCAMP (Sauro, 1993), Gepasi (Mendes, 1997), and MIST (Ehlde and Zacchi, 1995). Among these programs, user-friendly Gepasi is widely used for dynamic simulation as well as for common tasks, and Gepasi has recently been upgraded to version 3.30. DBSolve (Goryanin et al., 1999) provides an integrated environment for metabolic, enzymatic, and receptor-ligand binding simulation. As for whole cell simulation, the Virtual Cell (Loew and Schaff, 2001) and E-CELL (Tomita, 2001) have demonstrated the value of biological modeling in understanding propagation of *in silico* metabotropic calcium waves in human neuroblastoma cell and erythrocyte physiology, respectively.

6.6 Conclusion

Modeling and simulation of cellular process are invaluable for organizing and integrating available metabolic knowledge and designing the right experiments. Simulation of biological systems through metabolic modeling can provide crucial information concerning cellular behavior under various genetic and environmental conditions, thus suggesting various strategies for the development of efficient biotechnology processes. The current predictive power of biological simulation is, however, limited by insufficient knowledge of global regulation and kinetic information, and thus *in silico* design-based process development might seem to be unrealistic. However, considering the fact that the currently widespread simulation of electrical circuits and aircraft design had also been criticized for similar reasons in their emerging days, it is expected that increased accuracy and validity of biological simulation will be achieved in the near future; the accumulation of large amounts of global scale data from genomics advances in simulation methods will make this true.

Systems biotechnology is the way biotechnology should be developed and practiced from now hence. Upstream (strain, cell, and organism development), midstream (fermentation and other unit operations) and downstream processes of biotechnology will benefit significantly from adapting systems biotechnological approaches. The cases of mid- to down-stream bioprocesses resemble the systems engineering approach that has been successfully applied in chemical industries (the core subject of chemical engineering). Now it is time to adapt systems biotechnological approaches for developing upstream processes such as strain development, which will ultimately lead to successful biotechnology development when combined with systems engineering of mid- to down-stream processes. This is Systems Biotechnology!

Acknowledgements. Our work was supported by the Korean Systems Biology Research Program (M10309020000-03B5002-00000) of the Ministry of Science and Technology, by the IBM SUR program, and by the BK21 project.

References

Adam, P.J., Berry, J., Loader, J.A., Tyson, K.L., Craggs, G., Smith, P., De Belin, J., Steers, G., Pezzella, F., Sachsenmeir, K.F., Stamps, A.C., Herath, A., Sim, E., O'Hare, M.J., Harris, A,L. and Terrett. J.A. (2003) Arylamine N-acetyltransferase-1 is highly expressed in breast cancers and conveys enhanced growth and resistance to Etoposide in vitro. Mol. Cancer Res. 1:826-835.

Alur, R., Belta, C., Kumar, V., Mintz, M., Pappas, G.J., Rubin, H. and Schug, J. (2002) Modeling and analyzing biomolecular networks. Computing Sci. Eng. 4:20-31.

Amrolia, P., Sullivan, S.G., Stern, A. and Munday, R. (1989) Toxicity of aromatic thiols in the human red blood cell. J. Appl. Toxicol. 9:113-118.

Berkum, N.L. and Holstege, F.C. (2001) DNA microarrays: raising the profile. Curr. Opin. Biotechnol. 12:48-52.

Brent, R. (2000) Genomic biology. Cell 100:169-183.

Carlson, J.M. and Doyle, J. (2002) Complexity and robustness. Proc. Natl. Acad. Sci. USA 99:2538-2545.

Choe, L.H., Chen, W. and Lee, K.H. (1999) Proteome analysis of factor for inversion stimulation (Fis) overproduction in Escherichia coli. Electrophoresis 20:798-805.

Choi, J.H., Lee, S.J., Lee, S.J. and Lee, S.Y. (2003) Enhanced production of insulin-like growth factor I fusion protein in Escherichia coli by coexpression of the down-regulated genes identified by transcriptome profiling. Appl. Environ. Microbiol. 69:4737-4742.

Cornish-Bowden, A, and Hofmeyr, J.H. (1991) METAMODEL-A program for modeling and control analysis of metabolic pathways on the IBM PC and compatibles. Comput. Appl. Biosci. 7:89-93.

Dauner, M. and Sauer, U. (2001) Stoichiometric growth model for riboflavin-producing Bacillus subtilis. Biotechnol. Bioeng. 76:132-143.

Delneri, D., Brancia, F.L. and Oliver, S.G. (2001) Towards a truly integrative biology through the functional genomics of yeast. Curr. Opin. Biotechnol. 12:87-91.

Demmelmair, H., Sauerwald, T., Koletzko, B. and Richter, T. (1997) New insights into lipid and fatty acid metabolism via stable isotopes. Eur. J. Pediatr. 156:S70-S74.

Devos, D. and Valencia, A. (2001) Intrinsic errors in genome annotation. Trends Gen. 17:429-431.

Dongre, A.R., Opiteck, G., Cosand, W.L. and Hefta, S.A. (2001) Proteomics in the post-genome age. Biopolymers 60:206-211.

Drummelsmith, J., Brochu, V., Girard, I., Messier, N. and Ouellette, M. (2003) Proteome mapping of the protozoan parasite leishmania and application to the study of drug targets and resistance mechanisms. Mol. Cell Proteomics. 2:146-155.

Edwards, J.S. and Palsson, B.O. (2000) Metabolic flux balance analysis and the in silico analysis of Escherichia coli K-12 gene deletions. BMC Bioinformatics. 1:1-10.

Ehlde, M. and Zacchi, G. (1995) MIST: a user-friendly metabolic simulator. Comput. Appl. Biosci. 11:201-207.

Eisen, M.B., Spellman, P.T., Brown, P.O. and Botstein, D. (1998) Cluster analysis and display of genome-wide expression patterns. Proc. Natl. Acad. Sci. USA 95:14863-14868.

Endy, D. and Brent, R. (2001) Modeling cellular behavior. Nature 409:391-395.

Erasmus, D.J., van der Merwe, G.K. and van Vuuren, H.J. (2003) Genome-wide expression analyses: metabolic adaptation of Saccharomyces cerevisiae to high sugar stress. FEMS Yeast Res. 3:375-399.

Eymann, C., Homuth, G., Scharf, C. and Hecker, M. (2002) Bacillus subtilis functional genomics: global characterization of the stringent response by proteome and transcriptome analysis. J. Bacteriol. 184:2500-2520.

Fell, D.A. (1997) Understanding the control of metabolism. Portland Press.

Fraser, C.M., Eisen, J.A. and Salzberg, S.L. (2000) Microbial genome sequencing. Nature 406:799-803.

Fukuda, K. and Takagi, T. (2001) Knowledge representation of signal transduction pathways. Bioinformatics 17:829-837.

Glassbrook, N., Beecher, C. and Ryals, J. (2000) Metabolic profiling on the right path. Nat. Biotechnol. 18:1142-1143.

Gohar, M., Okstad, O.A., Gilois, N., Sanchis, V., Kolsto, A.B. and Lereclus, D. (2002) Two-dimensional electrophoresis analysis of the extracellular proteome of Bacillus cereus reveals the importance of the PlcR regulon. Proteomics. 2:784-791.

Goryanin, I., Hodgman, T.C. and Selkov, E. (1999) Mathematical simulation and analysis of cellular metabolism and regulation. Bioinformatics 15:749-758.

de Graaf, A.A., Eggeling, L. and Sahm, H. (2001) Metabolic engineering for L-lysine production by Corynebacterium glutamicum. Adv. Biochem. Eng. Biotechnol. 73:9-29.

Han, M.J., Jeong, K.J., Yoo, J.S. and Lee, S.Y. (2003) Engineering Escherichia coli for increased productivity of serine-rich proteins based on proteome profiling. Appl. Environ. Microbiol. 69:5772-5781.

Hanahan, D. and Weinberg, R.A. (2000) The hallmarks of cancer. Cell 100:57-70.

Hartwell, L.H., Hopfield, J.J., Leibler, S. and Murray, A.W. (1999) From molecular to modular cell biology. Nature 402:C47-C52.

Hatzimanikatis, V., Lee, K.H. and Bailey, J.E. (1999) A mathematical description of regulation of the G1-S transition of the mammalian cell cycle. Biotechnol. Bioeng. 65:631-637.

Hogenesch, J.B., Ching, K.A., Batalov, S., Su, A,I., Walker, J.R., Zhou, Y., Kay, S.A., Schultz, P.G., Cooke and M.P. (2001) A comparison of the celera and ensembl predicted gene sets reveals little overlap in novel genes. Cell 106:413-415.

Hong, S.H., Park, S.J., Moon, S.Y., Park, J.P. and Lee, S.Y. (2003) In silico prediction and validation of the importance of the Entner-Doudoroff pathway in poly(3-hydroxybutyrate) production by metabolically engineered Escherichia coli. Biotechnol. Bioeng. 83:854-863.

Hua, Q., Yang, C., Baba, T., Mori, H. and Shimizu, K. (2003) Responses of the central metabolism in Escherichia coli to phosphoglucose isomerase and glucose-6-phosphate dehydrogenase knockouts. J. Bacteriol. 185:7053-7067.

Hughes, T.R., Marton, M.J., Jones, A.R., Roberts. C.J., Stoughton, R., Armour, C.D., Bennett, H.A., Coffey, E., Dai, H., He, Y.D., Kidd, M.J., King, A,M., Meyer, M.R., Slade, D., Lum, P.Y., Stepaniants, S.B., Shoemaker, D.D., Gachotte, D., Chakraburtty, K., Simon, J., Bard, M. and Friend, S.H. (2000) Functional discovery via a compendium of expression profiles. Cell 102:109-126..

Ideker, T., Galitski, T. and Hood, L. (2001) A new approach to decoding life: systems biology. Annu. Rev. Genomics Hum. Genet. 2:343-372.

Jeong, H., Tombor, B., Albert, R., Oltvai, Z.N. and Barabasi, A.L. (2000) The large-scale organization of metabolic networks. Nature 407:651-654.

Jin, S., Ye, K. and Shimizu, K. (1997) Metabolic flux distributions in recombinant Saccharomyces cerevisiae during foreign protein production. J. Biotechnol. 54:161-174.

Jordan, J.D., Landau, E.M. and Iyengar, R. (2000) Signaling networks: the origins of cellular multitasking. Cell 103:193-200.

Karp, P.D. (2000) An ontology for biological function based on molecular interactions. Bioinformatics 16:269-285.

Kitano, H. (2002a) Computational systems biology. Nature 420:206-210.

Kitano, H. (2002b) Systems biology: a brief overview. Science 295:1662-1664.

Klamt, S., Stelling, J., Ginkel, M. and Gilles, E.D. (2003) FluxAnalyzer: exploring structure, pathways, and flux distributions in metabolic networks on interactive flux maps. Bioinformatics 19:261-269.

Kolpakov, F.A., Ananko EA, Kolesov GB, Kolchanov NA (1998) GeneNet: a gene network database and its automated visualization. Bioinformatics 14:529-537.

Lee, D.Y., Yun, H., Park, S. and Lee, S.Y. (2003) MetaFluxNet: the management of metabolic reaction information and quantitative metabolic flux analysis. Bioinformatics 19:2144-2146.

Lee, J.H., Lee, D.E., Lee, B.U. and Kim, H.S. (2003) Global analyses of transcriptomes and proteomes of a parent strain and an L-threonine-overproducing mutant strain. J. Bacteriol. 185:5442-5451.

Lee, K.H. (2001) Proteomics: a technology-driven and technology-limited discovery science. Trends Biotechnol. 19:217-222.

Lee, S.Y. (1996) High cell-density culture of Escherichia coli. Trends Biotechnol. 14:98-105.

Lee, S.Y., Papoutsakis ET (1999) Metabolic Engineering. Marcel Dekker.

Leerkes, M.R., Caballero, O.L., Mackay, A., Torloni, H., O'Hare, M.J., Simpson, A.J. and de Souza, S.J. (2002) In silico comparison of the transcriptome derived from purified normal breast cells and breast tumor cell lines reveals candidate upregulated genes in breast tumor cells. Genomics 79:257-265.

Leung, Y.F., Lam, D.S., Pang, C.P. (2001) In silico biology: observation, modeling, hypothesis and verification. Trends Genet. 17:622-623.

Li, J., Adrian, T.E. (1999) A factor from pancreatic and colonic cancer cells stimulates glucose uptake and lactate production in myoblasts. Biochem. Biophys. Res. Commun. 260:626-633.

Loew, L.M. and Schaff, J.C. (2001) The Virtual Cell: a software environment for computational cell biology. Trends Biotechnol. 19:401-406.

Marton, M.J., DeRisi, J.L., Bennett, H.A., Iyer, V.R., Meyer, M.R., Roberts, C.J., Stoughton, R., Burchard, J., Slade, D., Dai, H., Bassett DE, Jr., Hartwell, L.H., Brown, P.O. and Friend, S.H. (1998) Drug target validation and identification of secondary drug target effects using DNA microarrays. Nat. Med. 4:1293-1301.

Matthews, D.E., Pesola, G., Campbell, R.G. (1990) Effect of epinephrine on amino acid and energy metabolism in humans. Am. J. Physiol. 258:E948-956.

McAtee, C.P., Hoffman, P.S. and Berg, D.E. (2001) Identification of differentially regulated proteins in metronidozole resistant Helicobacter pylori by proteome techniques. Proteomics. 1:516-521.

Mendes, P. (1997) Biochemistry by numbers: simulation of biochemical pathways with Gepasi3. Trends Biochem. Sci. 22:361-363.

Nelson, K.E., Paulsen, I.T., Heidelberg, J.F. and Fraser, C.M. (2000) Status of genome projects for nonpathogenic bacterial and archaea. Nat. Biotechnol. 18:1049-1054.

Nielsen, J. and Olsson, L. (2002) An expanded role for microbial physiology in metabolic engineering and functional genomics: moving towards systems biology. FEMS Yeast Research 2:175-181.

Owens, G.E., Keri, R.A., Nilson and J.H. (2002) Ovulatory surges of human CG prevent hormone-induced granulosa cell tumor formation leading to the identification of tumor-associated changes in the transcriptome. Mol. Endocrinol. 16:1230-1242.

Phair, R.D., Misteli, T. (2001) Kinetic modeling approaches to in vivo imaging. Nat. Rev. Mol. Cell Biol. 2:898-907.

Phelps, T.J., Palumbo, A.V., Beliaev, A.S. (2002) Metabolomics and microarrays for improved understanding of phenotypic characteristics controlled by both genomics and environmental constraints. Curr. Opin. Biotechnol. 13:20-24.

Poland, J., Schadendorf, D., Lage, H., Schnolzer, M., Celis, J.E. and Sinha, P. (2002) Study of therapy resistance in cancer cells with functional proteome analysis. Clin. Chem. Lab. Med. 40:221-234.

Primiano, T., Baig, M., Maliyekkel, A., Chang, B.D., Fellars, S., Sadhu, J., Axenovich, S.A., Holzmayer, T.A. and Roninson, I.B. (2003) Identification of potential anticancer drug targets through the selection of growth-inhibitory genetic suppressor elements. Cancer Cell. 4:41-53.

Regan, L. and Gregory, M. (1995) Flux analysis of microbial metabolic pathways using a visual programming environment. J. Biotechnol. 42:151-161.

Roberts, C.J., Nelson, B., Marton, M.J., Stoughton, R., Meyer, M.R., Bennett, H.A., He, Y.D., Dai, H., Walker, W.L., Hughes TR, Tyers M, Boone C, Friend SH (2000) Signaling and circuitry of multiple MAPK pathways revealed by a matrix of global gene expression profiles. Science 287, 873-880.

Robinson, M., Jiang, P., Cui, J., Li, J., Wang, Y., Swaroop, M., Madore, S., Lawrence, T.S. and Sun, Y. (2003) Global genechip profiling to identify genes responsive to p53-induced growth arrest and apoptosis in human lung carcinoma cells. Cancer Biol. Ther. 2:406-415.

Ryu, D.D.Y. and Nam, D.H. (2000) Recent progress in biomolecular engineering. Biotechnol. Prog. 16:2-16.

Rzhetsky, A., Koike, T., Kalachikov, S., Gomez, S.M., Krauthammer, M., Kaplan, S.H., Kra, P., Russo, J.J. and Friedman, C. (2000) A knowledge model for analysis and simulation of regulatory networks. Bioinformatics 16:1120-1128.

Sahm, H., Eggeling, L. and de Graaf, A.A. (2000) Pathway analysis and metabolic engineering in Corynebacterium glutamicum. Biol. Chem. 381:899-910.

Sauer, U., Hatzimanikatis, V., Hohmann, H.P., Manneberg, M., van Loon, A.P. and Bailey, J.E. (1996) Physiology and metabolic fluxes of wild-type and riboflavin-producing Bacillus subtilis. Appl. Environ. Microbiol. 62:3687-3696.

Sauro, H.M. (1993) SCAMP: a general-purpose simulator and metabolic control analysis program. Comput. Applic. Biosci. 9:441-450.

Schuster, S., Fell, D.A. and Dandekar, T. (2000) A general definition of metabolic pathways useful for systematic organization and analysis of complex metabolic networks. Nat. Biotechnol. 18:326-332.

Seeber, F. (2003) Biosynthetic pathways of plastid-derived organelles as potential drug targets against parasitic apicomplexa. Curr. Drug Targets Immune Endocr. Metabol. Disord. 3:99-109.

Sherlock, G. (2000) Analysis of large-scale gene expression data. Curr. Opin. Immunol. 12:201-205.

Shimizu, T., Shima, K., Yoshino, K., Yonezawa, K., Shimizu, T. and Hayashi, H. (2002) Proteome and transcriptome analysis of the virulence genes regulated by the VirR/VirS system in Clostridium perfringens. J. Bacteriol. 184:2587-2594.

Simpson, T.W., Follstad, B.D. and Stephanopoulos, G. (1999) Analysis of the pathway structure of metabolic networks. J. Biotechnol. 71:207-223.

Somogyi, R. and Sniegoski, C.A. (1996) Modeling the complexity of genetic networks: Understanding multistage and pleiotropic regulation. Complexity 1:45-63.

Steele, D., Kertsburg, A and Soukup, G.A. (2003) Engineered catalytic RNA and DNA: new biochemical tools for drug discovery and design. Am. J. Pharmacogenomics 3:131-144.

Stein, R.C. and Zvelebil, M.J. (2002) The application of 2D gel-based proteomics methods to the study of breast cancer. J. Mammary Gland Biol. Neoplasia. 7:385-393.

Stelling, J., Klamt, S., Bettenbrock, K., Schuster, S. and Gilles, E.D. (2002) Metabolic network structure determines key aspects of functionality and regulation. Nature 420:190-193.

Stephanopoulos, G. and Vallino, J.J. (1991) Network rigidity and metabolic engineering in metabolite overproduction. Science 252:1675-1681.

Tomita, M. (2001) Whole-cell simulation: a grand challenge of the 21st century. Trends Biotechnol. 19:205-210.

Venter, J.C., Adams, M.D., Myers, E.W., Li, P.W., Mural, R.J., Sutton, G.G., Smith, H.O., Yandell, M., Evans, C.A., Holt, R.A., Gocayne, J.D., Amanatides, P., Ballew, R.M., Huson, D.H., Wortman, J.R., Zhang, Q., Kodira, C.D., Zheng, X.H., Chen, L., Skupski, M., Subramanian, G., Thomas, P.D., Zhang, J., Gabor, M.G.L., Nelson, C., Broder, S., Clark, A.G., Nadeau, J., McKusick, V,A., Zinder, N., Levine, A.J., Roberts, R.J., Simon, M., Slayman, C., Hunkapiller, M., Bolanos, R., Delcher, A., Dew, I., Fasulo, D., Flanigan, M., Florea, L., Halpern, A., Hannenhalli, S., Kravitz, S., Levy, S., Mobarry, C., Reinert, K., Remington, K., Abu-Threideh, J., Beasley, E., Biddick, K., Bonazzi, V., Brandon, R., Cargill, M., Chandramouliswaran, I., Charlab, R., Chaturvedi, K., Deng, Z., Di Francesco, V., Dunn, P., Eilbeck, K., Evangelista, C., Gabrielian, A.E., Gan, W., Ge, W., Gong, F., Gu, Z., Guan, P., Heiman, T.J., Higgins, M.E., Ji, R.R., Ke, Z., Ketchum, K.A., Lai, Z., Lei, Y., Li, Z., Li, J., Liang, Y., Lin, X., Lu, F., Merkulov, G.V., Milshina, N., Moore, H.M., Naik, A.K., Narayan, V.A., Neelam, B., Nusskern, D., Rusch, D.B., Salzberg, S., Shao, W., Shue, B., Sun, J., Wang, Z., Wang, A., Wang, X., Wang, J., Wei, M., Wides, R., Xiao, C., Yan, C., Yao, A., Ye, J., Zhan, M., Zhang, W., Zhang, H., Zhao, Q., Zheng, L., Zhong, F., Zhong, W., Zhu, S., Zhao, S., Gilbert, D., Baumhueter, S., Spier, G., Carter, C., Cravchik, A., Woodage, T., Ali, F., An, H., Awe, A., Baldwin, D., Baden, H., Barnstead, M., Barrow, I., Beeson, K., Busam, D., Carver, A., Center, A., Cheng, M.L., Curry, L., Danaher, S., Davenport, L., Desilets, R., Dietz, S., Dodson, K., Doup, L., Ferriera, S., Garg, N., Glucksmann, A., Hart, B., Haynes, J., Haynes, C., Heiner, C., Hladun, S., Hostin, D., Houck, J., Howland, T., Ibegwam, C., Johnson, J., Kalush, F., Kline, L., Koduru, S., Love, A., Mann, F., May, D., McCawley, S., McIntosh, T., McMullen, I., Moy, M., Moy, L., Murphy, B., Nelson, K., Pfannkoch, C., Pratts, E., Puri, V., Qureshi, H., Reardon, M., Rodriguez, R., Rogers, Y.H., Romblad, D., Ruhfel, B., Scott R., Sitter, C., Smallwood, M., Stewart, E., Strong, R., Suh, E., Thomas, R., Tint, N.N., Tse, S., Vech, C., Wang, G., Wetter, J., Williams, S., Williams, M., Windsor, S., Winn-Deen, E., Wolfe, K., Zaveri, J., Zaveri, K., Abril, J.F., Guigo, R., Campbell, M.J., Sjolander, K.V., Karlak, B., Kejariwal, A., Mi, H., Lazareva, B., Hatton, T., Narechania, A., Diemer, K., Muruganujan, A., Guo,

N., Sato, S., Bafna, V., Istrail, S., Lippert, R., Schwartz, R., Walenz, B., Yooseph, S., Allen, D., Basu, A., Baxendale, J., Blick, L., Caminha, M., Carnes-Stine, J., Caulk, P., Chiang, Y.H., Coyne, M., Dahlke, C., Mays, A., Dombroski, M., Donnelly, M., Ely, D., Esparham, S., Fosler, C., Gire, H., Glanowski, S., Glasser, K., Glodek, A., Gorokhov, M., Graham, K., Gropman, B., Harris, M., Heil, J., Henderson, S., Hoover, J., Jennings, D., Jordan, C., Jordan, J., Kasha, J., Kagan, L., Kraft, C., Levitsky, A., Lewis, M., Liu, X., Lopez, J., Ma, D., Majoros, W., McDaniel, J., Murphy, S., Newman, M., Nguyen, T., Nguyen, N., Nodell, M., Pan, S., Peck, J., Peterson, M., Rowe, W., Sanders, R., Scott, J., Simpson, M., Smith, T., Sprague, A., Stockwell, T., Turner, R., Venter, E., Wang, M., Wen, M., Wu, D., Wu, M., Xia, A., Zandieh, A., Zhu, X. (2001) The sequence of human genome. Science 291:1304-1351.

Verrills, N.M., Kavallaris, M. (2003) Drug resistance mechanisms in cancer cells: a proteomics perspective. Curr. Opin. Mol. Ther. 5:258-265.

Voit, E.O. (2000) Computational analysis of biochemical systems. Cambridge Univ. Press.

Waghray, A., Schober, M., Feroze, F., Yao, F., Virgin, J. and Chen, Y.Q. (2001) Identification of differentially expressed genes by serial analysis of gene expression in human prostate cancer. Cancer Res. 61:4283-4286.

Wiechert, W. (2002) Modeling and simulation: tools for metabolic engineering. J Biotechnol. 94:37-63.

Williams, K.L. (1999) Genomes and proteomes: towards a multidimensional view of biology. Electrophoresis 20:678-688.

Wittmann, C. and Heinzle, E. (2001) Application of MALDI-TOF MS to lysine-producing Corynebacterium glutamicum: a novel approach for metabolic flux analysis. Eur. J. Biochem. 268:2441-2455.

Wu, W., Hu, W. and Kavanagh, J.J. (2002) Proteomics in cancer research. Int. J. Gynecol Cancer. 12:409-423.

Yale, J. and Bohnert, H.J. (2001) Transcript expression in Saccharomyces cerevisiae at high salinity. J. Biol. Chem. 276:15996-16007.

Ye, R.W., Tao, W., Bedzyk, L., Young, T., Chen, M. and Li, L. (2000) Global gene expression profiles of Bacillus subtilis grown under anaerobic conditions. J. Bacteriol. 182:4458-4465.

Yoon, S.H., Han, M.J., Lee, S.Y., Jeong, K.J., Yoo and J.S. (2002) Combined transcriptome and proteome analysis of Escherichia coli during the high cell density culture. Biotechnol. Bioeng. 81:753-767.

Yoshida, K., Kobayashi, K., Miwa, Y., Kang, C.M., Matsunaga, M., Yamaguchi, H., Tojo, S., Yamamoto, M., Nishi, R., Ogasawara, N., Nakayama, T. and Fujita, Y. (2001) Combined transcriptome and proteome analysis as a powerful approach to study genes under glucose repression in Bacillus subtilis. Nucleic Acids Res. 29:683-692.

Zhang, S., Day, I.N. and Ye, S. (2001) Microarray analysis of nicotine-induced changes in gene expression in endothelial cells. Physiol. Genomics. 5:187-192.

7 Computational Modeling of Biological Processes with Petri Net-Based Architecture

Masao Nagasaki[1], Atushi Doi[2], Hiroshi Matsuno[2], Satoru Miyano[1]

[1] Human Genome Center, Institute of Medical Science,
University of Tokyo, 4-6-1 Shirokane-dai, Minato-ku,
Tokyo, 108-8639, Japan
e-mail: masao@ims.u-tokyo.ac.jp, miyano@ims.u-tokyo.ac.jp
http://genomicobject.net/
[2] Graduate School of Science and Engineering,
Yamaguchi University, 1677-1 Yoshida, Yamaguchi 753-8512, Japan
e-mail: atushi@ib.sci.yamaguchi-u.ac.jp, matsuno@sci.yamaguchi-u.ac.jp

7.1 Introduction

With the rapid increase in biological knowledge about cellular processes, systems biology inevitably requires computational environments in which we can understand a cell as a system and predict its behavior for hypothesis generation and further experimental investigation. Related to this, particularly needed is software with which users in the fields of biology and medicine can, by themselves, model and simulate biological processes in the cell by compiling biological knowledge and analyzing experimental data. Various biological processes have received attention for modeling and simulation. Especially, gene regulatory networks, metabolic pathways, and signal transduction cascades are considered important basic biological processes for systemic understanding.

In 1999, we anticipated the methodological change in biology and medicine due to the emergence of systems biology, and started a software development project which is to attain the following objective:

"To create concepts for modeling and develop a software environment with which large-scale complicated biological processes can be modeled, simulated and analyzed as easily as possible by users who are familiar with biological entities and processes but not necessarily familiar with the details of the modeling architecture."

In 2003, on the other hand, the US Department of Energy has started the Genomes to Life (GTL) project (http://www.doegenomestolife.org/.). It includes a goal similar to our stated objective to "develop the computational methods and capabilities to advance understanding of complex biological systems and predict their behavior". The GTL project shall surely enhance the computational strategy in systems biology and will prove that this direction is essential to biology.

In order to pursue the above objective, we investigated (i) modeling of biological processes, (ii) simulation of biological processes, (iii) visualization of their simulations, and (iv) integration of existing biological pathway databases for modeling, and obtained a series of results and software (Doi et al., 2004a, 2004b; Matsuno et al., 2000, 2001, 2003a, 2003b, 2003c; Nagasaki 2003, 2004, 2004a, 2004b, 2004c; Nakano et al., 2002; http://genomicobject.net/public/BiotechBook2004/code/;   http://Genomic Object.net/.; and http://www.doegenomestolife.org/.) that could achive our objective. Namely, we have developed the applications Genomic Object Net (GON) and GONML for (i) and (ii), GON Visualizer for (iii), and BioPathway Executer (BPE) and BPE Online System (BPEOS) for (iv). For modeling, we have defined the new concepts of hybrid functional Petri net (HFPN) and hybrid functional Petri net with extension (HFPNe) as the architecture for modeling, so that biological processes can be modeled and simulated in a suitable manner. GON employs the architecture of HFPNe for implementation. This paper presents some details of these contributions.

First, architecture is required for modeling and simulation of biological processes. In 1999, we investigated software tools and methods for modeling biological pathways to develop an architecture which is most suited to our objective. At that time, there were ODE-based attempts to modeling chemical reactions, e.g., Gepasi (Mendes, 1993), E-Cell (Tomita et al., 1999) and others, *e.g.* Lisp based architecture QSIM (Kuipers and Shults 1994) and the π-Calculus-based architecture Bio-Calculus (Nagasaki et al., 1999, and Onami et al., 2001). Unfortunately, applications based on these architectures are not considered acceptable for our objective. This is due not only to their poor GUI interfaces but also to some mathematical requirements arising from the architectures themselves that are not relevant to biology and not acceptable to users. However, we found that architectures based on Petri nets might be suited to our objective because of their intuitive graphical representation and their capabilities for mathematical analyses (Reisig and Rozenberg, 1998a, and Reisig and Rozenberg, 1998b).

At the initial stage of our research, we employed an existing Petri net called hybrid Petri net (HPN) (Alla and David, 1998, and Drath, 1998, 1999) and could successfully model and simulate the gene regulatory network of λ phage (Matsuno et al., 2000). HPN allows us to model this complicated regulatory network easily and intuitively. However, in the case of the glycolytic pathway of *Escherichia coli*, we found that HPN is not good at modeling the biological process intuitively. This motivated us to extend the HPN architecture to HFPN (Matsuno et al., 2000). With HFPN, we have modeled and simulated various biological processes, including the glycolytic pathway of *Escherichia coli*, the gene regulation of circadian rhythms in *Drosophila*, the boundary formation by notch signaling in *Drosophila* (Matsuno et al., 2003b), and the apoptosis induced by *Fas* ligand (Matsuno et al., 2003c; http://GenomicObject.net/.).

In HFPN, we assign an integer or real variable to a biological entity such as a protein to represent its quantity or density. The speed of a reaction between biological entities is specified as a function of the variables assigned to the entities. However, there are other biological processes which are not efficiently modeled with HFPN. For example, DNA sequences are not directly handled with HFPN since it does not allow us to assign a string variable. The investigation of more complex biological processes led us to extend the HFPN architecture to include data types such as `string`, `boolean`, `list`, `pair`, and `object`. This extension led to the concept of HFPNe. GON, with the HFPNe archtecture (Nagasaki et al., 2004b) makes it feasible to model and simulate biological processes such as the transcription process from DNA to mRNA in bacteria, the alternative splicing process in the DSCAM gene in *Drosophila*, the translation process from mRNA to protein of gene *trpL* in E. *coli*, the translation process with frameshift in HIV-1 RNA, complex carbohydrate synthesis, Huntington's disease model, and protein modification of gene *p53* (Nagasaki 2004, and Nagasaki et al., 2004a).

Modeling and simulation of complex biological processes can be well treated with GON. However, GON is not enough for our objective from the viewpoint of simulation analysis. For visualization, the simulation of a model created with a graphical model canvas can be viewed only as a 2D time course graph. The situation is more or less similar for other applications (see Table 7.13 for comparison). In contrast, sophisticated animations of simulation states are very informative for evaluating and tuning models. For this, we have developed the GON Visualizer (Nagasaki et al., 2004b). By writing an XML document for the GON Visualizer, users can realize a personalized animation for simulation.

With the GON and GON Visualizer, users can, for a target biological process, model, simulate, and create personalized visualization for biological process simulation. However, users need to create all the biological processes from scratch. On the other hand, pathway databases such as KEGG (Kanehisa and Goto, 2000) and BioCyc (Karp et al., 2002, 2002) compile a large number of static biological pathway models with biochemical information which are not directly simulatable. We have therefore developed a software BPE (Nagasaki et al., 2003, 2004c) that suitably reconstructs pathway information from KEGG and BioCyc for simulation. With this aim, we have developed a reconstruction method for biological pathways in KEGG and BioCyc by extensively using the HFPNe architecture for modeling and the flexible features in the graphical model editor on GON. We have also develop an online system of BPE called BPEOS (Nagasaki, 2004; http://bpe.genomicobject.net/).

Thus, the project started in 1999 has contributed to the development of a software environment mentioned in the objective[1]. These products have been used in some biology laboratories. This fact suggests that the software environment is useful for research in biology and medicine.

The outline of this chapter is as follows:

Section 7.2 surveys several kinds of Petri nets – Petri net (Reisig and Rozenberg, 1998a, 1998b), timed Petri net (Reisig and Rozenberg, 1998a, 1998b), continuous timed Petri net (David et al., 1987), and hybrid Petri net (Alla and David, 1998)) – and discusses the advantages and limitations when biological processes are modeled with these Petri nets. Then, in Sections 7.3 and 7.4, we define HFPN and HFPNe, which inherit the features of hybrid object net (Drath, 1998), hybrid Petri net (Alla and David 1998), and hybrid dynamic net (Drath, 1998) in order to model and simulate biological processes that are difficult to handle with other Petri nets.

In Subsections 7.5.1 through 7.5.4, we describe how we can use HFPN and HFPNe to model four biological processes – (a) translation of mRNA - alternative splicing, (b) translation of mRNA - frameshift, (c) Huntington's disease model, and (d) protein modification - *p53* – and show the usability of HFPN and HFPNe for modeling. The differences between HFPNe and other high-level Petri nets, OCP-nets (Maier and Moldt 2001), and Reference nets (Kummer, 2001) are discussed in Section 7.6.

Section 7.7 implements modeling/simulation software, Genomic Object Net (GON), with the HFPN/HFPNe architecture, and develops an XML format for modelings/simulation of biological processes named GONML. Subsections 7.7.3 and 7.7.4 compare other modeling and simulation software – Cell Designer (http://sbserv.symbio.jst.go.jp/), E-Cell (Tomita et

---

[1] GON and Visualizer have been commercialized in 2003 as Cell IllustratorTM and Cell AnimatorTM from Gene Networks Inc. (http://www.gene-networks.com/)

al., 1999), Virtual Cell (Schaff et al., 1997), Gepasi (Mendes, 1993), Path-Pursuit (http://www.scbio.co.jp/products/pathpursuit/index.html) – and XML formats of biological processes – SBML (Hucka et al. 2003) and CellML (http://www.cellml.org/) – and discusses the advantages of GON and GONML over the software and XML formats.

Section 7.8 introduces the importance of animations for biological processes that can easily and effectively visualize the simulation results, especially of GON in Section 7.7, develops animation software, Visualizer, for biological processes, and describes its usage with seven biological processes, transcription, translation, repression, expression, binding, degradation, and translocation. The last section discusses the effectiveness of Visualizer in education and research in molecular biology.

Section 7.9 discusses the importance of software that automatically creates executable models of biological processes from pathway databases. A new database is developed that sorts out and compiles existing pathway databases, KEGG, BioCyc, and BRENDA (Schomburg et al., 2002), and develops an application, Biopathway Executer (BPE), that creates executable pathways in the GONML format while inheriting the original customized pathway views of the databases. We also supply an online service with BPE, BPE Online Service (BPEOS).

Finally, Section 7.10 summarizes the sofaware environment that consists of applications (GON, GONML, GON Visualizer, BPE, BPEOS) with their architectures (HFPN/HFPNe), and describe future research issues.

7.2 Hybrid Petri Net and Hybrid Dynamic Net

Petri net is a mathematical model for representation and analysis of concurrent processes. The original Petri net was proposed in 1962 by Petri (Reisig and Rozenberg, 1998a), and since then various types of Petri nets have been proposed. In this section, we informally review the notions of the original Petri net, the timed Petri net (Reisig and Rozenberg, 1998a), the continuous Petri net (David and Alla, 1987), and the hybrid Petri net (Alla and David, 1998).

In general, a *Petri net* (PN) is a finite network consisting of the following four kinds of elements (see Fig. 7.1): (1) place, (2) transition, (3) arc, and (4) token. A *place* can hold *tokens* as its value, and we call their quantity the *mark* of the place. We denote the set of places by *E*. A *marking* of E is a mapping that assigns a mark (the quantity of tokens) to each place. An *arc* is assigned a nonnegative number called the *weight*. A *transition* has arcs coming from places and arcs going out from the transition to places. A transition with these arcs defines a *firing condition* in terms of the values of the places where the arcs are attached. After firing, the marks of the places are updated according to the weights assigned to the arcs.

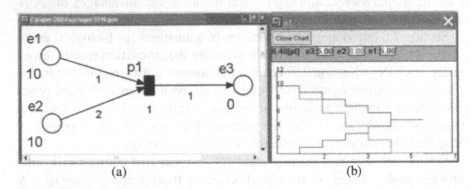

(a)   (b)

Fig. 7.1. A graphical representation of a TPN (left window) which is comprised of places e_1, e_2, and e_3, transition p_1, and three arcs, where place, arc, and transition are represented by the symbols for "circle", "arrow", and "filled rectangle", respectively. Places e_1 and e_2 have 10 tokens each and place e_3 has no token. The three arcs have weights 1, 2, and 1. The delay of transition p_1 is 1. The right window shows a 2D time series graph that plots the simulation result of this TPN started from the initial marks

A *timed Petri net* (TPN) is a Petri net which counts time and allows the *delay* in firing. Figure 7.1(a) shows an example of a TPN with which we shall explain some concepts related to TPNs. This TPN consists of three places, e_1, e_2, and e_3, one transition, p_1, and three arcs, (e_1, p_1), (e_2, p_1) and (p_1, e_3). The arcs are assigned constant values called weights, $w(e_1, p_1) = 1$, $w(e_2, p_1) = 2$, and $w(p_1, e_3) = 1$, respectively. Transition p1 is assigned a constant value called the *delay*, $d(p_1) = 1$. Since the time is counted in TPN, the marking is parametrized with time t as $M(t)$. Then, the mark of place e_i at time t is denoted as $M(e_i, t)$. The marking at time 0 is called the initial marking, and each mark at time 0 is called the initial *mark*. The initial marks of e_1, e_2, and e_3 are 10, 10, and 0, respectively. We say that transition p_1 is *triggered* at time t if the marks $M(e_1, t)$ and $M(e_2, t)$ of e_1 and e_2 at time t satisfy the firing conditions $M(e_1, t) \geq w(e_1, p_1)$ and $M(e_2, t) \geq w(e_2, p_1)$. The marking $M(t)$ at time t is calculated as follows for $t \geq 1$. Recall that $d(p_1) = 1$ for transition p_1. This means that p_1 can fire at $d(p_1)$ time after it is triggered. Formally, if transition p_1 is triggered at time $t - d(p_1)$, it can fire at time t, and the marks are updated at time t as $M(e_1, t) = M(e_1, t - d(p_1)) - w(e_1, p_1)$ and $M(e_2, t) = M(e_2 d(p_1)) - w(e_2, p_1)$, and the weight $w(p_1, e_3)$ is added into $M(e_3, t)$, i.e., $M(e_3, t) = M(e_3, t - d(p_1)) + w(p_1, e_3)$. For example, at time $t = 1$, the transition p_1 fires and all places that are connected to the transition change their marks, i.e., $M(e_1, 1) = M(e_1, 0) - w(e_1, p_1) = 9$, $M(e_2, p_1) = M(e_2, 0) - w(e_2, p_1) = 8$, and $M(e_3, 1) = M(e_3, 0) + w(e_3, p_1) = 1$. With similar steps, the marks of places at time t can be calculated and plotted, as in Fig. 7.1(b).

Using the delay mechanism, a biological process that consists of processes with various time intervals can be easily modeled. For example, in *E. coli* the transcription rate of a gene with strong promoter regions can be one mRNA molecule every two seconds, while the frequency of a gene with weak promoter regions can be one mRNA molecule every ten minutes (Berg et al., 2002).

With the concept of time in TPN, we can model some chemical reactions. But places of TPN can take only nonnegative integers for their marks. It is an unfavorable feature when biological transitions require some real numbers for their modeling. Thus, an enhanced Petri net that can deal with real numbers is necessary.

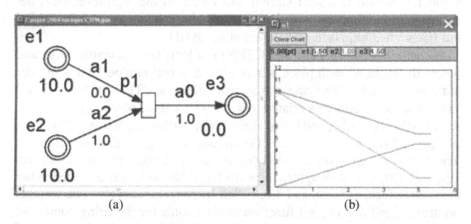

(a)   (b)

Fig. 7.2. A graphical representation of a CTPN (left window), comprised of places e_1, e_2, and e_3, transition p1, and three arcs, where place, arc, and transition are represented by "double circle", "arrow", and "unfilled rectangle", respectively. The marks of places e1and e2 are both 10.0, and the mark of place e_3 is 0.0. The weights of arcs (e_1, p_1), (e_2, p_1), and (p_1, e_3) are 0.0, 1.0, and 1.0, respectively, and their speeds are 1.0, 2.0, and 1.0, respectively. The right window shows a 2D time series graph that plots the simulation result of this TPN started from the initial marks

The Petri net was used to model metabolic pathways where places represent biological compounds (metabolites), transitions represent chemical reactions between metabolites that are usually catalyzed by a certain enzyme, and tokens indicate the presence of compounds (Reddy et al., 1993). This approach is based on the condition that event mechanisms and discussions are based only on *qualitative* aspects. That is, a place having tokens represents only the presence of the corresponding compound in the place, no matter how many tokens are contained in the place. This approach was expanded to model metabolic processes (Hofestädt, 1994). Hofestädt and Thelen (1998) tried to make *quantitative* simulations by using the self-modifying Petri net model (Valk, 1978) where the number of tokens in a place is used to represent the level of concentrations of the corresponding compound. The main feature of the self-modifying Petri net is that the value of a place can be used as a parameter to the formula describing the weight on the arc from the place that represents the threshold and consumption of tokens for firing. With this modification, biochemical processes are modeled with actual concentrations. Moreover, in order to represent more complex relations and conditions, they use the functional Petri net where the calculation of the dynamic biocatalytic processes can be realized by using functions for specifying the arc weight. By using Design/CPN, which is a well known tool based on the high-level Petri net technique, modeling and simulating of metabolic pathways can be carried out (Genrich et al., 2001, and Heiner et al., 2001).

A *continuous timed Petri net* (CTPN) is a Petri net that counts time, and where the mark of each place is a nonnegative real number and firing occurs continuously. We again use an example of a CTPN, in Fig. 7.2, for explaining some concepts related to it. There are three places, e_1, e_2, and e_3, which hold 10.0, 10.0, and 0.0 as their initial marks, respectively. Two arcs (e_1, p_1) and (e_2, p_1) go into transition p_1 and arc (p_1, e_3) goes out from p_1. These arcs, (e_1, p_1), (e_2, p_1), and (p_1, e_3) are assigned constant values 0.0, 1.0, and 1.0, called weights, respectively. They are also assigned other constant values, 1.0, 2.0, and 1.0, called speeds, respectively. The weights on arcs (e_1, p_1) and (e_2, p_1) function as thresholds for the firing condition. The weight on arc (p_1, e_3) means nothing. For transition p_1, the speeds of arcs (e_1, p_1), (e_2, p_1) are called the input speeds of p_1 and the speed of arc (p_1, e_3) is called the output speed of p_1. Transition p_1 fires as long as the conditions $M(e_1, t) \geq w(e_1, p_1)$ and $M(e_2, t) \geq w(e_2, p_1)$ are satisfied. While p_1 is firing, $M(e_3, t)$ is increased with speed 1.0 and $M(e_1, t)$ and $M(e_2, t)$ are decreased with speeds 1.0 and 2.0, respectively. Namely, $dM(e_1, t)/dt = -1.0$, $dM(e_2, t)/dt = -2.0$, and $dM(e_3, t)/dt = 1.0$. Figure 7.2 shows its simulation. In this definition of CTPN, the input speed and output speeds can be different for any transition. However, another definition of CTPN makes a restriction that the input speed and output speeds must be the same for every transition.

Ordinary differential equations (ODEs) are widely used to express biological phenomena such as biochemical reactions. CTPN can be used for modeling with this feature. If a biological process is modeled and represented as a large system of ODEs, it may be difficult to observe the whole process intuitively like a picture. On the other hand, the biological process modeled with CTPN may provide us an intuitive graphical representation that includes the network structure and biological knowledge of the process. Thus, it is more understandable.

Consider the glycolytic pathway and lac operon gene regulatory network (Doi et al., 2004a, 2004b). The lac operon gene regulatory network contains a switching mechanism that may be modeled with TPN. The mechanism of gene regulation usually consists of activation and repression. The glycolytic pathway is a cascade of enzyme reactions that may be modeled with CTPN. Furthermore, in an enzyme reaction, some quantity of the enzyme is required for reaction while the quantity of the enzyme itself is not decreased during the reaction, except for its degradation.

Some favorable features also have been introduced in Petri net theory. In addition to normal arc, *inhibitory arc* and *test arc* have been defined for convenience (Fig. 7.3). An inhibitory arc with weight r enables the transition to fire only if the value of the place at the source of the arc is less than or equal to r. An inhibitory arc can be used to represent the function of "repress" in gene regulation. A test arc does not consume any contents of the place at the source of the arc by firing. Test arcs can be used to model transcription processes and enzyme reactions since nothing is consumed by these processes.

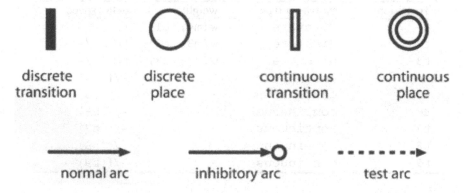

discrete   discrete   continuous   continuous
transition   place   transition   place

normal arc   inhibitory arc   test arc

Fig. 7.3. Basic elements of hybrid Petri net

As explained above, biological processes may involve both discrete and continuous features simultaneously. *Hybrid Petri net* (HPN) can deal with these features. Alla and David (1998) defined the concept of HPN by combining TPN and CTPN. In HPN, the speeds and weights assigned to arcs are constant. Instead of using a constant for representing the speed of an arc, Drath (Drath, 1998, and Hucka et al., 2003) has defined the concept of *hybrid dynamic net* (HDN) by assigning the speed of firing to a transition that depends on the values of places where the transition has arcs. This means that the arcs connected to the transition have the same speed, and this speed can be controlled as a function of the values of some specific places.

Figure 7.4 shows an HPN model which describes the transcription of two genes – gene1 and gene2 – on the same operon to mRNAs – mRNA1 and mRNA2, and their translations from mRNAs to proteins – protein1 and protein2. The types of the places and transitions in the model are summarized in Tables 7.1 and 7.2.

Table 7.1. Properties of entities in Fig. 7.4.

Place	place type	initial mark
m1	discrete	M(m1,0)
m2	discrete	M(m2, 0)
m3	discrete	M(m3, 0)
m4	continuous	M(m4, 0)
m5	continuous	M(m5, 0)
m6	continuous	M(m6, 0)
m7	continuous	M(m7, 0)

Table 7.2. Properties of transitions in Fig. 7.4.

Transition	transition type	weight	delay/speed
t1	discrete	w(m4; t1)	f(t1)/-
t2	discrete	w(m3; t2)	f(t2)/-
t3	discrete	w(m3; t3)	f(t3)/-
t4	continuous	-	-/f(t4)
t5	continuous	-	-/f(t5)
t6	continuous	-	-/f(t6)
t7	continuous	-	-/f(t7)
t8	continuous	-	-/f(t8)
t9	continuous	-	-/f(t9)

The initial mark of place m1 at time 0 (M(m1, 0)) is set to be one (this represents the RNA polymerase binding to the promoter of the operon), whereas the marks of other places, m2, m3, m4, m5, and m6, are zero. The delay f (t1) associated with the discrete transition t1 reflects the time needed for the transcription of gene1 by the RNA polymerase. Whenever the transcription of gene1 is finished, the mark of the continuous place m4, which represents the mRNA concentration of gene1, is increased by w(m4, t1). The degradation rate for mRNA of gene1 is given by f(t6).

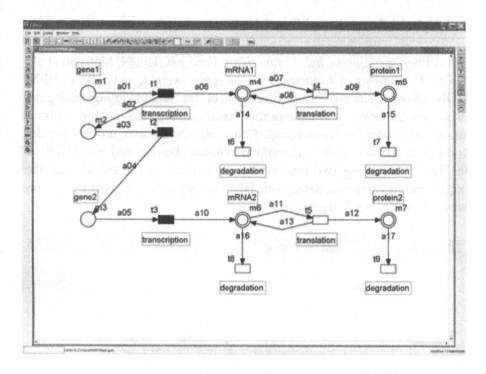

Fig. 7.4. An example of HPN. Discrete place and discrete transition are represented by symbols "single circle" and "filled rectangle", respectively. Continuous place and continuous transition are represented by symbols "double circle" and "unfilled rectangle", respectively. This example models biological transitions, transcriptions and translations of two genes, gene1 and gene2

The speed $f(t4)$ of the continuous transition t4 reflects the translation speed of gene1. The place m4 is simultaneously an input and an output of the transition t1 because it is required for translation but should not be consumed. For this modeling, we can also use a test arc. The increasing rate of gene1 protein (the mark of the place m2) is given by $f(t4)$. The degradation rate of gene2 protein is given by $f(t7)$. The delay $f(t2)$ of the transition t2 represents the time needed for the RNA polymerase to move from the end of gene1 to the beginning of gene2. When the mark of m3 becomes greater than $w(m3, t2) = 0$, RNA polymerase begins the gene2 transcription. Further comments on gene2 are omitted, since they are similar to the ones for gene1 described above.

7.3 Hybrid Functional Petri Net

We define the notion of *hybrid functional Petri net* (HFPN, Matsuno et al., 2003c) by allowing any functions for the speed, weight, and delay in HPN. HDN allows dynamic firing speed, favorable for modeling biological processes. However, it is unfavorable that the arc(s) connected to the transition must have the same speed. Consider a continuous process for decomposing a trimer to three monomers. This can be modeled with HDN, as in Fig. 7.5, by using two transitions, p1 and p2, and a test arc. On the other hand, it can be modeled with HPN, as in Fig. 7.5. This is the reason why we assign speed to each arc.

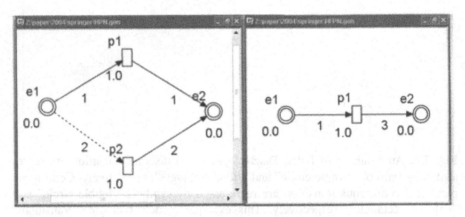

Fig. 7.5. A biological process of decomposing trimers to monomers is modeled with HDN and HPN

In addition to this feature, the dynamic feature is also necessary for modeling biological processes. Consider a chemical reaction $2CO_2 + H_2S + 2H_2O \rightarrow 2CH_2O + H_2SO_4$ that has stoichiometries, two for the compounds CO_2, H_2O, and CH_2O, and one for the compounds H_2S and CH_2O. In such a chemical reaction, the reaction rate depends on the masses of the stoichiometries. When modeling with HFPN, the input or output speed of an arc is proportional to the stoichiometry of a compound that represents the value of the place, e.g., the consumption speeds of CO_2 and H_2O are two times faster than that of H_2S, and the production speed of CH_2O is two times faster than that of H_2SO_4. Moreover, there are many ODE-based chemical kinetics, e.g., the Michaelis-Menten reactions, Hill kinetics, and Ping-Pong kinetics (Voet and Voet 1995).

One of the issues of our objective is to create a suitable architecture that can represent biological processes as easily as possible. Thus, this extesion of HPN/HDN is necessary for modeling these biological processes.

7.4 Hybrid Functional Petri Net with Extension

7.4.1 Definitions

For modeling more complex biological processes intuitively, we are required to deal with various kinds of biological information, e.g., the density of molecules, the number of molecules, sequences, molecular modifications, binding location, localization of molecules, etc. The purpose of this section is to formally define an extension of HFPN with which we can cope with this feature in biological system modeling.

First, we introduce *types* for biological entities and processes. The set T of *types* is defined by the following abstract syntax:

```
⟨type⟩ ::= boolean || integer || integer+ || real
        || real+ || string || pair (⟨type⟩,⟨type⟩)
        || list ⟨type⟩ || vector ⟨type⟩ || object
        (⟨type⟩, ··· , ⟨type⟩)
```

Then, for $\theta \in T$, we define the domain $D(\theta)$ of θ as follows:

1. $D(\texttt{boolean}) = \{\texttt{true, false}\}$, $D(\texttt{integer}) = Z$ (the set of integers), $D(\texttt{integer+}) = N$ (the set of nonnegative integers), $D(\texttt{real}) = R$ (the set of real numbers), $D(\texttt{real+}) = R^{\geq 0}$ (the set of nonnegative real numbers), $D(\texttt{string}) = S$ (the set of strings over some alphabet).
2. $D(\texttt{pair}(\theta_1, \theta_2)) = D(\theta_1) \times D(\theta_2)$.
3. $D(\texttt{list}\,\theta) = U_{K \geq 0}\, D(\theta)^K$.
4. $D(\texttt{object}(\theta_1, \cdots, \theta_n)) = D(\theta_1) \times \cdots \times D(\theta_n)$.

For convenience, we denote $D^* = U_{\theta \in T} D(\theta)$.

Let E be a finite set. A *type function* for E is a mapping $\tau : E \to T$. For $e \in E$, $\tau(e)$ is called the *type* of e. A *marking* of E is a mapping $M : E \to D^*$ satisfying $M(e) \in D(\tau(e))$ for $e \in E$. For $e \in E$, $M(e)$ called the *mark* of e. We denote by M the set of all markings of E. We can regard M as the set $\prod_{e \in E} D(\tau(e))$. Consider a function $f : M \to R$. For a subset $F \subseteq E$ and an element $v \in \prod_{e \in F} D(\tau(e))$, let $f[F = v] : \prod_{e \in E-F} D(\tau(e)) \to R$ be the function obtained from f by restricting the value for F to v, i.e. $f[F = v]$ $(z) = f(z, v)$ for $z \in \prod_{e \in E-F} D(\tau(e))$. Let F be a subset of E such that $e \in F$ satisfies $D(\tau(e)) = R$ or $R^{\geq 0}$. We say that the function f is *continuous for*

F if $f[E - F = v] : \prod_{e \in F} D(\tau(e)) \rightarrow R$ is continuous on $\prod_{e \in F} D(\tau(e))$ for any $v \in \prod_{e \in E \cdot F} D(\tau(e))$.

Based on the above terminology, we define the concept of hybrid func tional Petri net with extension (HFPNe). The basic idea of HFPNe is two-fold: to introduce types, with which we can deal with various data types to employ functions of marking $f(M)$ to determine weight, delay, speed, etc., that control the system behavior. In the following definition, we use differ-ent terms for place, transition, arc, etc., which are conventionally used in Petri net theory, since biological system modeling requires more intuitive terms for representing biological entities and processes.

Definition 1 We define a *hybrid functional Petri net with extension* (HFPNe) $H = (E, P, h, \tau, C, d, a)$ as follows:

1. $E = \{e_1, \cdots, e_n\}$ is a non-empty finite set of entities and $P = \{p_1, \cdots, p_m\}$ is a non-empty finite set of processes, where we assume $E \cap P = 0^2$.

2. $h : E \cup P \rightarrow \{\text{discrete, continuous, generic}\}$ is a mapping called the *hybrid function*, A process $p \in P$ with $h(p) = \text{discrete}$ (or con-tinuous or generic) is called a *discrete process* (or *continuous process* or *generic process*). An entity $e \in E$ with $h(e) = \text{discrete}$ (or con-tinuous or generic) is called a *discrete entity* (or *continuous entity* or, *generic entity*).

3. $\tau : E \rightarrow T$ is a type function for E such that $\tau(e)) = \text{integer+}$ if e is a discrete entity, and $\tau(e) = \text{real+}$ if e is a continuous entity.

4. $C = (EP, PE, a, w, u)$ consists of subsets $EP \subseteq E \times P$ and $PE \subseteq P \times E$. An element in $EP \cup PE$ is called a connector[3]. Each connector has a *connector type*, which is given by a mapping a : $EP \cup PE \rightarrow \{\text{proc-ess, associate, inhibitor}\}$ called the *connector type function* that satisfies the conditions: (i) $a(c) = \text{process}$ for $c \in PE$. (ii) All connec-tors $c = (e, p) \in EP$ satisfy the conditions in Table 7.3 (a) and all con-nectors $c = (p, e) \in PE$ satisfy the conditions in Table 7.3 (b). A con-nector $c = (e, p) \in EP$ is called a *process connector* (or an *associate connector* or an *inhibitory connector*) if $a(c) = \text{process}$ (or associate or inhibitor)[4]. For a connector $c = (p, e) \in PE$, $a(c) = \text{process}$ by definition, and we also call it a *process connector*. We say that a con-

---

[2] Terms "**entity**" and "**process**" correspond to place and transition, respectively.

[3] "Connector" corresponds to arc.

[4] "Process connector", "associate connector", and "inhibitory connector" corre-spond to *arc with weight*, *test arc* and *inhibitory arc*, respectively.

nector $c = (e, p) \in EP$ is *discrete* (or *continuous* or *generic*) if p is a discrete process (or a continuous process or a generic process). In the same way, we also say that $c = (p, e) \in PE$ is *discrete* (or *continuous* or *generic*) if p is a discrete process (or a continuous process or a generic process). Let M be the set of all markings of E and let F be the set of continuous entities in E. We define $D_{\text{discrete}} = \{ f \mid f : M \rightarrow N \}$, $D_{\text{continuous}} = \{ f \mid f : M \rightarrow R^{\geq 0}$ is continuous for $F \}$, $D_{\text{generic}} = \{ f \mid f : M \rightarrow D^* \}$, and $D_{\text{boolean}} = \{ f \mid f : M \rightarrow \{\text{true, false}\}$. Then, w and u are given as follows:

(a) $w : EP \rightarrow D_{\text{discrete}} \cup D_{\text{continuous}} \cup D_{\text{boolean}}$ is a function called the *activity function* such that for a connector $c \in EP$ (i) $w(c) \in D_{\text{discrete}}$ if c is discrete, (ii) $w(c) \in D_{\text{continuous}}$ if c is continuous, (iii) $w(c) \in D_{\text{boolean}}$ if c is generic. For a connector (e, p), $w(e, p)$ is used as a function giving the threshold in discrete and giving continuous cases and the condition in the generic case required for enabling the process p.

(b) $u : EP \cup PE \rightarrow D_{\text{discrete}} \cup D_{\text{continuous}} \cup D_{\text{generic}}$ is a function called the *update function* that satisfies the following conditions: for a connector $c \in EP \cup PE$, let $c = (e, p) \in EP$ or $c = (p, e) \in PE$. (i) $u(c) \in D_{\text{discrete}}$ if c is discrete. (ii) $u(c) \in D_{\text{continuous}}$ if c is continuous. (iii) If c is generic, then $u(c)$ is a function in D_{generic} such that $u(c)(M)$ is in $D(\tau(e))$ for any marking $M \in M$. For a connector $c = (e, p)$ or $c = (p, e)$, $u(c)$ is used as a function which will update the mark of e.

5. $d : P_{\text{discrete}} \rightarrow D_{\text{continuous}}$ is a mapping called the *delay*, where P_{discrete} is the set of discrete processes in P. For a discrete process p, $d(p) : M \rightarrow R^{\geq 0}$ is called the *delay function* of p.

6. $a > 0$ is a real number called the *generic time*. The generic time is used as the clock for generic processes.

For graphical representation, HFPNe inherits the tradition of other Petri nets as in Fig. 7.6.

We introduce a parameter $t \in R^{\geq 0}$, called the *time* to a hybrid functional Petri net with extension $H = (E, P, h, \tau, C, d, a)$. Given a marking I called the *initial marking*, we define a marking $M(t)$ called the *marking at time t* and a marking $M_r(t)$ called the *reserved marking at time t* for $t \geq 0$ in the following way. By convention, we denote $M(e, t) = M(t)(e)$ and $M_r(e, t) = M_r(t)(e)$ for $e \in E$. We define $\bar{M}(t)$ by $\bar{M}(e, t) = M(e, t) - M_r(e, t)$

for discrete and continuous entities and $\tilde{M}(e, t) = M(e, t)$ for generic entities e.

Table 7.3. (a) For a connector $c = (e, p) \in EP$, the entity type $h(e)$, the process type $h(p)$, and the connector type $a(c)$ must satisfy the given conditions, where $\sqrt{}$ means that the connection is allowed and $-$ means that the connection is not allowed. (b) For a connector $c = (p, e) \in PE$, the connector type $a(c)$ is a process by definition. The entity type $h(e)$ and the process type $h(p)$ must satisfy the given conditions, where $\sqrt{}$ means that the connection is allowed and $-$ means that the connection is not allowed.

connect type		process connector		
process type		discrete	continuous	generic
entity type	discrete	$\sqrt{}$	$-$	$\sqrt{}$
	continuous	$\sqrt{}$	$\sqrt{}$	$\sqrt{}$
	generic	$-$	$-$	$\sqrt{}$

connect type		associate or inhibitory connector		
process type		discrete	continuous	generic
entity type	discrete	$\sqrt{}$	$\sqrt{}$	$\sqrt{}$
	continuous	$\sqrt{}$	$\sqrt{}$	$\sqrt{}$
	generic	$\sqrt{}$	$\sqrt{}$	$\sqrt{}$

(a)

connect type		process connector		
process type		discrete	continuous	generic
entity type	discrete	$\sqrt{}$	$-$	$\sqrt{}$
	continuous	$\sqrt{}$	$\sqrt{}$	$\sqrt{}$
	generic	$\sqrt{}$	$\sqrt{}$	$\sqrt{}$

(b)

First, we define $M(0) = I$, and $M_r(e, 0) = 0$ for all discrete and continuous entities e. For all generic entities e, $M_r(e, t) = \text{null}$ (the empty list) for any $t \geq 0$. For $t > 0$, we define $M(t)$ and $M_r(t)$ as follows. For a process $p \in P$ at time t, if the following conditions are satisfied, then the process p is said to be *enabled* at time t. Otherwise the process is said to be *unenabled* at time t.

1. If p is a discrete process, then for all connectors $c = (e, p) \in EP$ the following conditions hold:
   (a) $\tilde{M}(e, t) \geq w(e, p)(M(t))$ if $a(c) \neq \text{inhibitor}$.
   (b) $\tilde{M}(e, t) < w(e, p)(M(t))$ if $a(c) = \text{inhibitor}$.

2. If p is a continuous process, then for all connectors $c = (e, p) \in EP$ the following conditions hold:

(a) $\tilde{M}(e, t) \geq w(e, p)(M(t))$ if $a(c) \neq$ inhibitor.

(b) $\tilde{M}(e, t) \leq w(e, p)(M(t))$ if $a(c) =$ inhibitor.

3. If p is a generic process, then for all connectors $c = (e, p) \in EP$ the following conditions hold:

(a) $w(e, p)(\tilde{M}(t)) =$ true if $a(c) =$ inhibitor.

(b) $w(e, p)(\tilde{M}(t)) =$ false if $a(c) =$ inhibitor.

If an unenabled process turns out to be enabled at time t, the process is said to be *triggered* at time t. If an enabled process turns to be unenabled or an unenabled process turns to be enabled at time t, the process is said to be switched at time t. If a discrete process p is triggered at time t, we say that the discrete process can be *fired* at time $t + d(p)(M(t))$. If a generic process p is triggered at time t, we say that the generic process can be *fired* at time $t + \alpha$.

For an entity $e \in E$ and time t, let $S_d(t)$ be the set of discrete processes that can be fired at time t, and let $U_d(t)$ be the set of discrete processes which are triggered at time t. For a discrete process p that can be fired at time t, we denote by $q(p, t)$ the time when p is triggered. Let $S_c(t)$ be the set of continuous processes that are enabled at time t. Let $S_g(t)$ be the set of generic processes that can be fired at time t.

Note that we can choose a sufficiently small $\varepsilon_t > 0$ such that in the interval $[t - \varepsilon_t, t)$, neither a discrete nor a generic process is triggered or can be fired, and no continuous process is switched.

Also, note the following facts:

1. $S_c(t - \varepsilon_t) = S_c(t')$ for any $t' \in [t - \varepsilon_t, t)$ since no continuous process is switched in the interval $[t - \varepsilon_t, t)$

2. $\tilde{M}(t')$ is constant on $E - E_{\text{continuous}}$ in the interval $[t - \varepsilon_t, t)$ since neither a discrete nor a generic process is triggered or can be fired in the interval $[t - \varepsilon_t, t)$ where $E_{\text{continuous}} = \{e \in E \mid e$ is continuous$\}$.

3. For any continuous connector c, $u(c)(\tilde{M}(t'))$ is continuous on $[t - \varepsilon_t, t)$ since by definition $u(c)$ is continuous for $E_{\text{continuous}}$ and $\tilde{M}(t')$ is constant on $E - E_{\text{continuous}}$ in the interval $[t - \varepsilon_t, t)$.

Then, $M(t)$ is defined by the following procedure:

1. $Tmp \leftarrow M\ (t - \varepsilon_t)$, $Tmp_r \leftarrow M_r(t - \varepsilon_t)$
2. **if** $t = \alpha k$ for some integer $k \geq 1$ **then**
    for each generic process $p \in S_g(t)$
      $Tmp' \leftarrow Tmp$
      for each $(e, p) \in EP$ with $a(e, p) = $ process
        $Tmp'(e) \leftarrow u(e, p)(Tmp)$
      for each $(p, e) \in PE$
        $Tmp'(e) \leftarrow u(p, e)(Tmp)$
      $Tmp \leftarrow Tmp'$
3. **for each** continuous process $p \in S_c(t - \varepsilon_t)$
    $Tmp' \leftarrow Tmp$
    for each $(e, p) \in EP$ with $a(e, p) = $ process
      $Tmp'(e) \leftarrow Tmp'(e) - \int_{t-\varepsilon t}^{t} u(e, p)(\tilde{M}(x))dx$
    for each $(p,e) \in PE$
      $Tmp'(e) \leftarrow Tmp'(e) + \int_{t-\varepsilon t}^{t} u(p, e)(\tilde{M}(x))dx$
    $Tmp \leftarrow Tmp'$
4. **for each** discrete process $p \in S_d(t)$
    $Tmp' \leftarrow Tmp$
    for each $(e, p) \in EP$ with $a(e, p) = $ process
      $Tmp'(e) \leftarrow Tmp'(e) - u(e, p)(\tilde{M}(q(p, t)))$
    for each $(p, e) \in PE$
      $Tmp'(e) \leftarrow Tmp'(e) - u(p, e)(\tilde{M}(q(p, t)))$
    $Tmp \leftarrow Tmp'$
5. $M(t) \leftarrow Tmp$

Then $M_r(t)$ is defined as follows:

6. **for each** entity e with $h(e) = $ discrete or continuous
    $Tmp_r(e) \leftarrow Tmp_r(e) - \sum_{\substack{p \text{ with } p \in S_d(t) \\ \text{and } (e,p) \in EP}} u(e, p)(\tilde{M}(q(p, t))) + \sum_{\substack{p \text{ with } p \in U_d(t) \\ \text{and } (e,p) \in EP}} u(e, p)(\tilde{M}(t - \varepsilon_t))$
7. $M_r(t) \leftarrow Tmp_r.$

We call $M(t)(t \geq 0)$ the *behavior* of H starting at the initial marking $M(0) = I$.

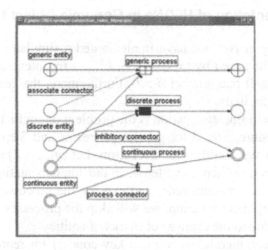

Fig. 7.6. Graphical notations of HFPNe components

7.4.2 Relationships with Other Petri Nets

HFPN $H = (E, P, h, \tau, C, d)$ is defined from HFPNe by deleting all matters with "generic" and by adding the restriction that $u(c) = w(c)$ for any discrete connector $c = (e, p) \in EP$. This condition means that the weight $w(c)$ of the connector is the same as the number of tokens $u(c)$ removed from the entity e by firing. This convention is traditionally employed in Petri net, as a weight. In our definition of HFPNe, however, we have separated these two notions. HPN $H = (E, P, h, \tau, C = (EP, PE, a, w, u), d)$ (Alla and David, 1998) is defined by adding the following restriction (i) to HFPN: $w(c)$, $u(c)$, and $d(p)$ are constants for any connector $c \in EP \cup PE$ and any process $p \in P$. HDN $H = (E, P, h, \tau, C = (EP, PE, a, w, u), d)$ [19, 20] is also defined by adding the following restriction (ii) to HFPN: For any continuous process p, it is assumed that $w(e, p) = u(p, e')$ for any process connectors $(e, p) \in EP$ and $(p, e') \in PE$.

If we delete all matters with "discrete" from HPN, we have the definition of CTPN. If we delete all matters with "continuous" from HPN, we have the definition of TPN. Furthermore, if we delete the matters with "delay" from TPN, we have the definition of the original Petri net. Thus, HFPNe is a highly abstract extension of the Petri net for biological process modeling that can involve PN, TPN, CTPN, HPN, and HFPN as special cases.

7.4.3 Implementation of HFPNe in Genomic Object Net

In Genomic Object Net, we have implemented a simulator of HFPNe by approximating the time t by $t = 0, \delta, \cdots, k\delta, \cdots$ for integers k by using an appropriately small real number $\delta > 0$. Furthermore, the generic time α is set to be δ for simplicity.

Another issue in implementation is the problem of conflict resolution. In the above procedure, Step 2 for generic processes and Step 4 for discrete processes may have conflicts for execution. Let $pi_1, \ldots, pi_t$ be processes which can be fired in Step 2 or Step 4. In our implementation, we arrange these processes in a random order and execute the processes according to this order. During this execution, we will skip the processes that cannot be fired any more due to the changes of marks of entities.

Needless to say, hierarchization is a key concept for representing complex network structures in an intuitive way (Matsuno et al., 2000). The hierarchical representation has been introduced in the HDN model by employing the object-oriented approach, and this model is called the hybrid object net (HON) (Drath, 1998, 1999). In Genomic Object Net, we have inherited this hierarchical representation schema for the HFPNe. Moreover, for describing HFPNe, we have developed an XML format called GONML, which will be discussed in Subsection 7.7.3.

7.5 Modeling of Biological Processes with HFPNe

In this section, we demonstrate that more biological processes can be easily modeled with HFPNe than HFPN. For this purpose, we select for modeling four biological processes that extensively use the HFPNe features. These biological processes are important activities in living cells and should be handled with application tools that aim to model and simulate biological systems. Our aim is not only to theoretically describe how to model biological processes, but also to provide a useful application tool to users in biology and medicine. In the following sections, we exemplify that complex biological processes can be modeled with GON, while illustrating snapshots of HFPNe models, as in Fig. 7.7(b), Fig. 7.8(a), Fig. 7.9, and Fig. 7.10. Other biological processes, e.g., complex carbohydrate synthesis and Xenopus cell cycle pathway including cell division processes, have been described (Matsui et al., 2004; Nagasaki, 2004; Nagasaki et al., 2004a).

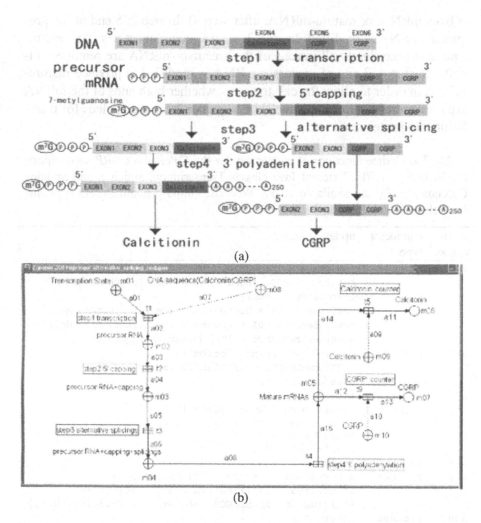

Fig. 7.7. (a) An alternative RNA splicing model of the *Calcitonin/CGRP* gene in Fig. 7.7(b). (b) An alternative RNA splicing model of the *Calcitonin/CGRP* gene with HFPNe

7.5.1 From DNA to mRNA in Eucaryotes – Alternative Splicing

The mechanism from DNA to mRNA in eucaryote is more complicated than that in bacteria. The major difference derives from eucaryotic genes that consist of two regions, i.e., exons and introns. As in Fig. 7.7(a), the mechanism consists mainly of four steps: step 1: transcription; step 2: 5 capping; step 3: RNA splicing; and step 4: 3 polyadenylation. In step 1, DNA is transcribed into precursor-mRNA (especially named to distinguish it from mRNA, or mature-mRNA, after step 4). In step 2, 5 end of the precursor- mRNA is modified. In step 3, each splicing event removes one intron, and accordingly all introns of the precursor-mRNA are removed. Finally, in step 4, 3 end of precursor-mRNA is modified to produce mature-mRNA in order to allow the cell to assess whether both ends of the mRNA are present before it exports the RNA sequence from the nucleus for translation into proteins.

Table 7.4. Update functions of connectors for the *Calcitonin/CGRP* transcription model in Fig. 7.7(b). External Java classes Transcription, Splicing, and Splicing CalcitoninCGRP are available at our Web site (http://genomicobject.net/public/BiotechBook 2004/code/).

conn-ector	connector type	update function

a01	process	import("gon.Transcription");
		 totalnum = m08.length(); num = m01.length();
		 if(totalnum > num){
		 nextcode = m08.substring(totalnum-num-1,totalnum-nu);
		 newsequence = m01 + Transcription::Trans(nextcode);}
		 else{new_sequence = "";} return newsequence;

a02	process	import("gon.Transcription");
		 if(Transcription::Finish(m01,m08)){return m01;}
		 else{return "";}

a03	process	return m02;

a04	process	import("gon.Transcription");
		 if(!m02.equals("")){return Transcription::Capping(m02);}
		 else{return "";}

a05	process	return "";

a06	process	import("gon.Splicing_CalcitoninCGRP");
		 if(m03.equals("")){return m03;} else{return
		 Splicing_CalcitoninCGRP::AlternativeSplicing(m03);}

a08	process	return "";
a10	process	return m10;
a11	process	num = 0; for(i=0;i<m05.length;++i){ if(m05[i].equals(m09)){num++;}} return num;
a12	process	return m05;
a13	process	num = 0; for(i=0;i<m05.length;++i){ if(m05[i].equals(m10)){num++;}} return num;
a14	process	return m05;

a15	process	import("gon.Transcription");
		 if(m04.equals("")){return m05;}
		 else{return
		 m05+[Transcription::Polyadenylation(m04)];}

In step 3, there is a eukaryote-specific splicing process named alternative RNA splicing. The alternative RNA splicing is to produce different mRNA from the same precursor-mRNA by splicing it in different ways.

The DNA to mRNA transcription with alternative RNA splicing was found in 1982 for *Calcitonin/CGRP* gene expression (Amara et al., 1982). We draw focus to modeling *Calcitonin/CGRP* gene expression while combining other recent biological knowledge (Coleman et al., 2003, Tran et al., 2003).

As in Fig. 7.7(a), the *Calcitonin* gene expression consists of four introns and five exons, and the transcription process progresses with step 1, step 2, step 3 and step 4. In step 3, by alternative splicing events, one of exon1/exon2/exon3/exon4 (say set1) or exon2/exon3/exon5/exon6 (say set2) is selected. If set1 (set2) is selected, the mature-mRNA is translated into *Calcitonin* (*CGRP*). The HFPNe model can faithfully realize these steps as generic processes and realize precursor-mRNA and mature-mRNA states as generic entities with the type string (see Fig. 7.7.(b)). In the model, the mature-RNAs, *Calcitonin* mRNA and *CGRP* mRNA, are represented by the generic entity m09 with the type list string. The generic entities m12, m13, m14, and m15 are used to inform which sequence should be spliced in the generic processes t03, t04, t05, and t06, respectively. These generic notions are necessary for modeling the four steps from DNA to mRNA. It is hard to model with HFPN [18] and other simulation tools [50, 77]. The detailed parameters and functions are described in Tables 7.4 and 7.5.

Table 7.5. Properties of entities for the *Calcitonin/CGRP* transcription model in Fig. 7.7(b).

entity	entity type	type	initial mark
m01/m02/m03/m04	generic	string	""
m05	generic	list string	( )
m06/m07	discrete	integer+	0
m08/m09/m10	generic	string	see [27]

In another example of alternative splicing, the *DSCAM* gene in *Drosophila*, four exons (A, B, C, and D) are selected and combined. Each precursor-mRNA contains 12 alternatives for exon A, 48 alternatives for exon B, 33 alternatives for exon C, and two alternatives for exon D (Webster et al., 2000). Thus, there are 38,016 possible mature mRNAs for the DSCAM gene. If the model is created with HFPN, we have to deal with 38,016 entities for the DSCAM transcription process. If the model is created with HFPN, 38,016 entities are necessary for the simple *DSCAM* transcription model.

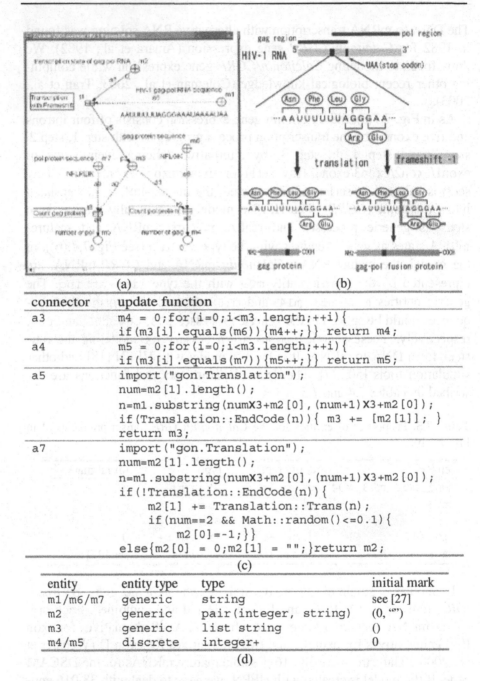

connector	update function
a3	`m4 = 0;for(i=0;i<m3.length;++i){` `if(m3[i].equals(m6)){m4++;}} return m4;`
a4	`m5 = 0;for(i=0;i<m3.length;++i){` `if(m3[i].equals(m7)){m5++;}} return m5;`

a5	`import("gon.Translation");`
	`num=m2[1].length();`
	`n=m1.substring(numX3+m2[0],(num+1)X3+m2[0]);`
	`if(Translation::EndCode(n)){ m3 += [m2[1]]; }`
	`return m3;`

a7	`import("gon.Translation");`
	`num=m2[1].length();`
	`n=m1.substring(numX3+m2[0],(num+1)X3+m2[0]);`
	`if(!Translation::EndCode(n)){`
	`    m2[1] += Translation::Trans(n);`
	`    if(num==2 && Math::random()<=0.1){`
	`        m2[0]=-1;}}`
	`else{m2[0] = 0;m2[1] = "";}return m2;`

(c)

entity	entity type	type	initial mark
m1/m6/m7	generic	string	see [27]
m2	generic	pair(integer, string)	(0, "")
m3	generic	list string	()
m4/m5	discrete	integer+	0

(d)

Fig. 7.8. (a) Ribosomal frameshifting in HIV-1 gag-pol. (b) Ribosomal frameshifting in HIV-1 gag-pol expressed with HFPNe. The characterization of ribosomal frameshifting was first described by Tyler (Jacks et al., 1988). (c) Update functions in (b). (d) Properties of entities in (b)

7.5.2 Translation of mRNA – Frameshift

Frameshift is also an important biological process that occurs during RNA translations. The frameshift is to skip or re-read some ribonucleotides when translating RNAs, and it is commonly used by many RNA viruses as programmed ribosomal frameshifting (Jacks et al., 1988).

For example, a model of ribosomal frameshifting in the human immunodeficiency virus (HIV-1) (gag-pol expression in Fig. 7.8(b)) can be modeled with HFPNe as in Fig. 7.8(a). As in Fig. 7.8(b), two proteins, gag and pol, are produced from one RNA sequence with the frameshift by re-reading a ribonucleotide, adenine (A), twice. In HFPNe, the generic entity e3 has the type pair(integer (i1), string (s1)) in order to express frameshifting states; i1 denotes how many ribonucleotides are skipped (+1) or re-read (-1) and s1 denotes the length of the current translated amino-acid sequence. The frameshifting occurs at a specific point. In addition, the probability of a re-read at the point is 0.1 in wild type (Jacks et al., 1988). Thus, in the model we assign an mRNA translation skip function with stochastic behavior to this specific point. The stochastic feature is already realized in HFPN, and HFPNe also inherits this feature. The detailed update functions are summarized in Fig. 7.8(c) and the initial marks and types of entities are summarized in Fig. 7.8(d). It is also not straightforward to represent the ribosomal frameshifting with HFPN.

7.5.3 Huntington's Disease

As an advanced pathway model with HFPNe, we selected a genetic disease called Huntington's disease. Disease pathway modeling and simulation are becoming the most important topics for treating the disease from the pathway level in biology and medicine. Huntington's disease is an autosomal dominant progressive neurodegenerative disorder that is characterized by chorea, psychiatric disturbances, and dementia (Martin and Gusella, 1986). The disease, in short, is the generic defects of *Huntingtin*. *Huntingtin* is a multi-domain protein with a polymorphic glutamine/proline (G/P)-rich domain at the N terminus (Huntington 1993). Polyglutamine (polyQ) sequences in unaffected individuals range from 11 to 34 glutamine residues, whereas those of *Huntingtin* disease patients contain 37 or more glutamine residues (more than 90) (Bates et al., 2002). The disease appears when a specific polyQ length is exceeded.

Based on the disease model proposed by Wellington et al. (Hickey and Chesselet, 2003), we created an HFPNe model for this disease, as shown in

Fig. 7.9. Our model uses the following known experimental facts found in the literature.

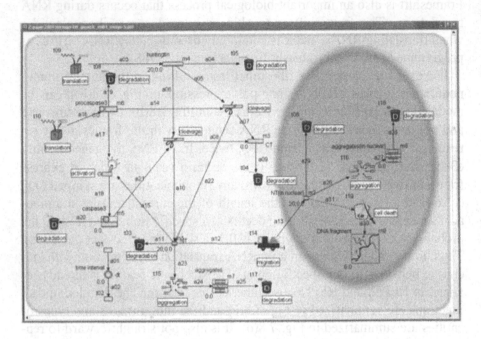

Fig. 7.9. Huntington's disease model with HFPNe. HFPNe components in this figure are replaced with suitable images that represent biological information

fact 1 *Huntingtin* can be cleaved by caspase-3 and yields two fragments, N terminal region (*NT*) that contains polyQ repeats in Huntingtin and C terminal region (*CT*) (Hickey and Chesselet, 2003).

fact 2 Both disease *Huntingtin* and normal *Huntingtin* can cleave, and the rates of fragmentation are the same (Wellington et al., 2002).

fact 3 *Procaspase-3* has low-level catalytic activity for disease *Huntingtin* and is capable of cleaving the same substrates, i.e., *NT* and *CT*, as activated *caspase-3* [71].

fact 4 When cleaved by *caspase-3*, *NT* has responsibility for cytotoxicity [36, 84].

fact 5 *NT* has the ability to form protein aggregates and can be found in the nucleus and in the cytoplasm (Roizin et al., 1979).

fact 6 The aggregate number of *NT* increases in proportion to the length of polyQ [74].

fact 7 NT fragments of mutant Huntingtin have the ability to induce *caspase-3* [11].

fact 8 Both disease and normal *NTs* can cross the nuclear membrane. The smaller the cleavage product, the greater the tendency of *Huntingtin* to cross [25, 85].

Table 7.6. Properties of connectors for Huntington's disease model in Fig. 7.9. The other property of process connectors, i.e., update function, is summzrized in Table 7.7.

connector	connector type	activity function
a02/a09/a19/a20	process	0.0
a04/a05/a06/a11	process	return true;
a12	process	return{ (m4[1]>20.0)?true:false;}
a14	associate	return{ (m4[0]>37&&m6>0.0)?true:false;}
a15	associate	return{ (m4[0]>37&&m1>0.0)?true:false;}
a17	process	20.0
a21	associate	return{ (m5[1]>0.0)?true:false;}
a23/a26/a29	process	return true;
a25/a28	process	1.0
a31	process	return{ (m2[1]>10.0)?true:false;}

Huntingtin and *NT* change their function depending on their polyQ length (**fact 3, fact 6, fact 7**). Thus, in our model, these proteins are represented with generic entities with the type pair(integer+, real+). The first attribute integer+, corresponds to the length of polyQ, and the second attribute, real+, corresponds to the quantity of the protein, i.e., *NT* or *Huntingtin*. In our model, *NT* and *Huntingtin* are represented with m1 and m4, respectively. The properties of connectors in the model are summarized in Tables 7.6 and 7.7. The properties of processes and entities are summarized in Tables 7.8 and 7.9. *Huntingtin* m4 is translated by the generic process t09 while *procaspase-3* m6 is translated by the continuous process t10. The *procaspase-3* m6 can cleave t12 disease *Huntingtin* (**fact 3**). Thus, the weight function of associate connector a14 has a function that depends on the length of Huntingtin m4 and the cleavage process t12 is not enabled for normal *Huntingtin*. The activity functions and types of connectors are summarized in Table 7.6. On the other hand, the *caspase-3* m5 can cleave normal *Huntingtin* and disease *Huntingtin* modeled with process t11 (**fact 2**). Thus, the weight of associate connector a21 has a function that does not depend on the length of *Huntingtin* m4. *Huntingtin* m4 is cleaved and separated into *CT* m3 and *NT* m1 (**fact 1**). *CT* does not contain the polyQ region and is represented by continuous entity m3 (**fact 1**).

Table 7.7. Update functions of connectors for the Huntington's disease model in Fig. 7.9. Update function must be defined for all process connectors that are connected with at least one generic process.

connector	connector type	update function
a01/a02	process	1.0
a03	process	m4[1] = m4[1]+1.0Xdt; return m4;
a04	process	m4[1] = m4[1] - (m4[1]Xdt)/200; return m4;
a05	process	m4[1] = m4[1]-0.0001Xm4[1]Xm6Xdt; return m4;
a06	process	m4[1] = m4[1]-0.001Xm4[1]Xm5Xdt; return m4;
a07	process	m3 = m3+0.0001Xm4[1]Xm6Xdt; return m3;
a08	process	m3 = m3+0.001Xm4[1]Xm5Xdt; return m3;
a09	process	m3/50
a10	process	m1[1] = m1[1]+0.001Xm4[1]Xm5Xdt; return m1;
a11	process	m1[1] = m1[1]-(m1[1]/100)Xdt; return m1;
a12	process	m1[1] = m1[1]-0.001Xm1[1]Xdt; return m1;
a13	process	m2[1] = m2[1]+0.001Xm1[1]Xdt; return m2;
a16	process	1.0
a17	process	m6 = m6 - 0.001Xm1Xm6Xdt; return m6;
a18	process	m5 = m5 + 0.001Xm1Xm6Xdt; return m5;
a19	process	m6/100
a20	process	m5/100
a22	process	m1[1]=m1[1]+0.0001Xm4[1]Xm6Xdt;return m1;
a23	process	m1[1]=m1[1]-(m1[1]X(m1[0]/1000))Xdt;return m1;
a24	process	m7=m7+(m1[1]X(m1[0]/1000))Xdt;return m7;
a25	process	m7/100
a26	process	m2[1]=m2[1]-(m2[1]X(m2[0]/1000))Xdt;return m2;
a27	process	m8=m8+(m2[1]X(m2[0]/1000))Xdt;return m8;
a28	process	m8/100
a29	process	m2[1]=m2[1]-(m2[1]/100)Xdt;return m1;
a30	process	m9+=0.001Xm2[1];return m9;

NT inherits the polyQ region. The length of NT relates to the activity of the process t13 that changes *procaspase-3* m6 into *caspase-3* m5 (fact7). To model it, the weight function of the associate connector a15 depends on the length of *NT* m1 and process t13 cannot be activated by normal Huntingtin.

NT in cytoplasm migrates to the nucleus (**fact 8**), and *NT* in nucleus m2 causes cell death t19 with cytotoxicity (**fact 4**). From **fact 5**, cell death can be prevented by the aggregation of *NT*. Moreover, the aggregation rate depends on the length of polyQ (**fact 6**). *NT* in nucleus m02 should therefore be denoted by generic entities, such as *Huntingtin* m04 and *NT* m01, in the cytoplasm. *NT* in the cytoplasm m01 and *NT* in the nucleus m02 connect to the aggregation process t15 and t16, respectively. The update functions of process connectors a23 and a26 represent aggregate speeds and depend on the length of polyQ in *NT* in nucleus m2 (**fact 6**). The update functions of connectors are summarized in Table 7.7.

With the model, we can simulate the *n* polyQ length huntingtin ($0 \le n \le 100$ (Bates et al., 2002)) by changing only the initial marks of m1, m2, and m4, as in Table 7.9. If the same disease model is created with HFPN, (i) at least one extra entity and (ii) many connectors, are necessary; this means (i) an entity (say e1) that denotes the length of Huntingtin, and (ii) associate connectors that point from e1 to every process that has more than one connector whose weight function or speed function depends on the value of e1. Thus, the HFPNe Huntingtin disease model is simpler than the HFPN model.

Table 7.8. Properties of processes for Huntington's disease model in Fig. 7.9.

Process	process type
t01/t02/t04/t06/t07/t08/t10/t17/t18	continuous
t03/t05/t09/t11/t12/t13/t14/t15/t16/t19	generic

Table 7.9. Properties of entities for the Huntingtin disease model in Fig. 7.9. The initial value *n* in m1, m2, and m4 denotes the length of Q repeats in the huntingtin protein and must be assigned an integer value when simulating the model.

entity	entity type	type	initial mark
dt	continuous	real+	0.0
m1/m2/m4	generic	pair(integer+,real+)	(n,0.0)
m3/m5/m6/m7/m8/m9	continuous	real+	0.0

7.5.4 Protein Modification – p53

The previous HFPNe models extensively use generic entities and generic processes. However, their types of generic entities are only simple ones, e.g. string, list real, list string, pair(integer, string). A generic entity can take more the advanced type object as its type. Under GON, an object corresponds to a Java *class*, and a *method* of an object is a specific function assigned to the object. If a generic entity has the type object, the entity can be initialized with an object with methods and variables, and these methods can be applied to update functions of connectors that join the generic entity and generic processes and to change the mark by updating variables of the entity.

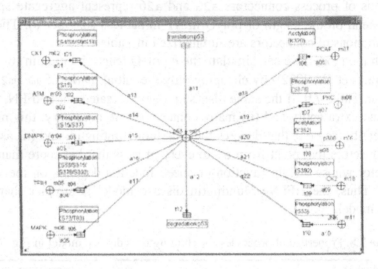

Fig. 7.10. A protein modification model of the *p53* protein with HFPNe. The generic entity in the center m01 is the modification target *p53*, and other generic entities m02, · · ·, m11 are enzymes that modify the *p53* entity. Generic processes t01, · · ·, t10 have connectors a01, · · ·, a10, and the modified state of *p53* in m01 is updated by their update functions

To show the effectiveness of generic entities with the type object, we deal with protein modification in biological processes with enzymes, e.g., phosphorylation, acetylation, and methylation. Specifically, the protein *p53* that can be modified by enzymes *CK1, ATM, DNAPK, TFIIH, MAPK, PCAF, PKC, p300, CK2*, and *JNK* is modeled (Table 7.10) [37]. By these enzymes, 18 positions of *p53* are modified. There are 2^{18} patterns. Thus, it is again hard to create a model with HFPN because 218 entities are necessary for the model with HFPN.

To model with HFPNe while using the type object for generic entities, Protein and Enzyme classes are created, and these classes are inherited in order to realize specific Protein class, e.g., p53, and specific Enzyme classes, e.g., CK1, ATM, DNAPK, TFIIH, MAPK, PCAF, PKC, p300, CK2, and JNK. As in Table 7.11, (i) the generic entity m01 takes a specific object

ProteinSet that is initialized with the p53 object that corresponds to the p53 class and inherits the Protein class, (ii) the generic entities m02, m03, m04, m05, m06, m07, m08, m09, m10, and m11 take specific objects whose classes inherit Enzyme classes CK1, ATM, DNAPK, TFIIH, MAPK, PCAF, PKC, p300, CK2, and JNK, respectively (a class name corresponds to an enzyme name). These objects are implemented with Java classes on GON. Code for these classes is available from http://genomicobject.net/-public/BiotechBook 2004/code/.

Table 7.10. The protein modification positions and type of *p53* enzymes [37].

enzyme	modification type	modification positions	
CK1	Phosphorylation	S4,S6,S9,S18	
ATM	Phosphorylation	S15	
DNAPK	Phosphorylation	S15,S37	
TFIIH	Phosphorylation	S33,S315 S378,S392	
MAPK	Phosphorylation	T73,T83	
PCAF	Acetylation	K320	
PKC	Phosphorylation	S378	
p300	Acetylation	K382	
CK2	Phosphorylation	S392	
JNK	Phosphorylation	S33	

Table 7.11. Properties of entities for the *p53* modification model in Fig. 7.10.

entity	entity type	type	initial mark
m01	generic	object	ProtenSet::Initialize(m01,p53::Initialize())
m02	generic	object	CK1::Initialize(m02)
m03	generic	object	ATM::Initialize(m03)
m04	generic	object	DNAPK::Initialize(m04)
m05	generic	object	TFIIH::Initialize(m05)
m06	generic	object	MAPK::Initialize(m06)
m07	generic	object	PCAF::Initialize(m07)
m08	generic	object	PKC::Initialize(m08)
m09	generic	object	p300::Initialize(m09)
m10	generic	object	CK2::Initialize(m10)
m11	generic	object	JNK::Initialize(m11)

To describe modification in biological processes by enzymes, the generic processes t01, ···, t10 are used. As in Table 7.12, the update functions a13, a14, a15, a16, a17, a18, a19, a20, a21, and a22 of the generic processes call the Modify method of the p53 class to simulate the modification in biological process by CK1, ATM, DNAPK, TFIIH, MAPK, PCAF, PKC, p300, CK2, and JNK, respectively. To describe translation and degradation biological processes of p53, the generic processes t11 and t12 are created, respectively. As in Table 7.12, processes t11 and t12 follow connectors with update functions a21 and a22 that call the Translation and Degradation methods of the p53 class to simulate the translation and degradation biological processes, respectively.

Table 7.12. Update functions of the p53 modification model with HFPNe in Fig. 7.10. All update functions are written in Pnuts language (http://www.pnuts.org/.). External java classes, CK1, ATM, DNAPK, TFIIH, MAPK, PCAF, PKC, p300, CK2, JNK, ProteinSet, Enzyme, and Protein are described at http://genomicobject. net/public/BiotechBook2004/code/. Connectors a01, · · ·, a10 ave connector type associate and update function does not exist.

connector	connector type	update function
a11	process	m01.Translate(); return m01;
a12	process	m01.Degradation();return m01;
a13	process	m01.Modify(m02); return m01;
a14	process	m01.Modify(m03); return m01;
a15	process	m01.Modify(m04); return m01;
a16	process	m01.Modify(m05); return m01;
a17	process	m01.Modify(m06); return m01;
a18	process	m01.Modify(m07); return m01;
a19	process	m01.Modify(m08); return m01;
a20	process	m01.Modify(m09); return m01;
a21	process	m01.Modify(m10); return m01;
a22	process	m01.Modify(m11); return m01;

At first glance, the HFPNe model of p53 modification biological processes seems complicated. However, as in Table 7.12, in the p53 model all update functions call a specific method, e.g., Modify, Translation, or Degradation. As in Table 7.11, all initial marks of generic entities are defined by calling a specific method, i.e., Initialize. Thus, if objects with suitable methods that correspond to biological processes are orgnaized as a biological process library, the majority of users, biological and medical scientists without programming skills, can create biological models. But with their expert knowledge of biological processes, they can create models by simply assigning a suitable object to a generic entity and a suitable method to the update function of the generic connector.

We can apply the same approach to the previous biological processes. In the previous example, generic entities can take type object whose class is DNA with transcription method or RNA with translation method instead of `string` primitive type. Thus, owing to the `object` extension of HFPNe, more complicated biological processes can be easily modeled than with HFPN.

On the other hand, the Gene Ontology (GO) Consortium is trying to produce a controlled vocabulary that can be applied to all organisms as knowledge of gene and protein roles in cells (Ashburner et al., 2000). By applying these gene ontology related vocabularies to names of objects and their methods, we can create a more standardized library for biological processes with HFPNe.

7.6 Related Works with HFPNe

In this section, a new versatile Petri net-based architecture HFPNe is demonstrated for biological process modeling and simulation. HFPNe introduces the notions of generic entities and generic processes to HFPN. In the HF- PNe architecture, generic entities can hold various kinds of types, including `object`. With feature and inherited features of HFPN, complex biological processes can be effectively modeled. Four biological processes, alternative splicing, frameshifting, Huntington's disease, and multi-domain modification process of *p53*, are employed to show the effectiveness of HFPNe.

From the theoretical point of view in the Petri net community, HFPNe can be one of the object-oriented Petri nets (OPN). This approach was first given by Becker and Colom [5]. In the community, two advanced Petri nets based on OPN architectures have been proposed, Objective Colored Petri Nets (OCP-nets) (Maier and Moldt, 2001) and Reference nets (Kummer 2001). OCP-nets are based on OPN enhanced by the fusion place concept of Hierarchical Colored Petri Nets (HCPNs). With this concept, OCP-nets can dynamically change (shrink or grow) the structure of their nets in simulation, a feature that does not exist in HFPNe. Reference nets are also based on OPN enhanced by the reference entities concept. With this concept, (i) an entity in a net (net1) can hold another net (net2), (ii) net2 can move to other entities in the net1 by firing, and (iii) net2 can change its state by firing. The differences between them are as follows: Reference nets can move the net in simulation processes but OCP-nets cannot. However, OCP-nets can create new connection rules in simulation processes. HFPNe does not support these OCP-nets and Reference nets features. On the other hand, the feature of delay function of HFPNe does not exist in the object-oriented Petri nets. However, in a cell various kinds of time scale biological processes exist, and to model these biological processes using one model the notion of delay is necessary. With delay functions, HFPNe can handle these biological processes efficiently. From a theoretical point of view, it may be easy to extend HFPNe to support OCP-net or Reference net features because an implementation of HFPNe GON has been already extended to support the feature to add/remove entities and processes during simulation.

For the reason mentioned in Subsection 7.5.4, we are trying to create a biological process library with HFPNe on GON. However, it is difficult to create all biological processes at once. Thus, as the first step, all processes in the Kyoto Model (Matsuoka et al., 2003) will be recompiled as a part of the library. The Kyoto Model is a ventricular cell model that functions by compiling classical electro-physiological findings. In the process, we will pursue efforts to locate the best approach to systematically reconstruct other existing biological process models that are like the Kyoto Model. Then we will apply a systematic approach to these other biological process models for enriching the library.

7.7 Genomic Object Net: GON

In 1999, we surveyed which architecture is suitable when modeling and simulating biological processes for biological and medical scientists. We concluded that Petri net-based applications are more suitable because of their intuitive graphical representation and their capabilities for mathematical analyses. The Petri nets community (http://www.daimi.au.dk/Petri Nets/tools/) has many implementations for Petri nets, but many of them can model only the DP or the CPN with a poor GUI while Petri net architectures are defined to be intuitive graphical representations. Fortunately, we have found one good tool, named VON++ [81]. VON++ is an application based on the HDN and implemented with Delphi [15]. The GUI is sophisticated and easy to use by users who know the architecture of the HDN.

However, when modeling and simulating biological processes, we found that the HDN architecture should be extended to HFPN for easy modeling, as described in Sections 7.2 and 7.3.

To deal with the extension from the HDN to HFPN, GON⁻ (GON Ver. 0.919) was released in 2001. This software is also implemented with Delphi, and the core architecture is HFPN. Using this software, we have shown that we can reorganize and represent various forms of biological process information, such as the glycolytic pathway of *E. coli* (Doi et al., 2004a), gene regulation of circadian rhythms in *Drosophila* ((Matsuno et al., 2003c), boundary formation by notch signaling in *Drosophila* (Matsuno et al., 2003b), and apoptosis induced by *Fas* ligand ((Matsuno et al., 2003c).

However, when modeling and simulating these biological processes, more extensions are needed for two purposes: the architecture and the GUI. The first demand for GON⁻ is that the core architecture HFPN should be extended to HFPNe as described in Sections 7.4 and 7.5. The second demand for GON⁻ is that the GUI should be more user friendly for the majority of users, who are experts in biological processes but are not experts in Petri nets, especially HFPN and HFPNe.

Thus, we have developed a new Genomic Object Net (GON Ver 1.0) [55] with Java from scratch. GON not only inherits basic ideas and concepts from GON⁻, but also enhances the modeling and simulation ability with its core architecture HFPNe. As in Section 7.5, these enhancements are useful for modeling and simulation of biological processes – *Calcitonin/CGRP* expression in Subsection 7.5.1, HIV-1 *gag-pol* expression in Subsection 7.5.2, Huntington's disease in Subsection 7.5.3, and protein modification of *p53* in Subsection 7.5.4. Moreover, the GUI design is developed so that users can intuitively model biological processes on GON.

Subsection 7.7.1 summarizes what kinds of HFPNe features are inherited in GON. Subsection 7.7.2 then describes the new GUI features useful when modeling and simulating biological processes, but not present, or insufficiently implemented, in GON⁻. When modeling and simulating biological processes in GON⁻, both expert knowledge of HFPN and biological processes were required. However, nearly all users of GON⁻ are biological and medical scientists. They have expert knowledge of biological processes but not of HFPN. Thus, Subsections *Graphical Model Canvas*, *Hierarchization and Item Collections*, and *Core Biological Process Library* describe new GUI features that are designed for these users to easily create and simulate models with GON. In addition, Subsection *Pnuts and Original Java Libraries* discusses another feature that aids users who have programming skills. The GUI feature in Subsections *Graphical Model Canvas* and *Hierarchization and Item Collections* are also important for large-scale modeling and simulation of biological processes such as BPE (Nagasaki et al., 2004c). Subsection 7.7.3 describes a newly developed XML format for modeling and simulation of biological processes, GONML. Subsection 7.7.4 compares related modeling and simulation application software of biological processes with GON.

7.7.1 GON Features That Derived from HFPNe Features

The architecture of GON is HFPNe. This extension was made from the viewpoint of modeling biological processes by identifying, inheriting, and resolving the merits and demerits of Petri nets, so far defined as follows:

1. The original Petri net deals with discrete quantities. It is suitable for rule-based simulation and other cases in which the quantities can be counted as integers. HFPNe inherits all aspects of the original Petri net.
2. The hybrid Petri net allows quantities to be continuous, in addition to supporting the ability of the original Petri net. Thus, biological processes with ODE-based kinetics can be realized.
3. The functional Petri net (Hofestädt and Thelen, 1998) allows dynamic changes of the network structure to some extent, but deals only with discrete quantities. HFPNe is defined to include the extension of this ability.
4. The hybrid object net (Drath, 1998) is defined by enhancing the Petri net with hierarchization in the network structure. The hierarchization (described in Subsection *Hierarchization and Item Collections*) is useful for describing large-scale network structures. This is inherited and extended in HFPNe.
5. HFPNe has more data "types" (integer, boolean, string, list, pair, and object) than the hybrid Petri net, the functional Petri net, and the hybrid object net. These types will be useful for modeling complex biological processes in Section 7.5.
6. The research on Petri nets, especially discrete ones, has a history of more than 30 years. It is mathematically well founded and practically well established. The simulation system of HFPNe can benefit from this Petri net research.

7.7.2 GON GUI and Other Features

Graphical Model Canvas

In GON, biological processes were modeled on the HFPN editor. On that editor, components of HFPN, entity, process, and connector, were drawn with simple figures, circle, rectangle, and arrow, respectively, as shown in Fig. 7.11(a). However, components of HFPN that model functions or biological elements in biological processes could have other biological information. Representation of this information on that editor will greatly assist users in intuitively understanding biological processes in the editor. Thus, in GON, an HFPNe editor called the *graphical model canvas* is developed.

The canvas has functions to include pictures to represent every component of HFPNe and its background picture for supplementary biological knowledge, and to attach text comments and URL links. In Fig. 7.11(a) and Fig. 7.11(b), the same biological processes, apoptosis induced by *Fas* ligand (Matsuno et al., 2003c; http://GenomicObject.net/), are modeled on the HFPN editor in GON⁻ and the graphical model canvas in GON. As shown in these figures, much biological information can be added to the graphical model canvas when modeling biological processes.

The core biological process library and BPE (Nagasaki, 2004, and Nagasaki et al., 2004c) extensively use these features of the graphical model canvas (suitable images, comments, and links being assigned to each item) as shown in Fig. 7.14 and Fig. 7.23.

Hierarchization and Item Collections

Hierarchization

Once a net is created, it is reusable by hierarchization, and a net with hierarchization is named *hierarchized* net. The hierarchization assigns a boolean flag, true or false, to all entities and processes in the net. If an entity is assigned true (or false), the entity is called a *published entity* (or an *unpublished entity*). If a process is assigned true (or false), the process is called a *published process* (or an *unpublished process*).

If a hierarchized net is loaded on a canvas, only published entities and processes can connect with processes and entities on the canvas. This means that unpublished processes, unpublished entities, and all connectors in the hierarchized net are hidden and cannot be accessed from components on the canvas as in Fig. 7.12. This notion was introduced by Drath (Drath 1998) to the Petri net community. The implementation of hierarchization in *GON* ⁻ was not complete. In GON, the function for entities is implemented and works well.

Item Collections

Users can register an item that consists of HFPNe components into the *item collections*, as in Fig. 7.13 (a) and Fig. 7.13 (b). Once registered, the item is reusable by choosing the item from the item collections, as in Fig. 7.13 (c) and Fig. 7.13 (d).

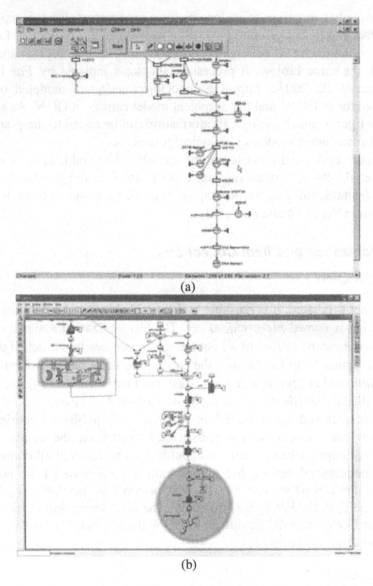

(a)

(b)

Fig. 7.11. Comparison between HFPN editor on GON⁻ and graphical model canvas on GON. The same biological processes, apoptosis induced by *Fas*, are modeled; (a) the biological processes on GON⁻ (Matsuno et al., 2003c); (b) the biological processes on GON (http://GenomicObject.net/)

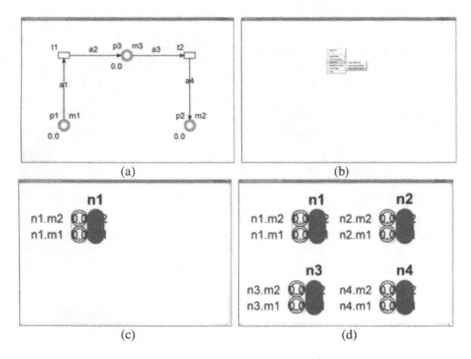

Fig. 7.12. Usage of the hierarchization. (a) Save a net (say net1) that will be hierarchized. Set to true entities that will be used on a canvas. Entities p1 and p2 are published in the figure. (b) Load net1 onto a canvas. (c) net1 is loaded to the canvas. Double circles denote published entities. When loading a hierarchized net to the canvas, names of variables in the net are automatically reassigned to avoid conflicts with variables of other components on the canvas. Unpublished entity p3 in the hierarchized net is hidden. (d) With the hierarchization feature, users can easily reuse already modeled biological processes

Comparison between a Hierarchized Net and an Item

Both a hierarchized net and an item in the item collection consists of components in HFPNe. The differences between them are as follows. When a hierarchized net is loaded on a canvas, only the published entities can connect with processes on the canvas, and no component in the hierarchized net is editable on the canvas, as in Fig. 7.12 (c) and Fig. 7.12 (d). In contrast, when an item is loaded on a canvas, all entities on the item can connect with processes on the canvas. In addition, all components are editable on the canvas, as in Fig. 7.13 (c) and Fig. 7.13 (d).

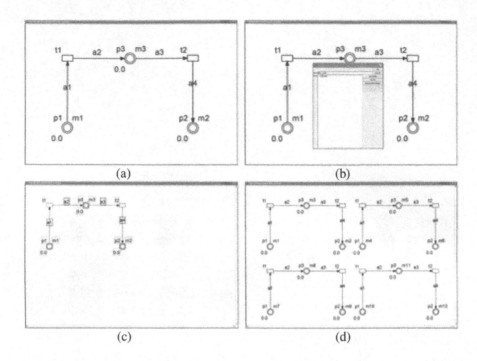

Fig. 7.13. Usage of the item collections. Users can register their favorite items into the item collections with two steps, (a) and (b), and can reuse the items as (c) and (d). (a) Select components that would like to register as an item. The net is the same as in Fig. 7.12(a). (b) Assign a unique name to the selected components onto the dialog in (b). (c) Select an item in the same dialog in (b), and then load the item is onto the canvas. (d) When loading an item onto a canvas, names of variables in the item are automatically reassigned to avoid conflicts with variables of other components on the canvas. With the item collections, users can easily create many copies of one item with short steps. The net on the canvas is the same as in Fig. 7.12(d), whereas the copies of entity p2 exist on this canvas but do not exist on the canvas in Fig. 7.12(d) because the entity p2 is unpublished. This is one of the differences between the hierarchization and the item collections

Because of these differences, their suitable applications are naturally different. A hierarchized net is useful when modeling biological processes whose internal components, except for published entities, are not necessary. A good example is a hierarchized net that is created from metabolic pathway maps of KEGG database with BPE (Nagasaki et al., 2004c). On the other hand, an item is useful if it should be edited by users. An example is the core biological process library in Subsection *Core Biological Process Library* In many cases, there are more than one hundred components in a hierarchized net, while the number of components in an item is less.

Core Biological Process Library

A *core biological process library* is a set of special items in the item collections that consists of various items indexed with biological processes, e.g., bind, repress, transcribe, translate, degrade, and translocale, as shown in Fig. 7.14. The library was developed (Doi et al., 2004b, Nagasaki et al., 2004b) with technical knowledge and skills acquired by modeling various kinds of biological processes, e.g., the glycolytic pathway of *E.* coli, gene regulation in *Drosophila*, boundary formation by notch signaling in *Drosophila* (Matsuno et al., 2003b), apoptosis induced by *Fas* ligand, *Calcitonin/CGRP* expression in Subsection 7.5.1, HIV-1 *gag-pol* expression in Subsection 7.5.2, Huntington's disease in Subsection 7.5.3, and protein modification of *p53* in Subsection 7.5.4.

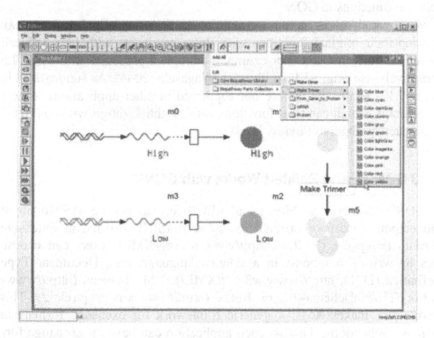

Fig. 7.14. Usage of the core biological process library. The snapshot is a sample pathway that consists of tree items, trimerization, transcription and translation, in the core biological process library

All items are also assigned valid parameters for simulation so as to match with their biological features, e.g., high/low degradation and high/low affinity. Owing to these valid assignments for parameters, users can create proper simulatable models for biological processes not mainly from HFPNe knowledge but from their biological knowledge, with the core biological process library as shown in Fig. 7.14.

Pnuts and Original Java Libraries

In GON, all functions in HFPNe, i.e., update function, activity function, and delay function, are realized with Pnuts (http://www.pnuts.org/). Pnuts is a script language for the Java environment with the following features: (i) simple and clean syntax (http://pnuts.org/snapshot/latest/doc/lang-TOC.html), (ii) an interactive interpreter, (iii) extensible through its module system, (iv) support for dynamic/static translation to JVM bytecode, (v) one of the fastest scripting language implementations on JVM, (vii) many advantages of Java (e.g., security, portability).

Pnuts also has a feature to handle basic arithmetic syntax. Thus, if targeting biological processes need to be modeled with basic kinetics, e.g., the mass action law, users without programming skills can assign these kinetics to functions in GON.

Moreover, if users have programming skills, especially Java, they can develop their original functions with Pnuts or classes with Java and call these functions in GON. For example, biological processes in Section 7.5 extensively use original Java libraries (Nagasaki, 2004). As summarized in Table 7.13, script add-ins are not supported in other applications, except PathPursuit, which can treat functions with MathML (http://www.scbio.co.jp/products/pathpursuit/index. html).

7.7.3 GONML and Related Works with GONML

In GON⁻, only original binary and ASCII formats can be used for input and output. Instead of original binary and ASCII formats, in Extensive Markup Language (XML) (http://www.w3.org/XML/) users can choose tags by writing a schema in a schema language, e.g., Document Type Definition (DTD; http://www.w3.org/XML/), XML-Schema (http://www-.w3.org/TR/xmlschema-0/), or Relax (http://www.xml.gr.jp/relax/). This architecture makes XML a generic framework for exchange formats in various applications. That is, each application can have an exchange format as a sublanguage of XML described by a schema, and all such applications can share generic tools and libraries for XML. Thus, adopting XML can reduce a large part of work common in software development. GON also adapts an XML format, GONML, as an input and output format of biological processes. GONML is the format of HFPNe and its graphical representations. GONML format is newly created by the authors, and the format with the XML Schema is given in Nagasaki (2004).

Table 7.13. A comparison of major software as of 2004. ++ (or +) means the feature is strongly implemented (or implemented) in the software.

GON	Cell Designer	E-Cell	Virtual Cell	Gepasi	Path Pursuit
Core Algorithm and method.					
HFPNe	ODE	ODE	ODE/PED	ODE	ODE
XML input and output.					
GONML	SBML	Original Format	Original Format	Original Format	Original Format
Data Export to CellML.					
+[1]	–	–	+[3]	–	–
Data Export to SBML.					
+[2]	++	–[7]	+[3]	+[3]	–
Simulation 2D Plotting.					
++	++	++	++	++	++
Advanced Simulation Views.					
++[8]	–	–	–	–	–
Pathway Editor.					
++	++	–	++	–	++
Metabolic Pathway Modeling and Simulation.					
++	++	++	++	++	++
Metabolic Pathway Analysis.					
+[4]	+[5]	–	–	++	–
Kinetic Based Signalling Pathway Modeling and Simulation.					
++	++	++	++	–	++
Rule (Discrete) Based Signalling Pathway Modeling and Simulation.					
++	–	–	–	–	+[6]
Rule (Discrete) and Kinetic Based Signalling Pathway Modeling and Simulation.					
++	–	–	–	–	+[6]
Signalling Pathway Analysis.					
+[4]	+[5]	–	–	–	–
Support Script Language.					
++ Pnuts	–	–	–	–	+MathML
Commercialized.					
++	–	–	–	–	++
Programming Language.					
Java	Java	C++	Java	C++	C++

[1]A subset of GONML can export to CellML format. [2]A subset of GONML can export to SBML format. [3]A function exists on the application but does not work. [4]We need other Petri net applications. [5]Need other SBW applications. [6]Some if-then rule-based modeling/simulation is possible. [7]SBML support in future. [8]Supported on GON Visualizer in Section 7.8.

As a major standardization project in the Petri net community, the Petri Net Markup Language (PNML) is known (Billington et al., 2003). The ongoing project is currently releasing a document type definition (DTD) only for basic Petri nets, i.e., DT, CT, CTN, and HPN. Thus, major high-level Petri net tools, e.g., Renew (Olaf and Frank, 2000) and Design/CPN (http://www.daimi.au.dk/designCPN/), are not equipped with the PNML format but with original XML-based file formats. HFPNe is one of the high-level Petri net tools. If GONML tries to support the PNML format, the PNML format needs to be extensively extended.

On the other hand, in the biopathway community, the Systems Biology Markup Language (SBML) and the Cell Markup Language (CellML) are the major modeling formats of biological processes. SBML aims at representing models of biochemical reaction networks, e.g., metabolic pathways, cell-signaling pathways, gene regulatory networks, and many other areas in systems biology. The CellML is another major project. The format mainly describes the chemical reactions in cells. Their notation can denote ODE-based metabolic networks with MathML (http://www.w3.-org/mathml/). However, currently SBML and CellML can denote ODE-based chemical kinetics in metabolic networks, but notations of other biological processes, i.e., cell-signaling pathways and gene regulatory networks, are not well organized. Thus, current SBML and CellML format can be a subset of GONML format (Nakano et al., 2002).

7.7.4 Related Works with GON

Several software packages for modeling and simulating metabolic and signaling pathways have been developed. We have selected six recent well known modeling/simulation applications: GON (Doi et al., 2004b, Nagasaki et al., 2004b), Cell Designer (http://sbserv.symbio.jst.go.jp/), E-Cell (Tomita et al., 1999), Virtual Cell (Schaff et al., 1997), Gepasi (Mendes 1993), and PathPursuit (http://www.scbio.co.jp/products/pathpursuit/index.html). Each application possesses some prominent features that are absent in others, as summarized in Table 7.13.

From the simulation viewpoint, many algorithms and methods employ ODEs. All have simulation graphic displays. From the modeling viewpoint, some have pathway drawing editors.

Gepasi is widely used for both research and education to simulate biochemical systems due to its powerful simulation engine and chemical kinetic library. E-Cell develops a system for representation and simulation with GUI. A system of reactions is represented with a spread-sheet compiling substances and reactions with ODEs. For reactions which cannot be represented with ODEs, it employs ad hoc user-defined C++ programs. E-Cell tries to model several biological processes, including biochemical reactions in human erythrocyte, signal transduction for bacterial chemotaxis, energy metabolism in mitochondria, and lytic-lysogenic switch network of λ phage (Tomita, 2001). Unfortunately, E-Cell and Gepasi have no user friendly modeling tools, and it is rather complicated to use these applications for modeling even simple biological processes for users. In Virtual Cell (Schaff et al., 1997), a model is defined as a collection where species (e.g., calcium and ATP), reactions (e.g., enzyme kinetics and receptor binding) and features (e.g., ER and cytosol), and ODEs for kinetic reactions and PDEs for diffusive objects are employed. Biological processes can be modeled on online pathway editors. Cell Designer also has a pathway graphic editor, enabling users to interactively draw biochemical networks. Via the System Biology Workbench (SBW) interface, ODE-based simulations are possible on other applications that support the SBW interface. PathPursuit also has a pathway graphic editor, enabling users to interactively draw biochemical networks, and ODE-based simulations are possible.

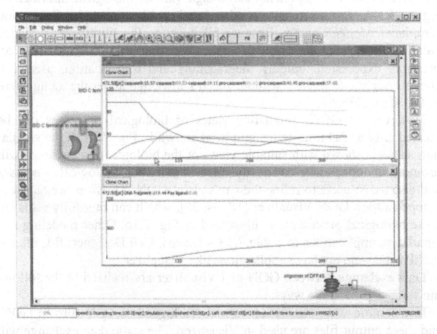

Fig. 7.15. One of signaling pathway models apoptosis induced by Fas in Fig. 7.11(b) is simulated in GON with 2D plotting graphs (http://GenomicObject.net/)

All these applications adapt different XML formats for their inputs/outputs. As in Table 7.13, some applications try to export SBML and CellML formats, but their output is inadequate or not yet implemented. The main reason is inadequate definition for biological processes in SBML and CellML formats, as mentioned in Subsection 7.7.3.

At the beginning of Section 7.7, we have started to develop modeling and simulation applications of biological processes with Petri nets because of their intuitive graphical representation and their capabilities for mathematical analysis. GON inherits these features directly (Subsection 7.7.1) and extends them (Subsection 7.7.2), and possesses various features better than other applications, as shown in Table 7.13.

7.8 Visualizer

In GON, when modeling biological processes, users can directly apply their biological knowledge on the graphical model canvas with the core biological process library of Subsection *Core Biological Process Library*, and HFPNe basic components can assign various biological information, e.g., mRNA/DNA sequence and related publications, in Subsection *Graphical Model Canvas*. Because all items in the library are assigned valid parameters for biological processes, *e.g.* transcription, translation, repression, expression, binding, degradation, and translocation, users can create simulatable models without much knowledge about the architecture of GON, i.e., HFPNe.

However, in GON, simulating states of biological processes can be viewed only as 2D time series graphs as shown in Fig. 7.15. If the simulation status is shown with suitable views of the biological processes, it will promote understanding of the dynamic activity for biological processes and also assist users to refine their models in GON. Therfore, we have developed a tool, GON Visualizer [18, 44, 55], which can faithfully visualize these biological processes, as illustrated in Fig. 7.16. Other modeling and simulation applications in Table 7.13 – Gepasi, Cell Designer, E-Cell, and PathPursuit – do not have applications like Visualizer.

Data exchange between GON and Visualizer are realized in the following static and dynamic ways.

In the static way, simulation results are logged as CSV files in GON, and these output files are used in Visualizer. The static data exchange will be used when simulation results in GON or other applications need to be repeatedly animated in Visualizer.

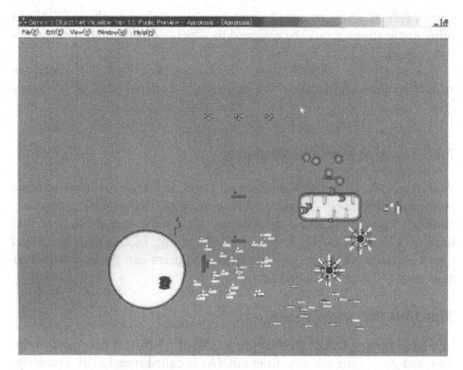

Fig. 7.16. The simulating data on GON in Fig. 7.15 is accessed via CORBA and animated on Visualizer

The dynamic data exchange is achieved with CORBA (http://www.-omg.org/) which is one of distributed object technologies. Thus, the simulation status in GON is directly displayed in Visualizer. In addition, simulation and visualization can be performed on separate computers. Currently, large-scale pathway models need to simulate in GON as BPEs (Nagasaki et al., 2004c), and a high performance computer is desirable. Users may also wish to compare dynamic simulation differences among pathways, such as a normal pathway simulation and a pathway with an overexpressed/knockout gene. To achieve this, multiple data connections between a set of GON applications and a set of Visualizer applications via CORBA are supported.

Visualizer adopts original XML format as its input. By writing XML files for Visualizer, users can realize personalized visualizations for data that are statically and dynamically generated in GON. The XML format of Visualizer is written by DTD format. In Nagasaki (2004), we described how to create basic animations on Visualizer with illustrations, while describing usages of tags and attributes of the XML in Visualizer. In short, the XML format consist of two parts; (i) firstly, the XML format defines actors with graphical images in an animation, and (ii) secondly, the XML format defines which output of simulation (simulating) results in GON and other applications should be assigned to which animation attributes in actors, e.g., speed, color, size, and number of actors.

Subsection 7.8.1 describes how to express basic biological processes with Visualizer. Subsection 7.8.2 discusses the related work with Visualizer.

7.8.1 Bio-processes on Visualizer

With the XML format of Visualizer in Nagasaki (2004), we express basic biological processes – transcription, translation, repression, expression, binding, degradation, and translocation – with XML, and illustrate animations on Visualizer in Fig. 7.18, Fig. 7.20, and Fig. 7.22. It should be noted that these animations are just examples, and users can freely create other animations of their own interests.

Transcription and Translation

In a cell, copying DNA sequences in a form of mRNAs is called *transcription*, and generating proteins from mRNAs is called *translation*. Transcription and translation states can be plotted on a 2D time series graph in GON, as in Fig. 7.15. However, applying the facts transcriptions occur in nucleus and translations occur at ribosomes in cytoplasms, better views can be created in Visualizer as shown in Figs. 7.18 (a)–(d) with the XML file in Fig. 7.17. Figs. 7.8(a)–(d) are arranged chronological order; the circle in the center is the nucleus and the rounded rectangle (excluding the portion of the circle) is the cytoplasm. In Fig. 7.18(b), to show that transcription of mRNA starts in the nucleus, wavy lines are displayed in the circle, and in Fig. 7.8(c), to show that translation of protein from mRNAs has begun, small circles are displayed. Because the number of the mRNA and the protein images on the window correspond to that of the data in GON, users can grasp the abstract number of these, as shown in Figs. 7.18(c) and (d). Both figures display mRNAs and proteins, but their numbers are different.

```
 1  <?xml version="1.0" encoding="UTF-8"?>
 2  <!DOCTYPE test SYSTEM "./GonVisTool.dtd">
 3  <test>
 4    <imageFile id="protein1" file="./images/protein1.png"/>
 5    <imageFile id="protein2" file="./images/protein2.png"/>
 6    <imageFile id="complex"  file="./images/complex.png"/>
 7    <imageFile id="cellbody" file="./images/cellbody.png"/>
 8    <imageFile id="nucleus"  file="./images/nucleus.png"/>
 9    <imageFile id="mRNA"     file="./images/mRNA.png"/>
10    <tableFile file="data.csv">
11      <placeName id="mRNA_data"     name="mRNA_data"/>
12      <placeName id="protein1_data" name="protein1_data"/>
13      <placeName id="protein2_data" name="protein2_data"/>
14      <placeName id="complex_data"  name="complex_data"/>
15    </tableFile>
16    <animation title="Transcription and Translation Simulation"
17              backColor="0 0 0">
18      <animeSingleObject id="cell" position="0 0 -2" >
19        <animeImage image="cellbody" size="800 522" />
20      </animeSingleObject>
21      <animeSingleObject id="nucleus" position="-100 0 -1" >
22        <animeImage image="nucleus" size="250 250" />
23      </animeSingleObject>
24      <animeMultiObject lowerBound="220 140 0" upperBound="260 100 0">
25        <animeImage image="protein1" size="10 10"/>
26        <animeMultiVisibility
27          event="protein1_data"
28          discretization="1"
29          threshold="0"/>
30      </animeMultiObject>
31      <animeMultiObject lowerBound="220 -140 0" upperBound="260 -100 0">
32        <animeImage image="protein2" size="10 10"/>
33        <animeMultiVisibility
34          event="protein2_data"
35          discretization="1"
36          threshold="0"/>
37      </animeMultiObject>
38      <animeMultiObject lowerBound="220 -20 0" upperBound="260 20 0">
39        <animeImage image="complex" size="10 10"/>
40        <animeMultiVisibility
41          event="complex_data"
42          discretization="1"
43          threshold="0"/>
44        <animeMultiMotion
45          event="complex_data"
46          motionPeriod="40"
47          type="oneway"
48          position="-100 0 0" />
49      </animeMultiObject>
50    </animation>
51  </test>
```

Fig. 7.17. An XML file that represents transcription and translation in a cell. Animations on Visualizer are shown in Fig. 7.18. The usages of tags and their attributes are described in Nagasaki (2004)

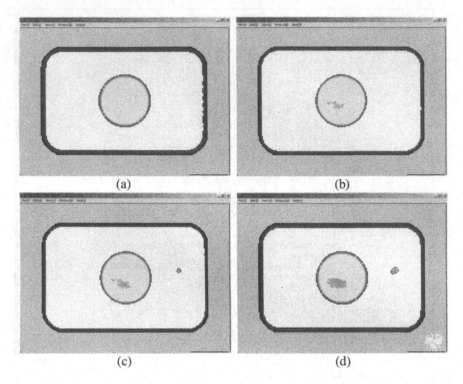

Fig. 7.18. Animations of the XML file in Fig. 7.17. Figs. (a)–(d) are arranged in chronological order. In these figures, a circle in the center illustrates a nucleus and a rounded rectangle, excluding the circle, illustrates a cytoplasm. Wavy lines on the nucleus in (b)–(d) are mRNAs, and small circles in the cytoplasm are translated proteins from the mRNAs. Transcription/translation starts between (a) and (b)/(b) and (c), respectively. As in (c) and (d), the number of mRNAs and proteins is increasing

Repression, Expression, and Binding

In biological processes, *repression* and *expression* are often used when a function of a protein, DNA, and mRNA is increased and decreased, respectively. These biological processes are sometimes realized with another biological process, bind. One of the meanings of "to *bind*" is that a protein tightly makes contact with a specific DNA sequence or with other proteins. For example, a protein binds to a specific DNA sequence and represses the transcriptional activity of an mRNA. The transcriptional activity can be measured with the 2D time series graph in GON by comparing simulation results with repressor proteins and without them. However, efficient visualization can be created on Visualizer with AnimeMultiObjects and

AnimeMultiMotion. AnimeMultiObjects can represent the mRNA and the protein. DNA AnimeMultiMotion can represent the binding status of the protein to the specific DNA sequences.

Figs. 7.20 (a)–(d) are arranged in chronological order. In these figures, a rectangle in the center illustrates DNA sequences and the subcomponent with a gray regin in the rectangle illustrates transcriptional DNA sequences. In (a), mRNAs are translated from the transcriptional place and displayed with wavy lines. In (b), repressor proteins appear (two proteins appear), and in (c) the repressor protein makes contacts with the transcriptional place and inhibits the activity of the mRNA transcription. After the event, mRNAs gradually degrade and, in (d), all mRNAs disappear.

```
1   <?xml version="1.0" encoding="UTF-8"?>
2   <!DOCTYPE test SYSTEM "./GenVisTool.dtd">
3   <test>
4   <imageFile id="DNA-image" file="./images/DNA_sequence.png"/>
5   <imageFile id="mRNA-image" file="./images/mRNA.png"/>
6   <imageFile id="repressor-image" file="./images/repressor.png"/>
7   <tableFile file="data.csv">
8   <placeName id="repressor-num-event" name="repressor_data"/>
9   <placeName id="mRNA-event" name="mRNA_data"/>
10  </tableFile>
11  <animation title="A protein binds and repress transcription
12    activity." backColor="0 0 0">
13    <animeSingleObject id="specific_DNA_position">
14        <animeImage image="DNA-image" size="200 20"/>
15    </animeSingleObject>
16    <animeMultiObject lowerBound="-100 20 0"
17        upperBound="100 100 0">
18      <animeImage image="mRNA-image" size="50 50"/>
19      <animeMultiVisibility event="mRNA-event"
20        discretization="1" threshold="1"/>
21    </animeMultiObject>
22    <animeMultiObject lowerBound="-100 20 0"
23        upperBound="100 100 0">
24      <animeImage image="repressor-image" size="20 20"/>
25      <animeMultiVisibility event="repressor-num-event"
26        discretization="3" threshold="3"/>
27      <animeMultiMotion event="repressor-num-event"
28        type="reversible" motionPeriod="4" period="-1"
29        threshold="10" reference="specific_DNA_position"
30        position="-30 10 0"/>
31    </animeMultiObject>
32  </animation>
33  </test>
```

Fig. 7.19. An XML file that creates animations in Visualizer. The XML file represents a transcription of mRNA from specific DNA sequences that is inhibited by a repressor protein in the nucleus. Animations on Visualizer are illustrated in Fig. 7.18. The usages of tags and their attributes are described in Nagasaki (2004)

Degradation

In a cell, nearly all mRNAs and proteins fragment into parts at certain speeds. This fragmentation activity is called *degradation*. In many cases, degradation speeds of proteins are regulated by other proteins that make contact with them. In these cases, the degradation status can be displayed with a 2D time series graph in GON. Intuitive visualization can be created in Visualizer with `AnimeMultiObject`, whose attribute `event` references the number of transcribed products, as illustrated in Figs. 7.20(c) and (d). In Fig. 7.20(c), a repressor protein binds to specific DNA sequences that are used to transcribe an mRNA. After the event, the mRNA cannot be translated from the sequences. As Fig. 7.20(d) shows, all mRNAs degrade and disappear from the cell.

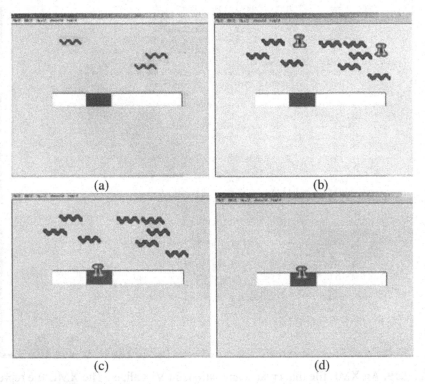

(a)   (b)

(c)   (d)

Fig. 7.20. Animations of the XML file in Fig. 7.19. Figs. (a)–(d) are arranged in chronological order. In these figures, a rectangle in the center illustrates a DNA sequence and the subcomponent with the gray regin in the rectangle is the transcriptional DNA sequence. In (a), mRNAs are translated from the transcriptional sequences and are displayed with twisted images (three mRNAs appear). In (b), (two) repressor proteins appear, and, in (c), the repressor protein makes contact with the transcriptional place and inhibits the mRNA transcription. After the event, mRNAs gradually degrade and, in (d), all mRNAs disappear

Translocation

In biological processes, *translocation* means that proteins, mRNAs, or other materials move from positions to other positions with regulations. For example, a protein can make contact with another protein, and the generated complex acquires the ability to translocate from the cytoplasm to the nucleus. In GON, it is difficult to analyze translocation activities with the 2D time series graph. However, easy visualization can be created on Visualizer with `AnimeMultiObject` and `AnimeMultiMotion`, whose attribute event references the number of the complex, as illustrated in Figs. 7.22(a)–(d) with the XML file in Fig. 7.21.

In (a)–(d), the circle in the center illustrates the nucleus, and the rounded rectangle (excluding the circle) is the cytoplasm. In (a), no protein exists. After short periods, as shown in (b), two types of protein appear; one protein with a small circle appears at the top right and the other with an small orange circle appears at the bottom right. These two types of proteins move and make a complex somewhere between the places where they appeared, as in (c). These complexes translocate from the contact position to the nucleus, as in (d).

7.8.2 Related Works with Visualizer

As shown in Table 7.13, several software packages for modeling and simulating biological processes have been developed. All applications have 2D plotting windows for visualizing simulation results, and many applications have graphical modeling editors.

However, none of the applications can create customized views to grasp the dynamic states for biological processes comparable to Visualizer in Figs. 7.16, 7.18, 7.20, and 7.22. From an information science point of view, Visualizer makes little contribution. However, we believe an animation tool for biological processes is useful because (i) it makes it easier for users to capture simulation results in GON, as in Subsection 7.8.1 and (ii) it is an effective communication medium, e.g., presentation and education in biological and medical fields.

Actually, well known textbooks for molecular biology, *Molecular Biology of the Cell* and *Molecular Cell Biology*, include animations of biological processes with Quicktime or Flash on CDROMs or online [51]. Part of these biological processes are already treated in Visualizer, as in Subsection 7.8.1. The difference between animations whether or not they are read only; once Visualizer XML files are created, Visualizer can create animations according to simulation results in simulators, especially in GON. Thus, once all biological processes in these textbooks are modeled in GON and Visualizer XML files are created as in the apoptosis models in Figs. 7.16., users can easily observe what will happen if the original biological processes, e.g., wild type, are modified, e.g., mutant and drug treatment, and we can improve our understanding of the mechanisms of biological processes in these textbooks.

```
 1  <?xml version="1.0" encoding="UTF-8"?>
 2  <!DOCTYPE test SYSTEM "./GonVisTool.dtd">
 3  <test>
 4    <imageFile id="protein1-image" file="./images/protein1.png"/>
 5    <imageFile id="protein2-image" file="./images/protein2.png"/>
 6    <imageFile id="complex-image"  file="./images/complex.png"/>
 7    <imageFile id="cellbody-image" file="./images/cellbody.png"/>
 8    <imageFile id="nucleus-image"  file="./images/nucleus.png"/>
 9    <imageFile id="mRNA-image"     file="./images/mRNA.png"/>
10    <tableFile file="data.csv">
11      <placeName id="mRNA_data"     name="mRNA_data"/>
12      <placeName id="protein1_data" name="protein1_data"/>
13      <placeName id="protein2_data" name="protein2_data"/>
14      <placeName id="complex_data"  name="complex_data"/>
15    </tableFile>
16    <animation title="Translocate Simulation " backColor="0 0 0">
17      <animeSingleObject id="cell" position="0 0 -2" >
18        <animeImage image="cellbody-image" size="800 622" />
19      </animeSingleObject>
20      <animeSingleObject id="nucleus" position="-100 0 -1" >
21        <animeImage image="nucleus-image" size="250 250" />
22      </animeSingleObject>
23      <animeMultiObject lowerBound="220 140 0" upperBound="260 100 0">
24        <animeImage image="protein1-image" size="10 10"/>
25        <animeMultiVisibility
26          event="protein1_data"
27          discretization="1"
28          threshold="0"/>
29      </animeMultiObject>
30      <animeMultiObject lowerBound="220 -140 0" upperBound="260 -100 0"
31        <animeImage image="protein2-image" size="10 10"/>
32        <animeMultiVisibility
33          event="protein2_data"
34          discretization="1"
35          threshold="0"/>
36      </animeMultiObject>
37      <animeMultiObject lowerBound="220 -20 0" upperBound="260 20 0">
38        <animeImage image="complex-image" size="10 10"/
39        <animeMultiVisibility
40          event="complex_data"
41          discretization="1"
42          threshold="0"/>
43        <animeMultiMotion
44          event="complex_data"
45          motionPeriod="40"
46          type="oneway"
47          position="-100 0 0" />
48      </animeMultiObject>
49    </animation>
50  </test>
```

Fig. 7.21. An XML file that creates animations in Visualizer. The XML file represents a translocation of a complex that consists of two proteins. These two proteins are generated in the cytoplasm. Animations on Visualizer are illustrated in Fig. 7.22. The usages of tags and their attributes are described in Nagasaki (2004)

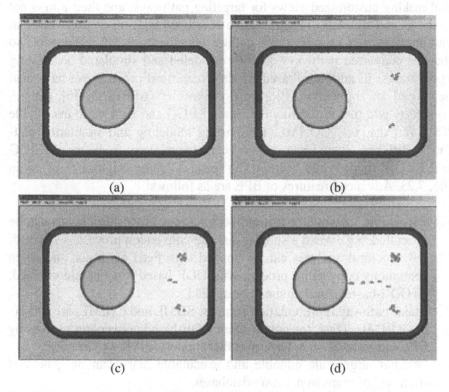

Fig. 7.22. Animations of the XML file in Fig. 7.21. In (a)–(d), the circle illustrates the nucleus, and the rounded rectangle, excluding the circle, illustrates the cytoplasm. In (a), no protein exists. After short periods, as shown in (b), two types of protein are created; one protein is represented with a small circle that appears at top right; the other is represented with a small circle that appears at the bottom right. These two types of proteins move and make a complex where between the places where they appeared, as in (c). These complexes translocate from the contact position to the nucleus, as in (d)

7.9 BPE

Several pathway databases are publicly available, such as the Kyoto Encyclopedia of Genes and Genomes (KEGG; Kanehisa and Goto, 2000), BioCyc (Karp et al. 2002, 2002), and WIT (Overbeek et al., 2000). On the other hand, there are many modeling and simulation applications, as described in Subsection 7.7.3. Unfortunately, these modeling and simulation applications cannot reuse pathway databases efficiently. Because the first aim of public pathway databases is to reorganize biochemical information for usage on computers for users, e.g., for searching interesting pathways and making customized views for targeting pathways, and their aim is not to model and simulate. Thus, we have developed conversion processes that can automatically convert these pathway databases to HFPNe models so that the converted pathways can be remodeled and simulated on existing applications. In addition, based on the conversion process, we have also developed an application, Biopathway Executer (BPE) [53, 56], that reconstructs two major pathway databases KEGG and BioCyc to executable XML formats, i.e., GONML, for existing modeling and simulation platforms. BPE can create large-scale executable pathways from sets of KEGG and BioCyc maps while keeping the features of the original maps, as in Fig. 7.23. Advanced features of BPE are as follows:

1. Executable metabolic pathways with various abstraction levels can be generated, e.g., when a simpler discrete conversion process is selected; DP structural analyses can be applied with Petri net tools; and when continuous conversion process with ODE-based kinetics are selected, an ODE-based simulation can be applied.
2. Major pathway representation formats, SBML and CellML, are subsets of GONML. Thus, the output of an ODE-based conversion process by BPE can be used on applications that support SBML or CellML.
3. Original large-scale editable and executable maps can be generated from sets of maps in pathway databases.
4. Starting from an executable metabolic model using BPE, users can construct finer models by themselves with biological knowledge and experimental data.
5. Applying hierarchization when generating a pathway with BPE, the pathway can always be automatically synchronized with recent original pathway databases.

We are also developing a public online service that extensively use BPE and GON, BPE Online Service (BPEOS). BPEOS consists of two services: (i) a download service that supplies XML files of GONML format for metabolic pathway maps in KEGG and (ii) a display service that supplies clickable image maps of all metabolic pathways in KEGG. The details of BPE and BPEOS are described in (Nagasaki, 2004, and Nagasaki et al., 2004c).

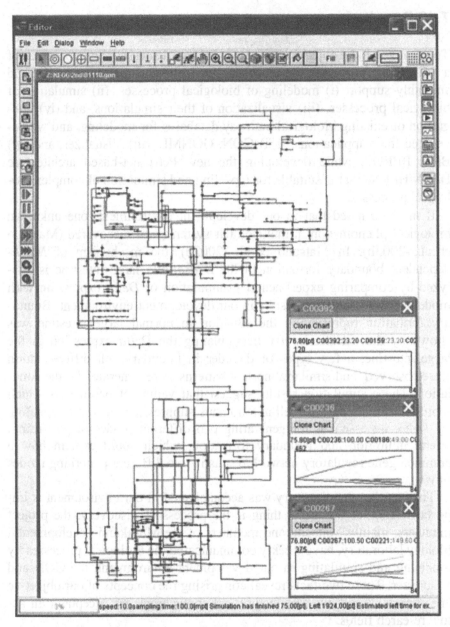

Fig. 7.23. A snapshot of the executable largescale metabolic pathway with 2D plotting graphs and animations using BPE. The map compiles 30 maps that are categorized into carbohydrate metabolism in KEGG. The executable map contains more than 10,000 HFPN components. Many substrates and products exist on the map but are not displayed, because they are also removed from the KEGG map for human readability

7.10 Conclusion

To accomplish the objective in Section 7.1, we discussed the importance of a biological processes development environment that can easily and smoothly support (i) modeling of biological processes, (ii) simulation of biological processes, (iii) visualization of their simulations, and (iv) integration of existing biological pathway databases for modeling, and we developed their applications, (i/ii) GON, GONML, (iii) Visualizer, and (iv) BPE, BPEOS, while developing the new Petri net-based architecture HFPN/HFPNe that is suitable for modeling and simulation of complex biological processes.

It must be noted that in our development environment, one unknown biological phenomenon in multicellular systems was discovered (Matsuno et al., 2003b). In Matsuno et al. (2003b), the mechanism of *Notch*-dependent boundary formation in the *Drosophila* large intestine is analyzed by comparing experimental manipulation of *Delta* expression with modeling and simulation results in our development environment. Boundary formation representing the situation in normal large intestine was shown by the simulation. By manipulating the *Delta* expression in the large intestine, a few types of disorder in boundary cell differentiation were observed, and similar abnormal patterns were generated by the simulation. These simulation results suggest that values of parameters which represent the strength of cell-autonomous suppression of *Notch* signaling by *Delta* are essential for generating two different modes of patterning; lateral inhibition and boundary formation, which could explain how a common gene regulatory network results in two different patterning modes *in vivo*.

The fact that the discovery was accomplished in our environment is important. Another important thing is the process of discovery; the project members, mainly Matsuno and members of the Murakami developmental biology laboratory, have weekly communicated the biological processes by modeling and simulating in our development environment, the GON and Visualizer. These two facts reveal comprising the concepts of our objective are important, and our architecture and applications are acceptable in actual research fields.

References

Alla, H. and David, R. (1998) Continuous and hybrid Petri nets. Journal of Circuits, Systems, and Computers 8:159–188.

Amara, S.G. and Jonas, V., Rosenfeld, M.G., Ong, E.S. and Evans, R.M. (1982) Alternative RNA processing in calcitonin gene expression generates mRNAs encoding different polypeptide products. Nature 298:240–244.

Ashburner, M., Ball, C.A., Blake, J.A., Botstein, D., Butler, H., Cherry, J.M., Davis, A.P., Dolinski, K., Dwight, S.S., Eppig, J.T., Harris, M.A., Hill, D.P., Issel-Tarver, L., Kasarskis, A., Lewis, S., Matese, J.C., Richardson, J.E., Ringwald, M., Rubin, G.M. and Sherlock, G. (2000) Gene ontology: tool for the unification of biology. The Gene Ontology Consortium. Nat. Genet. 25:25–29.

Bates, G., Harper, P. and Jones, L., eds 2002) untington's Disease. 3rd edn. Oxford University Press.

Becker, U. and Moldt, D. (1993) Object-oriented concepts for coloured Petri nets. In: IEEE International Conference on Systems, Man and Cybernetics. Volume 3., IEEE, pp 279–286.

Berg, J.M., Stryer, L. and Tymoczko, J.L. (2002) Biochemistry. 5th edn. W. H. Freeman.

Billington, J., Christensen, S., van Hee, K.M., Kindler, E., Kummer, O., Petrucci, L., Post, R., Stehno, C. and Weber, M. (2003) The Petri net markup language: concepts, technology, and tools. In: Applications and Theory of Petri Nets 2003, 24th International Conference (ICATPN). Volume 2679 of Lecture Notes in Computer Science., Springer-Verlag, pp 483–505.

BPEOS: http://bpe.genomicobject.net/.

Cell Designer: http://sbserv.symbio.jst.go.jp/.

CellML: http://www.cellml.org/.

Chen, M., Ona, V.O., Li, M., Ferrante, R.J., Fink, K.B., Zhu, S., Bian, J., Guo, L., Farrell, L.A., Hersch, S.M., Hobbs, W., Vonsattel, J.P., Cha, J.H. and Friedlander, R.M. (2000) Minocycline inhibits caspase-1 and caspase-3 expression and delays mortality in a transgenic mouse model of Huntington disease. Nat. Med. 6:797–801.

Coleman, T.P., Tran, Q. and Roesser, J.R. (2003) Binding of a candidate splice regulator to a calcitonin-specific splice enhancer regulates calcitonin/CGRP pre-mRNA splicing. Biochim. Biophys. Acta. 1625:153–164.

CORBA: http://www.omg.org/.

David, R. and Alla, H.: Continuous Petri nets. In: 8th European Workshop on Application and Theory of Petri Nets. Volume 340 of Lecture Notes in Computer Science., Springer-Verlag (1987) 275–294

Delphi: http://www.borland.com/delphi/.

Design/CPN: http://www.daimi.au.dk./designCPN/.

Doi, A., Fujita, S., Matsuno, H., Nagasaki, M. and Miyano, S. (2004) Constructing biological pathway models with hybrid functional Petri nets. In Silico Biology, Submitted.

Doi, A., Nagasaki, M., Fujita, S., Matsuno, H. and Miyano, S. (2004) Genomic Object Net:II. Modeling biopathways by hybrid functional Petri net with extension. Applied Bioinformatics 2:185–188.

Drath, R. (1998) Hybrid object nets: an object oriented concept for modeling complex hybrid systems. In: 3rd International Conference on Automation of

Mixed Processes: Hybrid Dynamical Systems (ADPM), Shaker Verlag, pp 437–442.

Drath, R, Engmann, U. and Schwuchow, S. (1999) Hybrid aspects of modeling manufacturing systems using modified Petri nets. In: 5th Workshop on Intelligent Manufacturing Systems. http://www.systemtechnik.tu-ilmenau. de/~drath/ download/Brasil98.ps.zip.

Extensible markup language (XML) (1998) http://www.w3.org/XML/.

Genomic Object Net (GON): http://GenomicObject.net/.

Genrich, H., Kuffner, R. and Voss, K. (2001) Executable Petri net models for the analysis of metabolic pathways. International Journal on Software Tools for Technology Transfer (STTT) 3:394–404.

GTL Scientific Plan: http://www.doegenomestolife.org/.

Hackam, A.S., Singaraja, R., Wellington, C.L., Metzler, M., McCutcheon, K., Zhang, T., Kalchman, M. and Hayden, M.R. (1998) The influence of huntingtin protein size on nuclear localization and cellular toxicity. J. Cell. Biol. 141:1097–1105.

Heiner, M., Koch, I. and Voss, K. (2001) Analysis and simulation of steady states in metabolic pathways with Petri nets. In: Third Workshop and Tutorial on Practical Use of Coloured Petri Nets and the CPN tools. pp 15–34 http://www.daimi.au.dk/CPnets/workshop01/cpnpapers/PB554.pdf.

HFPNe generic models: http://genomicobject.net/public/BiotechBook2004/code/.

Hickey, M.A. and Chesselet, M.F. (2003) Apoptosis in Huntington's disease. Prog Neuropsychopharmacol Biol Psychiatry 27:255–265.

Hofestädt, R. (1994) A Petri net application of metabolic processes. J. System Analysis, Modeling and Simulation 16:113–122.

Hofestädt, R. and Thelen, S. (1998) Quantitative modeling of biochemical networks. In Silico Biol. 1:39–53.

Hucka, M., Finney, A., Sauro, H.M., Bolouri, H., Doyle, J.C., Kitano, H., Arkin, A.P., Bornstein, B.J., Bray, D., Cornish-Bowden, A., Cuellar, A.A., Dronov, S., Gilles, E.D., Ginkel, M., Gor, V., Goryanin, I.I., Hedley, W.J., Hodgman, T.C., Hofmeyr, J.H., Hunter, P.J., Juty, N.S., Kasberger, J.L., Kremling, A., Kummer, U., Le Novere, N., Loew, L.M., Lucio, D., Mendes, P., Minch, E., Mjolsness, E.D., Nakayama, Y., Nelson, M,R., Nielsen, P.F., Sakurada, T., Schaff, J.C., Shapiro, BE., Shimizu, T.S., Spence, H.D., Stelling. J., Takahashi, K., Tomita, M., Wagner, J. and Wang, J. (2003) The systems biology markup language (SBML): a medium for representation and exchange of biochemical network models. Bioinformatics 19:524–531.

Jacks, T., Power, M.D., Masiarz, F.R., Luciw, P.A., Barr, P.J. and Varmus, H.E. (1988) Characterization of ribosomal frameshifting in HIV-1 gag-pol expression. Nature 331:280–283.

Kanehisa, M.and Goto, S. (2000) KEGG: kyoto encyclopedia of genes and genomes. Nucleic Acids Res. 28:27–30.

Karp, P.D., Riley, M., Paley, S.M. and Pellegrini-Toole, A.: The MetaCyc Database. Nucleic Acids Res. 30 (2002) 59–61.

Karp, P.D., Riley, M., Saier, M., Paulsen, I.T., Collado-Vides, J., Paley, S.M., Pellegrini-Toole, A., Bonavides, C. and Gama-Castro, S.: The EcoCyc Database. Nucleic Acids Res. 30 (2002) 56–58.

Kim, Y.J., Yi, Y., Sapp, E., Wang, Y., Cuiffo, B., Kegel, K.B., Qin, Z.H., Aronin, N. and DiFiglia, M. (2001) Caspase 3-cleaved N-terminal fragments of wild-type and mutant huntingtin are present in normal and Huntington's disease brains, associate with membranes, and undergo calpain-dependent proteolysis. Proc. Natl. Acad. Sci. U.S.A. 98:12784–12789.

Kohn, K.W. (1999) Molecular interaction map of the mammalian cell cycle control and DNA repair systems. Mol. Biol. Cell. 10:2703–2734.

Kuipers, B.J., Shults, B. (1994) Reasoning in logic about continuous systems. In: Principles of Knowledge Representation and Reasoning: Proceedings of the Fourth International Conference (KR94), Morgan Kaufmann, pp 391–402.

Kummer, O. (2001) Introduction to Petri nets and reference nets. Sozionik Aktuell 1:1–9.

Maier, C. and Moldt, D. (2001) Object coloured Petri nets - a formal technique for object oriented modeling. In: Concurrent Object-Oriented Programming and Petri Nets, Advances in Petri Nets. Volume 2001 of Lecture Notes in Computer Science., Springer-Verlag, pp 406–427.

Martin, J.B. and Gusella, J.F. (1986) Huntington's disease. Pathogenesis and management. N. Engl. J. Med. 315:1267–1276.

MathML: http://www.w3.org/mathml/.

Matsui, M., Fujita, S., Suzuki, S., Matsui, M.H.M. and Miyano, S. (2004) Simulated cell division processes of the Xenopus cell cycle pathway by Genomic Object Net. Journal of Integrative Bioinformatics 0001, Online Journal: http://journal.imbio.de/index.php?paper_id=3.

Matsuno, H., Doi, A., Hirata, Y. and Miyano, S. (2001) XML documentation of biopathways and their simulations in Genomic Object Net. Genome Informatics 12:54–62.

Matsuno, H., Doi, A., Nagasaki, M. and Miyano, S. (2000) Hybrid Petri net representation of gene regulatory network. Pacific Symposium on Biocomputing 5: 341–352

Matsuno, H., Fujita, S., Doi, A., Nagasaki, M. and Miyano, S. (2003) Towards biopathway modeling and simulation. In: 24th International Conference on Applications and Theory of Petri Nets (ICATPN 2003). Volume 2679., Lecture Notes in Computer Science, pp 3–22

Matsuno, H., Murakami, R., Yamane, R., Yamasaki, N., Fujita, S., Yoshimori, H. and Miyano, S. (2003) Boundary formation by notch signaling in Drosophila multicellular systems: experimental observations and gene network modeling by Genomic Object Net. Pacific Symposium on Biocomputing 8:152–163.

Matsuno, H., Tanaka, Y., Aoshima, H., Doi, A., Matsui, M. and Miyano, S. (2003) Biopathways representation and simulation on hybrid functional Petri net. In Silico Biol. 3:389–404.

Matsuoka, S., Sarai, N., Kuratomi, S., Ono, K. and Noma, A. (2003) Role of individual ionic current systems in ventricular cells hypothesized by a model study. The Japanese Journal of Physiology 53:105–123.

Mendes, P. (1993) GEPASI: a software package for modeling the dynamics, steady states and control of biochemical and other systems. Comput. Appl. Biosci. 9:563–571.

Molecular Cell Biology Media Resources: http://www.whfeeman.com/lodish/.

Nagasaki, M. (2004) A Platform for Biopathway Modeling/Simulation and Recreating Biopathway Databases Towards Simulation, Ph.D Thesis, The University of Tokyo, http://genomicobject.net/pub/nagasaki_phd.pdf.

Nagasaki, M., Doi, A., Matsuno and H., Miyano, S, (2003) Recreating biopathway databases towards simulation. In: Computational Methods in Systems Biology. Volume 2602 of Lecture Notes in Computer Science., Springer-Verlag, pp 191–192.

Nagasaki, M., Doi, A., Matsuno, H. and Miyano, S. (2004) A versatile Petri net based architecture for modeling and simulation of complex biological processes. Genome Informatics 14, Submitted.

Nagasaki, M., Doi, A., Matsuno, H. and Miyano, S. (2004) Genomic Object Net:I. A platform for modeling and simulating biopathways. Applied Bioinformatics 2:181–184.

Nagasaki, M., Doi, A., Matsuno, H. and Miyano, S. (2004) Integrating biopathway databases for large-scale modeling and simulation. In: The Second Asia-Pacific Bioinformatics Conference. Volume 29 of Conferences in Research and Practice in Information Technology., Australian Computer Society, pp 43–52

Nagasaki, M., Onami, S., Miyano, S. and Kitano, H. (1999) Bio-calculus: its concept and molecular interaction. Genome Informatics 10:133–143.

Nakano, M., Kitakaze, H., Matsuno, H. and Miyano, S. (2002) XML pathway file conversion between Genomic Object Net and SBML. Genome Informatics 13: 457–458.

Olaf. K., Frank, W. (2000) Renew - the reference net workshop. In: 21st International Conference on Application and Theory of Petri Nets. Volume 1825 of Lecture Notes in Computer Science., Springer-Verlag, pp 87–89 http://www.informatik.uni-hamburg.de/TGI/renew/renew.html.

Onami, S., Hamahashi, S., Nagasaki, M., Miyano, S. and Kitano, H. (2001) Automatic acquisition of cell lineage through 4D microscopy and analysis of early C. elegans embryogenesis. MIT Press.

Overbeek, R., Larsen, N., Pusch, G.D., D'Souza, M., Selkov, E.J., Kyrpides, N., Fonstein, M., Maltsev, N. and Selkov, E. (2000) WIT: integrated system for highthroughput genome sequence analysis and metabolic reconstruction. Nucleic Acids Res. 28:123–125.

PathPursuit: http://www.scbio.co.jp/products/pathpursuit/index. html.

Petri net community: http://www.daimi.au.dk/PetriNets/tools/.

Pnuts: http://www.pnuts.org/.

PnutsSyntax: http://pnuts.org/snapshot/latest/doc/lang-TOC.html.

Reddy, V.N., Mavrovouniotis, M.L, Liebman, M.N. (1993) Petri net representations in metabolic pathways. In: Proceedings First International Conference on Intelligent Systems for Molecular Biology. Volume 1., MIT Press, pp 328–336.

Regular language description for XML (Relax) (2000) http://www.xml.gr.jp/relax/.

Reisig, W. and Rozenberg, G., eds. (1998) Lecture on Petri nets I: Basic Models Lecture Notes in Computer Science. Volume 1491 of Lecture Notes in Computer Science. Springer-Verlag.

Reisig, W. and Rozenberg, G., eds. (1998) Lecture on Petri nets II: Applications Lecture Notes in Computer Science. Volume 1492 of Lecture Notes in Computer Science. Springer-Verlag.

Roizin, L., Stellar, S. and Liu, J.C. (1979) Neuronal nuclear-cytoplasmic changes in Huntington's chorea: electron microscope investigations. Raven Press, pp 95–122.

Roy, S., Bayly, C.I., Gareau, Y., Houtzager, V.M., Kargman, S., Keen, S.L., Rowland, K., Seiden, I.M., Thornberry, N.A., Nicholson, D.W. (2001) Maintenance of caspase-3 proenzyme dormancy by an intrinsic "safety catch" regulatory tripeptide. Proc. Natl. Acad. Sci. U.S.A. 98:6132–6137.

Schaff, J., Fink, C.C., Slepchenko, B., Carson, J.H. and Loew, L.M. (1997) A general computational framework for modeling cellular structure and function. Biophys. J. 73:1135–1146.

Schomburg, I., Chang, A. and Schomburg, D. (2002) BRENDA, enzyme data and metabolic information. Nucleic Acids Res. 30:47–49.

Senut, M.C., Suhr, S.T., Kaspar, B. and Gage, F.H. (2000) Intraneuronal aggregate formation and cell death after viral expression of expanded polyglutamine tracts in the adult rat brain. J. Neurosci. 20:219–229

The Huntington's disease collaborative research group (1993) A novel gene containing a trinucleotide repeat that is expanded and unstable on Huntington's disease chromosomes. Cell 72:971–83

Tomita, M. (2001) Whole-cell simulation: a grand challenge of the 21st century. Trends Biotechnol. 19:205–210

Tomita, M., Hashimoto, K., Takahashi, K., Shimizu, T.S., Matsuzaki, Y., Miyoshi, F., Saito, K., Tanida, S., Yugi, K. and Venter, J.C., Hutchison CA 3rd (1999) E-CELL: software environment for whole-cell simulation. Bioinformatics 15:72–84.

Tran, Q., Coleman, T.P. and Roesser, J.R. (2003) Human transformer 2beta and SRp55 interact with a calcitonin-specific splice enhancer. Biochim. Biophys. Acta. 1625:141–152.

Valk, R. (1978) Self-modifying nets, a natural extension of Petri nets. In: International Colloquium on Automata, Languages and Programming (ICALP). Volume 62 of Lecture Notes in Computer Science., Springer-Verlag, pp 464–476

Voet, D. and Voet, J.G. (1995) BIOCHEMISTRY. 2nd edn. John Wiley Sons, Inc.

VON++: http://www.systemtechnik.tu-ilmenau.de/~drath/visual_E.htm.

Webster, S.D., Cason, Z., Lemos, L.B. and Benghuzzi, H. (2000) Cytohistologic correlation in patients with clinical symptoms of postmenopausal bleeding. Biomed. Sci. Instrum. 36:367–372.

Wellington, C.L., Ellerby, L.M., Gutekunst, C.A., Rogers, D., Warby, S., Graham, R.K., Loubser, O., van, R.J., Singaraja, R., Yang, Y.Z., Gafni, J., Bredesen, D., Hersch, S.M., Leavitt, B.R., Roy, S. and Nicholson, D.W. and Hayden, M.R. (2002) Caspase cleavage of mutant huntingtin precedes neurodegeneration in Huntington's disease. J. Neurosci. 22:7862–7872.

Wellington, C.L., Ellerby, L.M., Hackam, A.S., Margolis, R.L., Trifiro, M.A., Singaraja, R., McCutcheon, K., Salvesen, G.S., Propp, S.S., Bromm, M., Rowland, K.J., Zhang, T., Rasper, D., Roy, S., Thornberry, N., Pinsky, L., Kakizuka, A., Ross, C.A., Nicholson, D.W., Bredesen, D.E. and Hayden, M.R. (1998) Caspase cleavage of gene products associated with triplet expansion disorders generates truncated fragments containing the polyglutamine tract. J. Biol. Chem. 273:9158–9167.

Wheeler, V.C., White, J.K., Gutekunst, C,A., Vrbanac, V., Weaver, M., Li, X.J., Li, S.H., Yi, H., Vonsattel, J.P., Gusella, J.F., Hersch, S., Auerbach, W., Joyner, A.L. and MacDonald, M.E. (2000) Long glutamine tracts cause nuclear localization of a novel form of huntingtin in medium spiny striatal neurons in HdhQ92 and HdhQ111 knock-in mice. Hum. Mol. Genet. 9:503–513.

XML Schema Part 0: Primer, W3C Working Draft (2000) http://www.w3.org/TR/xmlschema-0/.

8 Biological Sequence Assembly and Alignment

Wei Shi[1], Wanlei Zhou[1] and Yi-Ping Phoebe Chen[1,2]

[1] School of Information Technology
Faculty of Science and Technology, Deakin University
221 Burwood Hwy, Burwood, Vic 3125, Australia
[2] Australia Research Council Centre in Bioinformatics

8.1 Introduction

Computing technologies have played an increasingly important role in biology since the launch of Human Genome Project (Carol and Robert, 1996). Parallel computing, which acts as an effective way to speed up biological computing, has been used in many biological applications. Sequence assembly and sequence alignment are the most computing intensive parts of biological computing. They have benefited immensely from parallel computing, and will benefit more from further research on parallel biological computing. This chapter introduces recent developments in parallel sequence assembly and alignment.

Sequence assembly (Myers, 2002), also called fragment assembly, is used to recover fragments and build the original sequences. This is a very important step in DNA sequencing. Due to the large amount of biological data, it will take a very long time to assemble the fragments of a middle-sized genome such as rice. A parallel Euler sequence assembly approach is discussed in this chapter. This approach stores all the genomic data in the form of distributed hash table so as to assemble this data as a whole. This eliminates errors incurred by approximately partitioning the fragments into groups and assembling them into groups, as in other approaches. Further, our system can be run on networks of workstations or an supercomputers. It is particularly suitable for those having no access to supercomputers but to other computing resources such as workstations and PCs that are connected by a local network. This is the first effort to parallelize the Euler sequence assembly algorithm to assemble a large-scale genome. Sequence alignment (Liming et al., 2000) is also an important research area in bioinformatics. There are innumerable biological sequences with unknown structure and function. The alignment of these sequences to known sequences will yield insight into the unknown sequences if the two are similar. Sequence alignment can be further divided into multiple sequence alignment (MSA) and pair wise sequence alignment. The main purpose of an alignment is to propose homologies between sites in two or more sequences, but it is also a necessary step in judging homology between sequences or genes. The use of pair wise alignments is usually aimed at latter, while multiple alignments are used to assess homology between sites in many sequences.

Pairwise sequence alignment has the following significance:

- It can used to categorize and classify the DNA or protein sequences. The comparison between an unknown sequence and a known sequence can yield an insight into whether the two sequence are in the same category.
- Evolutionary relationships can be obtained by pair wise sequence assembly that identify the common parts of the two sequences.
- The DNA sequence can be aligned with the protein sequence to determine the function of the DNA sequence. The function of the unknown DNA sequence can also be known by comparing this sequence to known DNA sequences.
- The three dimensional structures of the protein sequence can be predicted by comparing it with the sequence of known dimensional structures.
- Pair wise sequence alignment is helpful in sequencing new genes. Multiple sequence alignment has shown significance in the following scopes:
- The shared homological regions of multiple sequences can be identified by taking advantage of MSA, which is very important for research in genetic diseases.
- MSA is often used to determine the consensus sequence of several aligned sequences.

- Secondary and tertiary structures of an unknown sequence can be predicted by comparing this sequence with multiple known sequences.
- MSA is a preliminary step in molecular evolution analysis using phylogenetic methods for constructing phylogenetic trees.

We parallelize the most used sequence alignment tools. For pair wise sequence alignment, we parallelize the Smith-Waterman algorithm (Temple and Michael, 1981). We also parallelize the Clustal W (Julie et al., 1994) multiple sequence alignment tool. These parallelizations, not only speed up biological computing, but also reduce the overall memory requirement by making use of the parallel computing technologies we develop.

The introduction to parallel sequence assembly and alignment is given in Section 1. Section 2 discusses issues with the parallel sequence assembly, including the Euler approach, parallel algorithms, determination of coverage, and implementation. Parallel pair wise sequence alignment is introduced in Section 3. Smith-Waterman algorithm and its parallelization are described. In Section 4, we present the parallelization of the Clustal W multiple sequence alignment tool. Load balancing and communication overhead, which play important roles in parallel computing, are discussed in Section 5. This chapter concludes with a discussion on the areas of research that need be focused on in the future.

8.2 Large-Scale Sequence Assembly

8.2.1 Related Research

Sequence assembly is used to recover the fragments that are broken from DNA sequences and assemble them into the original sequences. Currently, the most widely used approach for breaking DNA sequences is whole genome shotgun (WGS), which is less expensive and quicker than other approaches (Weber and Myers, 1997). The WGS fragments the genome into many pieces of various sizes. This fragmentation can be done in several ways, such as physically shaking the DNA and cutting it with restriction enzymes. The following is an example that illustrates the basic idea behind WGS. In real genome sequencing, both the genome and the read will be much longer than the genome and the read in the example.

Example:
Genome:
ATGC**GTAG**CTGTAGTGATCGAGGTCCAA**GTAG**CTGT
Reads from first copy:
ATGCGTAG, CTGTAGTG, ATCGAGGT, CCAAGTAG,
Reads from second copy:
GTAGCTGT, AGTGATCG, AGGTCCAA, **GTAGCTGT**

This example gives a simple and ideal whole genome shotgun. There are only two copies of the genome, and all the reads are of same size. There is no sequencing error, and all the nucleic acids have been identified. Each copy is broken into many reads. We cannot assemble the reads from one copy into the original genome because of lack of the information about their relative positions, called "context". At least two copies of the genome are therefore required to have context information available among the reads. We can see an example of this information by observing that the suffix of the first read from the first copy **"ATGCGTAG"**, and the prefix of the first read from the second copy **"GTAGCTGT"**, are the same. This overlap between the two reads can let them be joined into **"ATGCGTAGCTGT"**. A very challenging problem for sequence assembly is the "repeat" problem. That is, the assembler cannot distinguish well between the overlap and the repeats of reads. **"GTAG"** is an overlap between the two reads above, but it is also a repeat as shown in the genome in the example (the nucleic acid in boldface). Although the suffix of the first read from the first copy **"ATGCGTAG"** is the same as the prefix of the last read from the second copy, **"GTAGCTGT"**, this is *not* the overlap we have seen between the reads **"ATGCGTAG"** and **"GTAGCTGT"**. An assembly error will be produced if the two reads are joined together with repeat rather than overlap. It should be noted that in real genome sequencing the suffix and prefix of two reads with overlap or repeat are not necessarily exactly the same. Our example tries to explain this problem in a simple way.

The "repeat" problem had not been solved well until a new sequence assembly approach was proposed (Pavel et al., 2001). This approach reduces the sequence assembly problem to a variation of the classical Eulerian path problem, which has been demonstrated to be more accurate than other approaches. This Euler approach has a polynomial computing complexity rather than the exponential complexity of other approaches. Other sequence assembly programs fall into the "overlap-layout-consensus" paradigm, which was abandoned in Pevzner's approach. The following is a description for the three stages of the "overlap-layout-consensus" paradigm (Myers, 2002; and Kececioglu and Myers, 1995):

- Overlap – finding potentially overlapping fragments.
  The overlap problem is to find the best match between the suffix of one sequence and the prefix of another. If no sequencing errors occur, simply find the longest suffix of one string that exactly matches the prefix of another string. Because errors often occur in the process of sequencing, a common practice is to use the filtration method and to filter out pairs of fragments that do not share a significantly long common substring.

- Layout – finding the order of fragments.
  Many algorithms select a pair of fragments with the best overlap at every step. The selected pair of fragments with the best overlap score is checked for consistency. If this check is accepted, the two fragments are merged. At later stages of the algorithm, the collections of fragments (contig) – rather than individual fragments – are merged. The difficulty with the layout step is in deciding whether two fragments with a good overlap really overlap (i.e., their differences are caused by sequencing errors) or represent a repeat in a genome (i.e., their differences are caused by mutations).

- Consensus – deriving the DNA sequence from the layout.
  The simplest way to build a consensus is to report the most frequent character in the substring layout that is implicitly constructed after the layout step is completed. The weakness of this paradigm is that it cannot effectively solve the problem of fragment repeat, i.e., it cannot distinguish between fragment overlap and fragment repeat. It is a NP-hard problem to assemble the fragments under this paradigm. The software under this paradigm includes Phrap (Green, 1999), TIGR (Sutton et al., 1995), CAP3 (Huang and Madan, 1999), and Celera Assembler (Bonfield et al., 1995).

- Phrap – Phrap ("phragment assembly program", or "Phil's revised assembly program") is a program for assembling shotgun DNA sequence data. Some of its key features are: (1) allowing use of the entire read, not just the highest quality part; (2) using a combination of user supplied and internally computed data quality information to improve accuracy of assembly in the presence of repeats; (3) constructing contig sequences as a mosaic of the highest quality parts of reads.

- TIGR – The TIGR Assembler is a sequence fragment assembly program building contigs from small sequence reads. It uses a greedy algorithm and heuristics to build contigs, find repeat regions, and target alignment regions. Sequence overlaps are detected and scored using a 32-mer hash. Sequence alignment and merging is done using a Smith-Waterman algorithm. Gap penalties and score values corresponding to the bases and their quality values are predefined and hard coded into the program.

- CAP3 – CAP3 uses base quality values in the computation of overlaps between reads, construction of multiple sequence alignments of reads, and generation of consensus sequences. It also uses forward-reverse constraints to correct assembly errors and link contigs.
- Celera Assembler – Celera Assembler accepts an overlap only if there is no other sequence in the genome with $\geq 94\%$ sequence identity. Accordingly, fewer true overlaps are accepted in the initial assembly stage. In later stages of the Celera assembly, contigs are linked together by using mate-pair information, and the resulting gaps are then filled by various methods that may use sequences not included in the initial stages.

It is well known that one of the challenges to biological computing is the large amount of biological data and the colossal computing capacity required to process this data. Although Euler sequence assembly algorithm has a lower computing complexity than other approaches, it still needs a lot of time to assemble those biological fragments for small or middle sized genomes. Parallel computing is an efficient way to solve computing-intensive problems, and sequence assembly has shown good parallelism that can be exploited (Rajkumar, 1999; Terry et al., 2003; and Wei and Wanlei, 2003). In fact, parallel computing has been used in the current sequence assembly, for example, in sequencing the genome of the human being in the Human Genome Project. Many computing nodes have participated in the process of assembling fragments from the human genome. But this is not "real" parallel computing for sequence assembly because, in this approach, all fragments have to be first partitioned into many groups whose size is suitable for assembling in a single computing node. Fragments from one group can be assembled only with other fragments within the same group. So, each computing node can assemble the fragment only from perspective of a group, and not the whole genome. The partition of the fragments is conducted sequentially and may produce errors. These errors will result in incorrect sequence assembly because the assembly is confined to individual groups and cannot cross these groups.

But, in our approach, the parallel sequence assembly is carried out by each computing node from the view of the whole genome. Each fragment can be visited by each computing node. Each node can assemble any fragment into its local assembly result. The assembly is conducted by all the computing nodes in parallel. This is a "real" parallel sequence assembly approach because it is genome oriented, not group oriented. We are the first to propose such a real parallel approach.

8.2.2 Euler Sequence Assembly

The Euler sequence assembly approach was proposed by Pavel A. Pevzner (Pavel et al., 2001). The main contribution of the Euler assembly approach is that it transforms the biological sequence assembly problem into an Euler path problem that has a polynomial solution, which is a solution to the notorious "repeat" problem.

In the Euler sequence assembly approach, tuples are the minimal units to be assembled, rather than the reads as in other approaches. Tuples are generated from reads. Tuples from one read are all the substrings of that read with the same length, which is normally 20. All the tuples generated form a debruijn graph. The vertices of the graph are the tuples. Supposing the length of a tuple is l, if the last l-1 nucleotide acids of one tuple are the same as the first l-1 nucleotide acids of another tuple, there will be a directed edge in the graph which connects these two adjacent tuples. The Euler assembly approach is to find all the Euler paths in the graph. Each path is in fact a contig. The core of the Euler approach is the consistency analysis rule which solves the problems of path selection for branches when looking for Euler paths in a graph. The details for the consistency analysis rule can be found elsewhere (Pavel et al., 2001).

8.2.3 PESA Sequence Assembly Algorithm

Biological sequence assembly often costs a lot in computing time even for small or medium sized genomes because of the large magnitude of iterative computing. But most of the current assemblers are sequential programs. Biological data has to be partitioned before applying these programs to assemble the genome. The participation is conducted according to similarities. This process is not accurate. So errors could be introduced by the participation. These errors cannot be corrected by the assemblers. Thus, the sequential assembler cannot meet the requirements demanded by sequence assembly. The research on the parallel sequence assembler is just at its beginning. Our parallel sequence assembler is the first to use the parallel Euler approach. This section introduces the algorithm and implementation of our PESA sequence assembler.

Main idea

The PESA (Parallel Euler Sequence Assembly) algorithm we proposed is an effective parallelization of the Euler sequence assembly approach that includes data distribution and computation distribution. The data distribution is conducted first. Tuples are generated from all the reads and stored in a distributed hash table. A distributed hash table will take maximal advantage of the memory resources of a parallel computing platform. With more computing nodes or memory added to the computing platform, the hash table can accordingly become larger and accommodate more genome data. This table is evenly distributed over multiple computing nodes, and each node is responsible for its own part of the hash table. No single hash table containing all the data will eliminate the bottleneck for storing a large amount of genome data.

We use the djb2 hash algorithm to calculate the hash values for all tuple strings. Given a tuple string s, we calculate its hash value $h = djb2(s)$. Supposing the number of computing nodes is p and the size of the hash table is t; the size of the partial hash table on each node is t/p. The number of the computing node to which s will be assigned is $h\%(t/p)$. Each tuple will be stored in the corresponding partial hash table on some computing node. We use linked list to deal with the collision occurring in the hash table. Tuples with the same hash value will be put into the same linked list of the hash table in their processing order. After storing all the tuples in the hash table, we need to calculate the multiplicity of each tuple, which will determine how many times the tuple will appear in the final contigs. Multiplicities of all the tuples will be used to judge when the assembly process should finish. Only when the number of times that each tuple is visited equals its multiplicity will the assembly finish. This means all the tuples, not including their copies, have been assembled into contigs.

Based on the tuples stored in the local hash table, each computing node will start to assemble the tuples. The parallel assembly algorithm is described as follows:

Input: hash table and reads
Output: contigs

1. Take the first tuple t from the local hash table whose counter is bigger than 0. t is an initial contig.
2. Look for tuples adjacent to t on the right. If there is only one such tuple, and this tuple is on the same computing node, join the tuple directly to t. If this tuple is on some other computing node, this computing node will communicate with the remote computing node to request this tuple. If the counter of this tuple is bigger than 1, it can be joined into the current contig. It is the responsibility of the remote computing node to decrease the counter for this tuple by 1. If the number of tuples adjacent to t is more than 1, apply a consistency analysis rule to determine if there exists one, and only one, tuple that can be joined to the

contig. If so, join the tuple to the current contig if it is located on the same computing node. If it is located on another computing node, communicate with that node to join the tuple with the current contig, if possible.

3. Check if there are requests from other computing nodes and serve them if found.

4. Repeat (2) and (3) until the current contig cannot be extended any longer to the right because of no more tuples being available, counters of adjacent tuples becoming 0, or consistency analysis failing to determine which path the current contig should follow.

5. Look for tuples adjacent to t on the left, and deal with these tuples in the same way as described in (2), (3), and (4).

6. If there are tuples in the local hash table whose counters are bigger than 0, go to (1). Otherwise, the assembly process on this computing node finishes and the contigs generated will be sent to the master computing node.

7. The master computing node merges the contigs from all the nodes into the final contigs.

The counter for each tuple is initialized to be the multiplicity of the tuple, which describes how many times the tuple will appear in the final assembly result. The details for the counter can be seen in Section 3.2. Our parallel sequence assembly approach will extend the contigs from both the right direction and left direction, as shown in (2) and (5). This will help increase the lengths of the contigs generated by individual computing nodes, and thus reduce the computation to be carried out by the merging process, which merges all the partial contigs from all computing nodes. The reduced computation is in fact distributed over each computing node and executed in parallel.

The computing nodes involved assemble the tuples according to their local hash tables and generate contigs in parallel. Each node needs to communicate with others because the tuples to be joined to the current contig will possibly lie in other computing nodes. Details of communications among the computing nodes can be seen from (2) and (3). After one tuple is processed, each node will serve the request from other nodes so as to ensure that other nodes will not waiting for a long time to receive the response. This will produce a better utilization of the parallel system.

Finally, the master computing node will collect all the contigs from the slave nodes to assemble them further into the final result. The master node has no difference from other nodes except for the merging process. The merging process will also use a consistency analysis rule to assemble the current contigs into longer ones. The process is very similar to the assembly process discussed above. The tuples on both ends of every contig will be analyzed to see if they can be concatenated with other contigs. The merging process continues to assemble contigs until no more contigs can be joined.

Determination of coverage

The completion of the parallel Euler sequence assembly process depends on the coverage of the genome to be sequenced. Supposing the coverage of some genome is m, the number of a tuple that appears only once in the genome will ideally be m. The number of a tuple that appears more than once in the genome will ideally be a multiple of m. The number of a tuple appearing in the final assembly result should be the number of its appearing in the genome divided by m, i.e., multiplicity. We set a counter for each tuple that is initialized to its multiplicity. Each time a tuple is assembled, its counter will be decreased by 1. The parallel assembly process will finish when the counters of all tuples become zero.

In order to calculate the multiplicities of all the tuples, we have to know the coverage of the genome, which is in fact the number of copies of the genome to be sequenced. Generally, we can not get this information directly. In our approach, we calculated the coverage of the genome from statistics of all kinds of tuples with different numbers of their appearing in all the reads to be assembled. We define S_i as a set of tuples within which all tuples appear i times in all the reads. Among all the sets, there must exist a set $S_{coverage}$ in which all tuples have no repeats in the genome. The number of these tuples appearing in all the reads will be equal to the coverage of the genome. $|S_{coverage}|$ is larger than any other $|S_i|$, $i \neq coverage$ because in the genome the amount of tuples with multiplicity equal to 1 is more than the amount of tuples with multiplicity equal to 2, 3, or more. So, we can easily identify the set $S_{coverage}$ from all sets of tuples. The subscripting value of $S_{coverage}$ is just the coverage of the genome.

We compute statistics for four species from TIGR Benchmark (The Institute for Genomic Research, 2003). The result is shown as Figures 8.1 through 8.4 (the X axis represents the appearing number of tuples and the Y axis represents the number of tuples having some appearing number). From these figures, we can clearly see that there is a peak in each curve. The peak indicates the largest amount of tuples whose appearing number is just equal to the coverage of the genome. But there exists an error between experimental coverage of the genome and its real coverage, as discussed above. This is because some unqualified reads (too long or too short) have been removed from the chemical experiments for sequencing (Shamir and Tsur, 2002). So, the experimental coverage will be slightly smaller than the real value. When implementing the system, we will augment the experimental coverage and use it to calculate the multiplicity of each tuple.

Our next work is to conduct large-scale experiments to demonstrate our parallel assembly approach. The experiments will be carried out at the Australian Partnership for Advanced Computing National Facility, which owns a powerful AlphaServer SC with more than 500 CPUs and 700 GB RAM and a Cluster with 600 CPUs and 150 GB RAM.

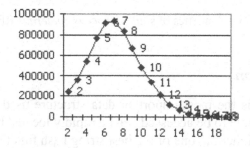

Fig. 8.1. Statistics of brucella suis

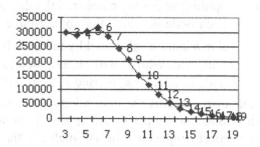

Fig. 8.2. Statistics of wolbachia sp

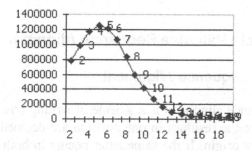

Fig. 8.3. Statistics of shewanella oneidensis

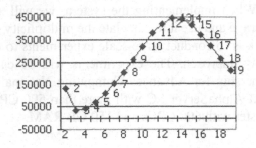

Fig. 8.4. Statistics of *staphylococcus epidermis* RP62A

Implementation

The hash table is the most important data structure used by sequence assembly. The *l*-tuple to be accessed can be rapidly located by using the hash table. The *djb2* function, one of the best string hash functions, is used here. The hash table is evenly distributed over each computing node. Assuming that the size of the hash table is n and the number of computing nodes available is p (the computing nodes are numbered 0,1,2,...,p-1), the size of partial hash table on each node is $\lceil n/p \rceil$. For some *l*-tuple generated from some read, its hash value h can be calculated by the hash function with the string of *l*-tuple as input. This *l*-tuple will be assigned to the computing node numbered $h\%\lceil n/p \rceil$. A linear list is used to deal with the hash conflict. The hash table also contains the multiplicity of each *l*-tuple that determines how many times the *l*-tuple would appear in the assembly result. The repeat and non-repeat *l*-tuples will be assembled at the same time. The parallel assembly will finish when the multiplicities of all the *l*-tuples are decreased to zero.

8.3 Large-Scale Pairwise Sequence Alignment

8.3.1 Pairwise Sequence Alignment

A pairwise sequence alignment is a scheme of writing one sequence on top of another, where the residues in one position are deemed to have a common evolutionary origin. If the same letter occurs in both sequences, then this position has been conserved in evolution. If the letters differ, it is assumed that the two derive from an ancestral letter (which could be one of the two or neither). Homologous sequences may have different lengths, though, which is generally explained through insertions or deletions in sequences. Thus, a letter or a stretch of letters may be paired with dashes in the other sequence to signify such an insertion or deletion. In such a simple evolutionarily motivated scheme, an alignment mediates the definition of a distance for two sequences. One generally assigns 0 to a match, some negative number to a mismatch, and a larger negative number to an indel. By adding these values along an alignment, one obtains a score for this alignment. A distance function for two sequences can be defined by looking for the alignment that yields the minimum score. Luckily, using dynamic programming, this minimization can be effected without explicitly enumerating all possible alignments of two sequences.

The idea of assigning a score to an alignment and then minimizing over all alignments is at the heart of all biological sequence alignment. However, many more considerations have influenced the definition of the scores and made sequence alignment applicable to a wide range of biological settings. First, note that one may either assign a distance or a similarity function to an alignment. The difference lies more in the interpretation of the values. A distance function will define negative values for mismatches or gaps and then aim at minimizing this distance. A similarity function will give high values to matches and low values to gaps and then maximize the resulting score. The basic structure of the algorithm is the same for both cases. In 1981, Smith and Waterman showed that for global alignment, i.e., when a score is computed over the entire length of both sequences, the two concepts are in fact equivalent. Thus, it is now customary to choose the setting that gives more freedom in appropriately modeling the biological setting than one is interested in. In the similarity framework, one can easily distinguish among the different possible mismatches and also among different kinds of matches. For example, a match between two tryptophanes is usually seen to be more important than a match between two alanines. For amino acids, scoring matrices have been defined to assign a score to each possible pair of amino acids.

The Smith-Waterman algorithm (Temple and Michael, 1981) is the optimal algorithm for pairwise biological sequence alignment; it gives the optimal local alignment of two sequences in a mathematical sense. Two sequences to be compared are placed on the top and at the left of a similarity matrix SM, and each element of SM is calculated using equation (8.1):

$$SM \; [i, j] = \begin{cases} SM \; [i, j-1] + gp \\ SM \; [i-1, j-1] + ss \\ SM \; [i-1, j] + gp \\ 0 \end{cases} \qquad (8.1)$$

The value of one element of *SM* is determined by the left, left upper and upper, elements. *gp* is the gap penalty for inserting a space into the sequence and *ss* is the value obtained by comparing two letters. It is often negative if the two letters are different. *gp* and *ss* can be reset by users. There will be one or more than one element with the maximum value after calculating values of all elements. Tracing back the path of each element it follows to get the maximum value, the algorithm gives one or more than one optimal local alignment between the two sequences.

8.3.2 Large Smith-Waterman Pairwise Sequence Alignment

Algorithm

The approach to parallelizing the pairwise sequence alignment is to distribute the computation along the diagonals of the similarity matrix, because the computation of element values along one diagonal is independent of that along other. But there is dependency between neighboring diagonals because the calculation of one element value relies on the values of its left, left upper and upper elements. So the parallel alignment is executed in a wavefront way, computing first the values along the first diagonal in parallel, then along the second diagonal in parallel, and so forth, through the last diagonal in parallel.

While the parallel calculation goes on, selection for the element with the highest score is also conducted, so that only the elements in the last diagonal are required to be rememberered. This greatly reduces the memory requirement.

The computing granularity can be changed to achieve the best performance according to the size of the similarity matrix and number of computing nodes available. There will be a trade-off between the granularity and load balancing. Larger granularity will reduce the communication overhead; this will improve the performance but, at the same time, it is more likely to incur load imbalance, which will degrade performance.

Implementation

Supposing we align sequences X and Y with the lengths m and n, respectively, and partition the similarity matrix into blocks, as shown in Table 8.1. The number of columns of each block is k, and the number of rows is l. Each block will be assigned to a computing node. The blocks on different nodes will be calculated in parallel. A computing node needs to get $k+l+1$ elements from left, left upper, and upper blocks when it calculates some block, and $k+1$ elements are needed from another node. By partitioning the matrix into blocks, each computing node will calculate more data (a block) after receiving the adjacent elements at one time. So, the granularity is increased and communication frequency is reduced. The values of k and l should be set according to the network bandwidth available. But the granularity should not be too large or the parallelism would be damaged.

Table 8.1. The distribution of similarity matrix over computing nodes

Sequence X

	0	1	2	...	$\lceil m/k \rceil$-1	P1
S e q u e n c e Y	$\lceil m/k \rceil$	$\lceil m/k \rceil$+1	$\lceil m/k \rceil$+2	...	$2\lceil m/k \rceil$-1	P2
	$2\lceil m/k \rceil$	$2\lceil m/k \rceil$+1	$2\lceil m/k \rceil$+2	...	$3\lceil m/k \rceil$-1	P3
	...	...	...	...	...	...
	$(t-1)\lceil m/k \rceil$	$(t-1)\lceil m/k \rceil$+1	$(t-1)\lceil m/k \rceil$+2	...	$t\lceil m/k \rceil$-1	Pt
	$t\lceil m/k \rceil$	$t\lceil m/k \rceil$+1	$t\lceil m/k \rceil$+2	...	$(t+1)\lceil m/k \rceil$-1	P1
	...	...	...	...	...	...
	$(\lceil n/l \rceil$-1$)\lceil m/k \rceil$	$(\lceil n/l \rceil$-1$)\lceil m/k \rceil$+1	$(\lceil n/l \rceil$-1$)\lceil m/k \rceil$+2	...	$\lceil n/l \rceil\lceil m/k \rceil$-1	$P\lceil n/l \rceil\%t$

8.4 Large-Scale Multiple Sequence Alignment

8.4.1 Multiple Sequence Alignment

Multiple sequence alignment is known to be NP-complete. Given a number of sequences of symbols from an alphabet, the aim is to build an alignment matrix that maximizes some function. Gaps may be introduced between symbols, and in some multiple sequence alignment formulations, the objective function includes a measure of the number and lengths of gaps.

The aim of multiple alignment is to find the sites that are homologous in all the sequences. This is a very active area of research and numerous approaches are being proposed, with varying degrees of performance depending on the nature of the sequences aligned. Most of the methods are based on a concept called progressive alignment. The methods work by constructing successive pairwise alignments; initially, two sequences are selected and aligned by pairwise methods, and the alignment is fixed. Then, a third sequence is selected and aligned with the first alignment, and this procedure is repeated until all sequences are aligned. Most methods use a "guide tree" to determine the order in which to add sequences.

Clustal W (Julie et al., 1994) is one of the most widely used multiple sequence alignment programs. This does not mean that it is ideal for all situations; it performs well with protein and protein-coding DNA sequences but is less suited to sequences like rRNA sequences.
The algorithm proceeds as follows:

1. Construct a distance matrix of all the $n(n-1)$ sequence pairs
2. Construct a guide tree by the neighbor-joining method based on the distances from the previous step
3. Progressively align sequences at the nodes in order of decreasing similarity, using sequence-sequence, sequence-alignment, and alignment-alignment alignments

There are three main parameters that can (and should) be varied when using Clustal W; the substitution cost matrix, the gap opening cost, and the gap extension cost. It is also possible to provide a user guide tree, skipping directly to step three in the procedure.

8.4.2 Large-Scale Clustal W Multiple Sequence Alignment

Algorithm

The parallelization of Clustal W is conducted in all its three stages. For the first stage, we will have two levels of parallelization. The first level of parallelization lies in the calculation conducted on the whole $n(n-1)$ pairs of sequences. Because the calculation on different sequence pair is completely independent, we get a very high degree of parallelism. The second level of parallelization lies in the pairwise sequence alignment. For achieving load balancing across all the computing nodes, we will partition all the computing nodes into groups with similar computing capacities. In the first level of parallelization, all sequence pairs will be distributed into the computing groups according to each pair's computing load, which can be estimated in terms of the length of each sequence in the pair. The second level of parallelization will be achieved in each group, i.e., parallel pairwise sequence alignment for each pair, conducted in the group the pair of sequences belongs to.

For the second stage, the calculation of the minimal value of each row in the distance matrix can be parallelized. Then, the minimal value of the matrix can be calculated according to each computing node's result. Finally, for the third stage, we exploit the parallelism that exists in the iterative loops.

Implementation

Different computing granularities can be adopted at different stages of the Clustal W algorithm in its implementation in a distributed computing environment. All sequence alignments conducted in the first stage of Clustal W are independent. They can be theirfore parallelized with smaller granularity so as to achieve maximal parallelism. But, for the second and third stages, the granularity should be bigger because there are more dependencies among the computing nodes. Smaller granularity will bring about greater communication overhead, which will offset the benefit gained from parallelism.

8.5 Load Balancing and Communication Overhead

Load balancing is a big problem for parallel computing. Load on the computing nodes with limited computing power will make other processes wait; thus, resources are wasted and performance is degraded. Since the communication overhead is relatively high in distributed systems, the interaction frequency between computing nodes should be as low as possible.

As for parallel sequence assembly and alignment, load distribution algorithms developed before can still be used to improve their performance. But they should be modified so as to be as effective as possible for load balancing in parallel biological computing. Factors this should be considered by these algorithms are communication overhead, and heterogeneity.

The interaction among computing nodes in a parallel sequence assembly algorithm is not trivial. Computing nodes have to request the l-tuples from other nodes. If one request is sent per l-tuple, there will be too many communication requests that will bring about a large amount of overhead, incurred mainly by the communication startup. So, these single requests should have to be incorporated to a request set that will be sent once. A similar situation occurs in sequence alignment, and a similar approach can be applied.

8.6 Conclusion

It is a worthwhile exercise to conduct large-scale biological sequence assembly and alignment by parallel computing to take advantage of its vast storage and computing capability. This chapter gives strategies for parallelization of the Euler sequence assembly, pairwise sequence assembly, and multiple sequence assembly and their implementation. Effective task scheduling and good computing granularity will boost the performance of biological applications running on a distributed computing environment. Good preliminary experimental results have been achieved when conducting parallel sequence assembly and alignment on clusters. However we should do more to take advantage of parallel computing. The load balancing discussed in this chapter is static, i.e., load distribution takes place at the beginning of calculation. In future work, we will investigate dynamic load balancing to adjust the load assigned to the computing nodes dynamically to be adaptable to the fluctuation of the distributed computing environment.

References

Bonfield, J.K., Smith, K.F., and Staden, R. (1995) A New DNA Sequence Assembly Program. Nucleic Acids Research 23:4992-4999.

Carol, A. Dahl, Robert, L. and Strausberg (1996.1) Human Genome Project: Revolutionizing Biology Through Leveraging Technology. Proceedings of SPIE - The International Society for Optical Engineering, pp 190-201.

Green, P. (1999) Documentation for Phrap and Cross-Match (Version 0.990319). http://www.genome.washington.edu/UWGC/analysistools/Phrap.cfm

Huang, X., Madan, A. (1999) CAP3: A DNA Sequence Assembly Program. Genome Research 9:868-877.

Julie, D.T., Desmond, G.H., Toby, J.G. and Clustal, W. (1994) Improving the Sensitivity of Progressive Multiple Sequence Alignment Through Sequence Weighting, Position-Specific Gap Penalties and Weight Matrix Choice. Nucl. Acid Res. 22: 4673–4680.

Kececioglu, J. and Myers, E. (1995) Combinatorial Algorithms for DNA Sequence Assembly. Algorithmica 13:7-51.

Liming, C., David, J. and Evgueni, L. (2000) Evolutionary Computation Techniques for Multiple Sequence Alignment. Proceedings of the IEEE Conference on Evolutionary Computation. San Diego 7:829–835.

Myers, E.M. (2002) Toward Simplifying and Accurately Formulating Fragment Assembly. Journal of Computational Biology 2(2):275-290.

Pavel, A., Pevzner and Haixu, T. and Waterman, S. (2001) An Eulerian Path Approach to DNA Fragment Assembly. Proceedings of National Academy of Sciences of the United States of America 98(17): 9748-9753.

Rajkumar, B. (1999) High Performance Cluster Computing. Vol.1, Architecture and Systems, Vol.2, Programming and Applications, Prentice Hall, Upper Saddle River, New Jersey, USA.

Shamir, R. and Tsur, D. (2002.5) Large Scale Sequencing by Hybridization. Proceedings of the Annual International Conference on Computational Molecular Biology, pp 269-277.

Sutton, G., White, O., Adams, M. and Kerlavage, A. (1995) TIGR assembler: A New Tool for Assembling Large Shotgun Sequencing Projects, Genome Science and Technology 1:9-19.

Temple, F.S. and Michael, S.W. (1981) Identification of Common Molecular Subsequences. J. Mol. Bio. 147:195–197.

Terry A Braun, Todd E Scheetz, Gregg Webster, Abe Clark, Edwin M Stone, Val C Sheffield, Thomas L Casavant (2003) Identifying Candidate Disease Genes with High-Performance Computing. The Journal of Supercomputing 26(1):7-24

The Institute for Genomic Research (2003) Benchmark Data for Genome Assembly. http://www.tigr.org/tdb/benchmark/

Weber, J. and Myers, G. (1997) Whole Genome Shotgun Sequencing. Genome Research 7:401-409.

Wei, S and Wanlei, Z. (2003.12) Large-Scale Biological Sequence Assembly and Alignment by Using Computing Grid, Lecture Notes in Computer Science, Springer-Verlag.

9 Modeling for Bioinformatics

Scott Mann and Yi-Ping Phoebe Chen

School of Information Technology
Faculty of Science and Technology
Deakin University
221 Burwood Highway, Melbourne Campus, VIC3125, Australia

9.1 Introduction

A model represents something that may be either an abstract or a concrete entity. Modeling is the process of creating a model. In science, it is normally carried out using a mathematical representation. Modeling in bioinformatics means any representation that simulates a biological process. This chapter deals with the important modeling approaches used in bioinformatics, namely, 1) Hidden Markov Model (HMM), 2) comparative modeling, 3) probabilistic modeling, and 4) molecular modeling.

Hidden Markov Model (HMM) gained ground in bioinformatics after having been applied to speech recognition. HMM will be elaborately discussed in this chapter. Comparative modeling is based on the characteristic conservation at the gene product and genomic levels. Comparative protein and comparative genomic modeling will be subsequently presented. The important probabilistic modeling approaches, namely, Bayesian networks and Stochastic Context-Free Grammars (SCFGs) will also be discussed. Finally, the molecular modeling techniques such as visualization of simple 3D molecules and analysis and simulation of large complex protein molecules will be discussed.

9.2 Hidden Markov Modeling for Biological Data Analysis

The Hidden Markov Model (HMM) is a dynamic statistical profile built from the analysis of a "training" dataset. Its major focus is on states and their transitions, and it can be visualized as a finite state machine. Probabilities are then assigned to each state (emissions) and between states (transitions). The term "hidden" arises from the fact that the state of the model at any time is a function of the input string.

Three primary roles of Hidden Markov Modeling in biological sequence analysis are discussed. They are:

- Sequence Identification
- Sequence Classification (PHMM), and
- Generation of Multiple Alignments (PHMM)

9.2.1 Hidden Markov Modeling for Sequence Identification

The applicability of the HMM to sequence identification arises from its ability to distinguish target sequences from the background of biological data. The goal of the Hidden Markov Model is to differentiate sequences that match the consensus from those that do not match. Figure 9.1 demonstrates this process clearly in a very simplified form.

Example Hidden Markov Model

- Arrows indicate transition probabilities
- Boxed data indicates emission probabilities

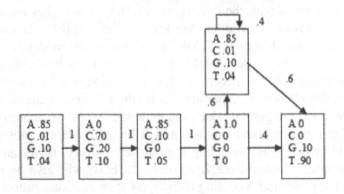

Fig. 9.1. Simplified Hidden Markov Model

In order to show the discrimination ability of such a model, two sequences are scored, "acaaat" which matches the consensus and "ttcttg", which deviates significantly from the consensus. The emission probabilities are multiplied with transition probabilities to form the score for the sequence, as can be seen below. The determination of the emission and transition probabilities is derived from alignments of target sequences comprising the training dataset.

$$P(acaaat) = 0.85*1*0.7*1*0.85*1*1*0.6*.85*0.6*0.9$$
$$\approx 1.39*10^{-1}$$

$$(9.1)$$

$$\textbf{P(ttcttg)} = 0.04*1*0.1*1*0.1*1*1*0.6*0.04*0.6*0.1$$
$$= 5.76*10^{-7}$$

$$(9.2)$$

The sequence that matches the consensus has a score 241,319 times greater than the sequence that deviates from the consensus. The ability to distinguish target sequences against non-targets is the primary role of the HMM.

Having a model that scores target regions against random nucleotide sequences would be a further improvement for more accurate discrimination. By scoring against a random sequence, the scores can be given a meaning in relation to a random sequence of nucleotides. For each nucleotide (A, C, G, and T) there is a 25% likelihood of the particular base being present at any given location. Thus, a target sequence of length n would have a probability of 0.25^n random nucleotides.

To score a sequence against this *null* model, a generic logarithmic function called "log-odds" can be applied to the frequency data in the probability matrix (Krogh, 1998). This matrix data is derived from the analysis of a training dataset. This function is essentially a ratio where the log function is applied to achieve computational efficiency as well as an additive scoring scheme. Another benefit of using the logarithm function is to avoid underflow issues arising from the computation of very small probabilities.

$$\text{Positional Score} = \ln \frac{weighting}{0.25}$$

$$(9.3)$$

With a scoring scheme implemented, attention can be devoted to model development.

The form, length, and location of the target sequence will define the structure of the HMM used for its identification. As Hidden Markov Modeling is a generic approach to sequences identification, detailed study of the target sequence must be performed before model development.

Two forms of target sequence become apparent, namely,1) regional identification and 2) specific short sequence identification. The former target category is concerned with the location of relatively large regions of genetic code; an example is the gene promoter region. The latter target category forms a small subsequence; an example is a basal promoter element within a gene sequence or a restriction enzyme site. These two forms of targets dictate the structure and complexity of the HMM.

The identification of regional targets in genomic sequences involves the construction of a trained model via sequence alignment of known target regions. Identification procedures are based on distinguishing trained targets against non target sequences. The Hidden Markov Model would contain three categories of states, namely, main, insert, and delete, that depend on the target sequence composition.

The main state represents non-gapped regions of the sequences; the insert state represents regions not conferring with the consensus sequence; and the delete state represent no emissions. Diagrammatic representation of these three states can be seen in Fig. 9.2.

The identification of short sequences presents a significant challenge; a series of generic steps is described for the construction and implementation of this approach.

Once a target has been decided upon and a draft model developed, emission and transition probabilities can be assigned via observations obtained from an appropriately large training dataset. To aid understanding, the basal promoter element called the TATA Box will be used for demonstration purposes.

A critical step is the detailed understanding of the target sequence of the TATA Box before any model development can begin. Intense research has led to the realization that this sequence has a consensus sequence of TATAAAA and exists with lengths of 5, 6, 7, and 8 nucleotides. The initial model can be seen in Fig. 9.2, prior to allowing length variability.

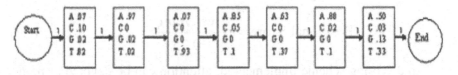

Fig. 9.2. Initial HMM with Probabilities Assigned

It can also be seen that the initial model is linear in form, with no branches, and with the transition probabilities set to 1, indicating a complete non-branching traversal. To alter this model for length variability, premature terminations were included, as shown in Fig. 9.3.

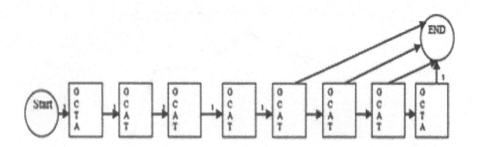

Fig. 9.3. Length Independent HMM

The inclusion of premature termination paths allows modeling of length variability. This is a generic process for any short target that varies in length. Once a model has been developed, probabilities are assigned via analysis of a training dataset. Data comprising the training set can be sourced from various locations. The NCBI Nucleotide database was queried for our case study with the search string "TATA_signal 'Homo Sapiens'". The results returned were human gene sequences containing the TATA Box annotation. By selecting the TATA_signal link on the Gen-Bank page, sequence composition could be discovered together with its position in the parent gene sequence. It is imperative that the training dataset be sufficiently large and represent true observations, and not be biased by the database search method. In general, the more representative the training dataset, the more effective the HMM will become.

By further investigating the properties of the target sequence, trends impacting the scoring scheme can be identified, as can be seen Fig. 9.4. The first five bases show a close match to the consensus, as does the sixth base; however, variation from consensus is clearly apparent beginning with the seventh base. Given the length variability beginning with the fifth base and sequence composition variability beginning with the seventh base, it was theorized that these regions would score poorly, perhaps masking the correct target sequence.

To negate the effects of scoring the latter portion of the TATA Box sequence poorly, reducing the sequences' overall score, the "Cumulative/Single Calculation" algorithm was applied.

Assigning the most highly conserved region's scoring significance to the region of highest variability would have masked the correct target site; the solution was to score these two regions differently.

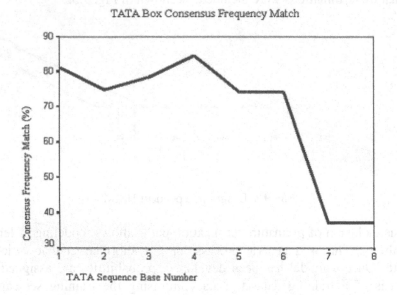

TATA Box Consensus Frequency Match

Fig. 9.4. Training Sequence TATA Box Consensus Match

Greater scoring significance is given to the first five bases, which score highly if correct. Less importance is attributed to the last three bases, as the variability incurred in scoring these regions may mask potentially correct scores from the first five bases. To score these regions appropriately, cumulative scoring can be applied to the first five bases. Variability within this region greatly impacts the cumulative score, which is a desirable attribute given that this region matches the consensus closely and variation is unwanted.

For the last three bases, which represent considerable variability, the single highest state score is used to represent the score for this region. This allows for the observed variation, but without penalizing the scores of the prior five bases.

The scores for the most conserved region are added together with the highest score from the remaining three bases to equal the final score for the potential TATA Box sequence.

This generic scoring optimization can be applied to any target sequence where deviation from the consensus occurs at a distinct level within the sequence, as seen in Fig. 9.4. Implemented as a computational scheme, the appropriate algorithm is outlined as follows

START:
> *While not at end of file*
>> *For each base*
>>> *Get substring of 8 bases*
>>>> **Calculate 5 base cumulative score**
>>>> **Calculate highest score of last 3 bases**
>>>> **Add the two scores together**
>>> *Return the highest scoring sequence*

END.

To effectively model deviation from the consensus occurring in the most highly conserved region, an optimization called consensus blurring can be applied to the scoring scheme. To implement this scheme, the score of the most highly conserved base position has its weighted score inverted. A consensus match grater than 95% at the nucleotide position is considered acceptable for consensus blurring. The effect of inverting the score of the most conserved base allows for target sequences varying in this position to score higher. Inverting or lowering the score of other bases would not necessarily lead to an improvement in correct target identification. Except the highest consensus matching base, others should not have their scores modified, as the variability from the consensus would be too wide, resulting in a high degree of false positive identification.

The steps involved in the short sequence identification method can be summarized as follows:

1. Gain a clear understanding of the target for identification
   - Length
   - Composition
   - Location
   - Deviation trends
2. Use the most representative dataset available
3. Model Length Variability, if applicable
4. Implement "Cumulative-Single" Scoring, if applicable
5. Implement consensus blurring, if applicable

In addition to these scoring optimizations, the co-location algorithm can be applied if the target sequence is located in known proximity to another highly conserved sequence. The goal of this algorithm is to reduce the number of false positive results by placing the scores into a positional context. This approach uses n HMMs developed for each marker sequence. When the sequences are scored, the highest scores are compared to a positional consensus framework to identify the correct target. Graphically these optimizations are presented in a flow diagram, as seen Fig. 9.5.

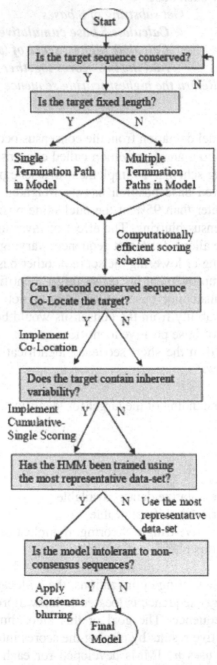

Fig. 9.5. Flow Chart for Short Target Sequence Model Development

When applying Hidden Markov Models to nucleic acid sequence identification, limitations are prominent.

The biological data under analysis is limited to a very small alphabet {A,C,T,G}. The greater yhe number of possible paths, the more accurate recognition of target matching sequences will become. Given only four bases per state, there is a 25% likelihood of a random occurrence matching the consensus base. As a consequence, a consensus base per state has a comparable background likelihood of 25% at each state. This value represents a very high background to distinguish a consensus score.

When applied to protein analysis, the alphabet is expanded by default to 20, accounting for each amino acid. This increase in the size of the alphabet significantly lowers the random likelihood of a unit matching the target at each state of the HMM.

The larger the alphabet, the lower the likelihood of random occurrences matching the consensus sequence under analysis. This is especially pertinent for sequences of considerable length. Protein analysis, having a five fold larger alphabet than nucleic acid, is better suited to HMM processing in this form.

To highlight these limitations using the case study, the TATA Box consensus sequence of length seven bases was chosen. When compared to the number of bases within the genes under analysis, the seven base TATA Box sequence has a $1/4^7 = 1/16384$ base probability of occurring; considering the typical length of human genes, the likelihood of encountering more than one matching sequence is quite high. This assumption is based on a GC content of 50%. Much work has centred around using HMMs for modeling large sequences of proteins. As an analogous example, a small polypeptide chain of seven amino acids has a $1/20 = 1/1.28 \times 10^9$ amino acid likelihood; the occurrence magnitude is significantly smaller than the seven base DNA sequence analysis.

In summary, the greater the target length and the larger the alphabet, the less likely that the target sequence will occur in the data under analysis.

As mentioned earlier, regional identification solves one of these limitations, namely, overcoming the short target sequence. With target regions in tens to hundreds of nucleotides in length, the chance of locating more than one target in the parent sequence is diminished significantly.

The effectiveness of short sequence identification is constrained by these two limitations; however, regional identification is less affected by short target lengths.

The approaches presented up to this point provide a platform for future improvement of current HMM identification techniques. The combination of regional analysis and short sequence "local" analysis would generate a multiple layer HMM process. Initially, a large model developed for regional identification would be enacted on the data. Once candidate regions have been identified, a second layer of processing would be executed, leading to the location of conserved markers in a positional framework using co-ocation, as discussed earlier. This second level of processing would add a higher degree of accuracy to the regional location.

This scheme mutually benefits both the regional and the local model. Improvements in accuracy to both models can be achieved, as can be seen Fig. 9.6.

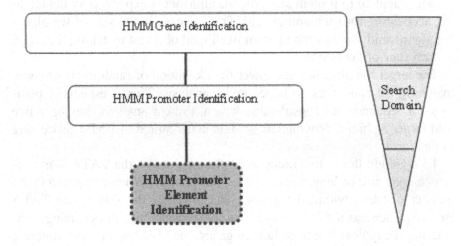

Fig. 9.6. Hierarchical Framework for Identification (not to scale)

Fig. 9.6, shows the relationship among three levels of identification. The top HMM is concerned with gene identification within genomic data, acting as a local model. A HMM promoter identification itself has a local model for promoter element identification. This scheme begins with a search domain encompassing the genome of the organism. At each successive stage, this search domain decreases as more locally significant smaller target sequences are located. The dotted box in Fig. 9.6 represents the end target for analysis. As discussed previously, the limitation of the short target sequence is diminished at each stage with the decrease in the search domain. The likelihood of more than one consensus matching target is therefore low. In this manner, the regional model is made more accurate by its associated dependent local HMM sub-models. The local models are also benefited by the identification using the shortened search domain.

A comparison of HMM techniques is presented in table 9.1.

The key outcomes presented in Table 9.1 highlight the benefits of using the combinational framework. First, the combined model has the ability to

identify targets independent of length. The allowance for regional and local identification can resolve sequences of both length categories. The
combined model is least affected by the limitations imposed by HMMs on
nucleic acid sequence identification. The short target length limitation is
overcome by the narrowed search domain, and the alphabet limitation is
lessened by the accuracy obtained via this multilayered approach to improve identification. Flexibility is most apparent in the regional model, as
the opportunity to model variation from the consensus of a large sequence
length is available. The combined model incorporates both the regional
and the local model; as such, there is a balance between the flexibility of
the regional model and the rigidity of the local model. The predicted outcomes of these techniques results in a combined model that offers greater
accuracy through multiple layers of identification and verification.

Table 9.1. HMM Form Analysis

Criteria / HMM Form	Local	Regional	Combined
Length of Target	Small 5-20 bases	Large 20-200 bases	Any length
Limitations	Alphabet, short target length	Alphabet	Low
Flexibility of Consensus	None	Some	Little
Predicted Accuracy	Domain Range Dependent else Low	Average	Good

HMMs represent a viable approach to sequence identification with the
applicability to both nucleic acid and amino acid analysis. Presented in this
chapter is the application of HMMs to sequence identification, primarily
focusing on nucleic acid sequences; however, this is a generic approach
applicable to many nucleic acid search routines and has good correlations
to protein analysis. The approaches presented here represents a foundation
for further development of Hidden Markov Modeling for sequence identification.

9.2.2 Hidden Markov Modeling for Sequence Classification

Sequence classification is generally concerned with the identification of
protein domains. Specifically, these domains are classified as conserved
structures, or behaving as discrete functional units.

In order to model family identification, Profile Hidden Markov Models
(PHMMs) are introduced. A generalized structure of the PHMM that

shows the main components is presented in Fig. 9.7. PHMMs follow the conventions of HMMs with the term "Profile" being attributed to its trained structure representing a profile of the target under analysis.

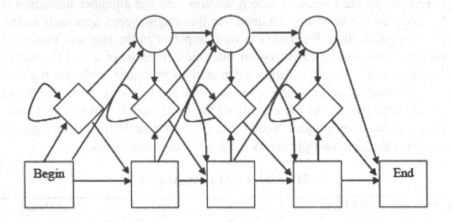

Fig. 9.7. Sample HMM Profile

Figure 9.7 demonstrates the main features of the HMM profile. The PHMM is derived from multiple alignment. The details of an appropriate multiple alignment portion of Fig. 9.7 are provided in Table 9.2 with three consensus columns.

Each node in Fig. 9.7 corresponds to a column in Table 9.2. It has a main state (box), an insert state (diamond), and a delete state (circle). The main states (boxes) represent data appearing in the columns in Table 9.2. The delete states (circles) represent non-existing (silent residue) data alignment gaps. The insert states (diamonds) represent additional data allowing sequences to include data between the columns of Table 9.2. The circular arrow to the insert state indicates that more than one such insertion of data is permissible.

Table 9.2. Amino Acid Data to Construct PHMM

Sequence Position		
1	2	3
D	W	W
D	W	W
E	W	W
G	W	T
D	W	W

Practical applications of this approach are realized while modeling a domain. Figure 9.8 shows the details of the SH3 domain in the extracted data (Krogh, 1998).

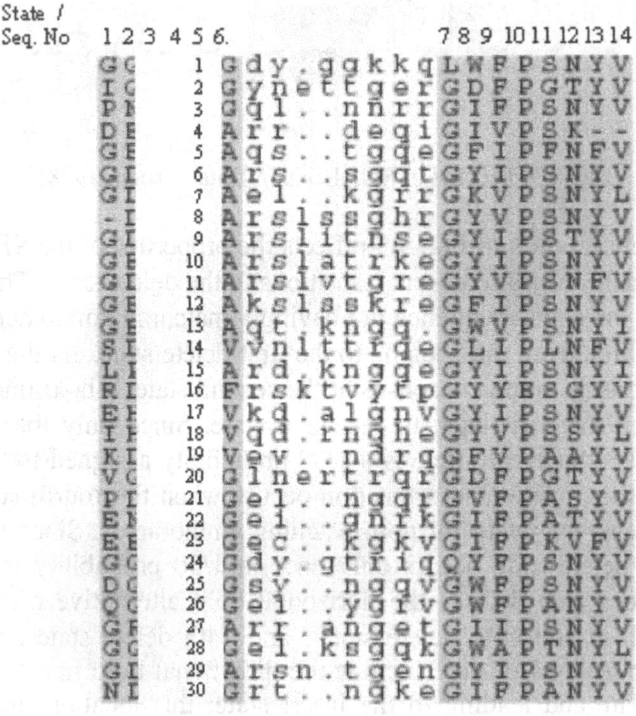

```
State /
Seq. No    1 2 3 4 5 6.                    7 8 9 10 11 12 13 14
G G    1   G d y . g q k k q L W F P S N Y V
I G    2   G y n e t t g e r G D F P G T Y V
P N    3   G q l . . n n r r G I F P S N Y V
D E    4   A r r . . d e q i G I V P S K - -
G E    5   A q s . . t g d e G F I P F N F V
G I    6   A r s . . s g q t G Y I P S N Y V
G I    7   A e l . . k g r r G K V P S N Y L
- I    8   A r s l s s g h r G Y V P S N Y V
G I    9   A r s l i t n s e G Y I P S T Y V
G E   10   A r s l a t r k e G Y I P S N Y V
G I   11   A r s l v t g r e G Y V P S N F V
G E   12   A k s l s s k r e G F I P S N Y V
G E   13   A q t . k n q q . G W V P S N Y I
S I   14   V v n l t t f d e G L I P L N F V
L I   15   A r d . k n g q e G Y I P S N Y I
R I   16   F r s k t v y t p G Y Y E S G Y V
E F   17   V k d . a l q n v G Y I P S N Y V
I F   18   V q d . r n q h e G Y V P S S Y L
K I   19   V e v . . n d r q G F V P A A Y V
V G   20   G l n e r t r q r G D F P G T Y V
P I   21   G e l . . n q q r G V F P A S Y V
E N   22   G e l . . g n r k G I F P A T Y V
E E   23   G e c . . k g k v G I F P K V F V
G G   24   G d y . g t r i q Q Y F P S N Y V
D G   25   G s y . . n g q v G W F P S N Y V
Q G   26   G e l . . y g r v G W F P A N Y V
G F   27   A r r . a n g e t G I I P S N Y V
G G   28   G e l . k s q q k G W A P T N Y L
G I   29   A r s n . t g e n G Y I P S N Y V
N I   30   G r t . . n g k e G I F P A N Y V
```

Fig. 9.8. SH3 Domain Amino Acid Alignment

In Fig. 9.8, the shaded regions represent the most conserved portions of the sequence, with the white lower case regions showing the most variability. When constructing a PHMM to suit this data, the main states are shown with a shade and the insert states are shown in the white background. The PHMM model constructed (Krogh, 1998) using the SAM software package (UCSC February 2004) is shown in Fig. 9.9.

The PHHM in Fig. 9.9, can be interpreted as bold nondirectional lines indicating horizontal traversal, with directional lines indicating traversal to the insert state (after the sixth state). Dashed lines indicate a traversal of low probability to the delete state. Main states are represented as rectangles, and correspond to the shaded regions of Fig. 9.8. Insert states are diamond shaped, with circular delete states showing the state number annotation.

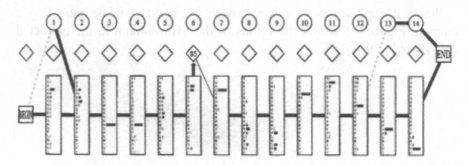

Fig. 9.9. PHMM of SH3 Domain Data (Krogh, 1998)

Further observation of Fig. 9.9 reflects the properties of the SH3 domain data. The dashed lines represent transitions to the delete state. The first one arises from the eighth sequence not having a matching amino acid, leading to the transition from the "begin" to the first delete state. As the eighth sequence conforms to the consensus at the second state, a bold line is drawn to indicate a traversal back to the main state. Since only the eighth sequence shows this trend there is a 1/30 probability assigned to this transition. The other delete state transition occurs when the fourth sequence at state 13 begins two states of non-matching amino acids. Since this transition to the delete state occurs only once, a 1/30 probability is assigned. This sequence also defines the horizontal bold alternative traversals between the 13th and 14th delete states, and 14th delete state and the end state. Other features of note include the directional bold line arising from the sixth state and leading to the insert state; this location indicates the transition from the main state (shaded in Fig. 9.8) to the variable insert state (white in Fig. 9.8). The number "85" located in the diamond indicates the probability in percentage terms of self insert transitions occurring in the insert region of the sequence.

As mentioned previously, the largest and most representative training dataset will benefit the effectiveness of the HMM. Related to this statement is the issue of over-fitting, whereby the model is trained with little evidential training data, resulting in diminished value of the result. Overfitting is an issue when model parameter data is obtained from a limited dataset. Datasets containing amino acids of a narrow range will mask the recognition of valid sequences containing variations from those in the training set. An example would be a state containing amino acids that have emission probabilities G, S and L. If a candidate sequence was scored, and contained an amino acid that differed from G, S, L, there would be an occurrence probability of 0. This problem, defined as over-fitting, makes the trained model inflexible with regard to data differing from the training dataset.

To partially solve this issue, techniques classified as regularization (Karchin, 1999) have been developed. One such technique, called pseudocounting, involves inserting false occurrences into the training dataset. These counts are added to amino acids regardless of occurrence in the columns of the training dataset. Given that there exist 20 distinct amino acids along with the existing amino acids in the columnar data for the state in the model, there will exist $(20x + n)$ counts, where n is defined as the number of rows (number of sequences) in the training dataset and x represents the pseudocount number. For a training dataset of five sequences with pseudocount 1, there will exist $20 \times 1 + 5 = 25$ amino acids for the column. The inclusion of pseudocounts affords the model greater flexibility when encountering valid candidate sequences deviating from the training dataset. The act of adding a count to all amino acids assumes that each amino acid is equally likely to be present in that state. This assumption does not hold true for many sequences, and an appropriate solution would be to adjust the counts relative to the observed amino acids in the sequences.

A more complicated and representative method, called Dirichlet mixtures (Sjolander et al., 1996), relies upon statistical analysis of the amino acid positional distributions within a dataset of protein sequences. The Dirichlet density forms the basis of the Dirichlet mixtures, and is defined as the probability density of the entire set of possible amino acid combinations at a specified position. The assignment of differential probabilities to characteristic distributions enables a distinction to be made. Differential probabilities can be assigned to amino acids that present a common identifying feature, namely, hydrophobic behavior (Karchin, 1999). The importance of such approaches embeds detailed protein structural data into the parameter elicitation process of constructing the HMM. Once identified, Dirichlet densities are combined with the observed values to equal the pseudocount for the amino acid.

The profile applicability of Hidden Markov Models is suited to many situations and is primarily involved with classification of protein sequences into an encompassing family. The word "profile" applies to the structure of the model, which acts as an identification mechanism capturing the key features of the family under analysis. The profile contains specific information relating to sequence composition, insert and delete regions, regions of conservation, and the categorization of residues associated with their positions. This has been highlighted in Fig. 9.9, which shows a profile for the SH3 Domain. Practical examples of Hidden Markov Modeling for family recognition can be found in the literature

(Baldi et al., 1994) for the identification of the globin, immunoglobulins, and kinase family members.

The essential elements that form the basis of PHMM generation for the identification of protein family members are discussed in this chapter. In nutshell, this process involves the model development for sequence identification, where parameters are obtained from alignments that constitute the training dataset. Issues concerning overfitting have been discussed in view of possible solutions. The major steps used in PHMM generation are summarized below:

1. Gain a clear understanding of the target domain for identification
   • Length
   • Composition
   • Location
   • Deviation trends
2. Use the most representative dataset available
3. Model the variability insert regions and consensus regions as main states
4. Use pseudocounts if necessary
5. Apply Dirichlet techniques for more complex sequences

The resultant PHMM that evolved out of these steps will serve as the basis for classification of sequences based on the trained model. Using this framework, the assignment of candidate sequences to protein families may give contextual insights into their functions.

9.2.3 Hidden Markov Modeling for Multiple Alignment Generation

The generation of multiple alignments is a task of great significance, with correlations to homology studies. The alignment process maybe applied to gather sequences of similar structure and function. Using HMMs for this purpose represents a significant improvement over traditional human meditated approaches.

In order to implement multiple alignment using profile HMMs, many algorithms are to be considered; however, the Viterbi algorithm is principally chosen to align candidate sequences to the pre-constructed model. The Viterbi algorithm is well suited to this task, as an optimal path is found using efficient recursive techniques.

The Viterbi algorithm is best described through an example, as shown in Fig. 9.10.

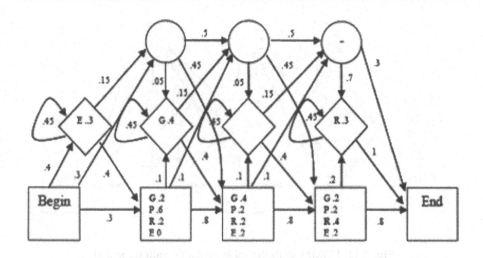

Fig. 9.10. PHMM with multiple paths for EGGR

Given a candidate sequence of EGGR, there exists more than one path through the model. To resolve the most likely path through the model, the Viterbi algorithm is applied; its component matrix is shown in Table 9.3. The columns represent states from the model and the rows represent the candidate sequences' amino acids.

Table 9.3. Viterbi Matrix Probability Data

	I_0	I_1	M_1	I_2	M_2	I_3	M_3
E	0.12						
G		0.003	0.08				
G					0.16		
R						0.021	0.32

The steps invoved in Viterbi Algorithm used is given below:

1. $P(E_{I0}) = (Start_{trans} \times E_{I0emiss})$ as the first element
2. $P(G_{I1}) = ((I_0 \rightarrow D_0)_{trans} \times (D_0 \rightarrow I_1)_{trans} \times (G_{I1emiss}))$ & $P(G_{M1}) = ((I_0 \rightarrow M_1)_{trans} \times (G_{M1emiss}))$
3. $P_{MAX}(I_1,M_1)$ back pointer set to I_0
4. Repeat (2)-(3) substituting amino acids until matrix complete

The resultant most probable path is shown in Fig. 9.11 in bold.

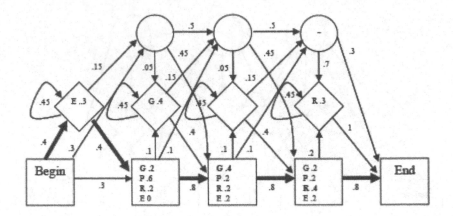

Fig. 9.11. PHMM with the most probable path indicated

When the back trace has been completed, the sequence aligns effectively with the PHMM. Consequently, the multiplication of probability data results in a score for the sequence. The magnitude of this score determines the status of the sequence being included in a multiple alignment.

The key steps in this process are listed below:

1. Develop a trained model by studying preformed multiple alignments consisting of the training dataset.
2. Use dynamic programming techniques to score candidate sequences using the Viterbi algorithm.
3. Include the candidate as part of the multiple alignment generated depending of the score from the Viterbi output.

9.2.4 Conclusion

The HMM represents a framework for identification and classification of biological data. There exist several limitations to HMMs besides the limited alphabet and short target sequences discussed earlier. Statistically, the multiplicative product of the sequence probability states defines the score for the sequence where the composition of each state acts independently of the others'. This assumption of independence is not necessarily true. For example, the amino acids of similar properties are clustered together, and hydrophobic regions highlight this problem. Identification of biologically significant chain interactions within the polypeptide chain cannot be carried out with models in this form, As a result, internal interactions representing hydrogen bonding or disulphide bridging cannot be predicted.

This section has highlighted three applications of HMMs for biological sequence data analysis. The HMM represents a valuable tool for sequence identification at multiple levels of length and complexity. The modeling of a target family represents a generic profile allowing for the classification of candidate sequences. Multiple alignment generation is considered to be highly time consuming but can be executed efficiently using the PHMM. These topics have been discussed at the introductory level, and insights into their operation and applicability serve as a basis for their use and future development.

9.3 Comparative Modeling

Comparative modeling is a computational technique associated with characteristic conservation at the gene product and genomic levels. Major applications include the discovery of structural/functional characteristics of a polypeptide product and cross-genome organizational studies. The rationale behind such studies relates the gap between known protein sequences (750,000) and known structures (17,000) (Westhead, 2004). With structural knowledge, functional insights can be gained. Additionally, development of drugs via structural design can be achieved. Not only can protein structures be predicted, but evolutionary trends can also be identified; this specifically applies to divergent evolutionary studies, and is achieved by comparing the novel sequence with sequences of known "template" or structural/functional characteristics and inferring such characteristics. In the case of the genome, the principle of comparison is still used on a much larger scale.

In this chapter, techniques used in comparative modeling of protein products and comparative genomics will be discussed at a high level.

9.3.1 Protein Comparative Modeling

A major prediction task that arises from the application of comparative modeling to protein analysis is the elucidation of structural and functional characteristics. Differential complexities in characteristic identification may indicate that structural features are easier to identify from functional characteristics (Westhead, 2004). It is suggested that protein structure is relatively conserved, irrespective of the functional changes. e.g., altered enzyme specificity or major changes from enzyme to structural protein.

The steps to be followed to create an experimental framework for protein comparative modeling are presented below:

1. Begin with a novel "target" sequence.
2. Collate "template" sequences of a similar known structure with the target.
3. Perform multiple alignments of the template sequences with the target.
4. Make predictions of structurally conserved regions and insert/delete regions.
5. Create a model of the predicted region(s) in step 4 that accounts for insert/delete modifications.
6. Add side chains to the model in step 5.
7. Evaluate and refine the model.

The target novel sequence forms the basis of the comparative process. However, the goal is to discover properties of this sequence by comparison with known "template" sequences. The collation of template sequences is based on sequence comparison methods, including the Position-Specific Iterated (PSI)-BLAST method, or via sequence-structure threading methods that utilise fold assignment and alignment, as stated by Baker and Sali (2001).

A simple method for collation is also available (Conteras-Moreira and Bates, 2002). It includes similarity searching against a database of protein structures such as the PDB (Berman et. al., 2000) using a nonredundant sequence database adjunct to the PDB (Bates and Sternberg, 1999). To improve sequence collation via the PSI-BLAST method, Conteras-Moreira and Bates have developed an approach called Domain Fishing to remove false templates and return higher quality template sequences.

Once a set of templates has been created, multiple alignment can be conducted through the use of online tools. Model development follows the multiple alignment task and is required to understand the three-dimensional structure of protein that confers biological functions. Modeling can be used in protein engineering for the design of proteins for therapeutic applications (Kemp, 2004). Construction of the model is based on the protein core, loops, and side chains. This is one of the methods used in construction. Another method is based on calculation of atom coordinates from approximately conserved template atoms (Levitt, 1992). A third method is based on the distance geometry optimizations that seek to satisfy the spatial restraints of the sequence-template alignment (Havel and Snow, 1991; Sali and Blundell, 1993; and Kolinski et al., 2001). After the model is created, further necessary refinements can be made by including bond geometry using energy minimization techniques.

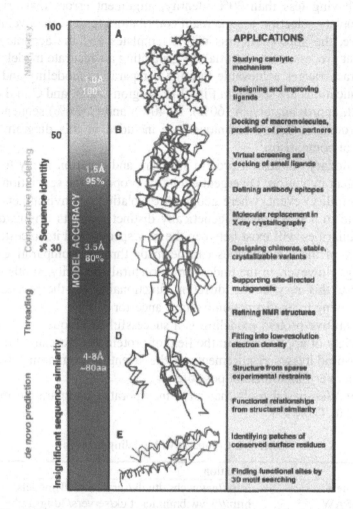

Fig. 9.12. Protein Model Accuracy and Application (Baker 2001)

The accuracy of the resultant model is dependent on a number of factors. The sequences can be grouped into categories based on model errors and a category defines the application of the model (Baker and Sali, 2001), as shown in Fig. 9.12. High accuracy models are regarded as those with the target sequence having greater than 50% identity with the template sequences. Models in this category have 1Å root mean square (RMS) error for the main chain atoms. Errors are primarily attributed to incorrect side chain packing and shifts/distortions of the main chain atoms and loops. Medium accuracy models represent 30% to 50% of sequence identity and have 90% of the main chain atoms with 1.5Å RMS error. Alignment faults also contribute to the errors. Low accuracy models are defined by the sequence having less than 30% identity; alignment errors that arise from poor template selection are the main contributors toward the overall error. Therefore, the appropriateness of the templates and the accuracy of the alignment processes are essential for generating an accurate model.

Accuracy ranges achievable through comparative modeling and associated applications are shown in Fig. 9.12. Regions A, B, and C in the figure represent, approximately, A (60%), B (40%), and C (30%) sequence identities. Protein modeling techniques are included in this diagram for the purpose of comparison.

Evolutionary studies on protein structure and function apply to studies of divergent evolution. Divergent evolution proposes the speciation (sexual incompatibility) event, where geographic isolation or environment factors contribute to a new species genetically distinct from its originators. Genetic similarities will exist between the new species and its ancestors. The discovery of these similarities can be made through comparative protein modeling. However, in the underlying structural similarity, subtle changes may exist; this may confer different functionality on the resultant gene product owing to its distinction from its ancestors.

Comparative protein modeling is a successful technique and it offers a wide variety of applications in the field of protein structure and functionality. It also addresses requirements of the scientific community when experimental verification is not possible.

Useful Web-based tools that have incorporated comparative modeling are listed in Table 9.4.

Table 9.4. Comparative Modeling Servers

Name	Location
CPHmodels	http://www.cbs.dtu.dk/services/CPHmodels/
3D-JIGSAW	http://www.bmm.icnet.uk/servers/3djigsaw/
SWISS-MODEL	http://www.expasy.ch/swissmod/

9.3.2 Comparative Genomic Modeling

Comparative genomic studies center on discovering functionally and evolutionarily significant information by comparing genomes. The identification of cross-genome protein fmilies may lead to targeting drugs better when the targets appearing in bacterial genomes do not correlate with the human genome, leading to antibiotic targets. Gene classification can be further enhanced with the availability of evolutionary groupings. This enables tracing structure/functionality back to a single ancestral gene; therefore, classification of the target gene is derived from its ancestral form.

Comparative genomics can be conducted at two levels, namely, 1) the DNA sequence level and 2) the protein level. At the DNA sequence level, it is done by comparing intergenic regions, whereas at the protein level it is done by comparing the coding sequences.

The main feature of comparative genomics is the alignment of genomes. This process maps nucleotides from one genome to another genome, and includes gaps to allow a greater degree of alignment. Precompiled alignments are listed in Table 9.5. These resources allow the researcher to perform comparative studies without the computational power involved in the alignment of two entire genomes.

Table 9.5. Precompiled Genome Alignments

Server / Browser	Included Genomes	URL
VISTA Genome Browser	human, mouse, rat	http://pipeline.lbl.gov
UCSC Genome Browser	mammals, worms	http://genome.ucsc.edu
EnteriX & GALA	enteric bacteria/human, mouse, rat	http://bio.cse.psu.edu
Ensembl	worms, fish, insects, mammals	http://www.ensembl.org

Alignment algorithms include the recursive hierarchical alignment of genomes at extended match locations used in the GLASS method (Batzoglou et al., 2000) and the decomposition of the genome into small overlapping segments for alignment used in the Wobble Aware Bulk Aligner (WABA) method (Kent and Zahler, 2000).

When studying coding regions specifically, understanding the terms ortholog and paralog is very important. As defined by Tatusov et al. (1997), orthologs are genes in different species that have evolved from a common ancestral gene via speciation. Paralogs are defined as genes related by duplication within the genome. Orthologs differ from paralogs in that the functionality of orthologs is partially retained, while paralogs generally develop new functionality. Graphically, this relationship is shown in Fig. 9.13. The identification of orthologs is the primary goal in comparative genomics, allowing for prediction of gene function, phylogenetic tree mapping, and comparative genome organization.

The identification of orthologs is associated with the location of clusters of orthologous groups (COGs). Each COG consists of orthologous genes or orthologous groups of paralogs from three or more phylogenetic lineages. Thus any two proteins from different lineages that belong to the same COG are orthologous, while each COG is thought to have evolved from a single ancestral gene. The identification of COGs was implemented by Tatusov using pairwise sequence alignments of 17,967 sequences from seven complete genomes, and forms the basis of the NCBI COG Database.

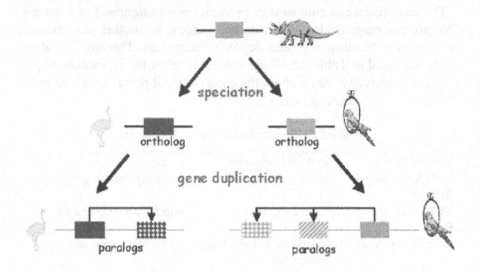

Fig. 9.13. Evolutionary Relationships (Suter-Crazzolara and Kurapkat 2001)

As an outcome of comparative genomics, specifically, of eukaryote studies, the identification of human disease genes has been made (Purdue, 2000). Orthologs of human disease genes can be seen in Table 9.6. Mutual identification schemes are possible with this approach. Cloned human disease genes can be used to search other eukaryote genomes. Alternatively, eukaryote disease genes can be used to search for orthologs in the human genome.

This chapter has briefly introduced the various aspects of comparative modeling that point to a promising and bright future for bioinformatics research. As discussed earlier, these processes offer a method for deciphering a novel protein structure and functionality. As a result, evolutionary paths can be identified in relation to the ancestral forms. Comparative modeling on the genomic scale has shown the ability to classify proteins, highlight differences in genome structure, locate antibiotic targets for new drug treatments, show evolutionary changes at the genomic level, and provide the ability to identify human disease genes. Comparative modeling has therefore been shown to be one of the most powerful techniques in bioinformatics, with a broad and diverse range of applications that may offer future research very promising results.

Table 9.6. Proposed Orthologs of Human Disease Genes (Purdue 2000)

Disease (gene)	Yeast	C. elegans	D. melanogaster
Ataxia telangiectasia (ATM)	+	+	+
Glycerol Kinase Deficiency (GK)	+	+	+
Hereditary non-polyposis colon cancer (MLH1 or MSH2)	+	+	+
Wilson Disease (WND)	+	+	+
Duchene muscular Dystrophy (DMD)	-	+	+
Marfan Syndrome (FBN1)	-	+	+
Neurofibromatosis type 2 (NF2)	-	+	+
Polycystic Kidney Disease type 2 (PLK2)	-	+	+
Multiple cancers (p53)	-	-	+
Multiple Endocrine Neoplasia type 1 (MEN)	-	-	+
Neurofibromatosis type 1 (NF1)	-	-	+
Juvenile Parkinson's Disease (parkin)	-	-	+

9.4 Probabilistic Modeling

Enforced by the nonconforming variable nature of biological sequences, probabilistic modeling is an essential element of data analysis. Many probabilistic approaches exist in the emerging field of bioinformatics. A brief overview that covers a limited subset of this modeling family is provided.

9.4.1 Bayesian Networks

Bayesian networks offer a combination of graph and probability theory; in the bioinformatics context, these networks can represent probabilistic connections between genes. The modeling of regulatory links is an application of Bayesian networks. For a regulatory link between two genes, knowing the value of one gene allows the prediction of the value of another gene in the system. As an example, a link from gene X to gene Y may indicate that if gene X is high, gene Y has 80% chance of being high, 17% chance of being medium, and 3% chance of being low. Based on the ability of these networks to represent probabilistic connections between genes, Bayesian networks have been used to analyze expression data (Friedman et al., 2000). The advent of microarray chips and the massive amount of data relating to the genomic complement of gene expression that can be retrieved simultaneously have made such processes a necessity. Once a model is developed, questions relating to gene expression level under different experimental conditions, and gene interrelationships via direct and indirect dependencies, can be answered.

9.4.2 Stochastic Context-Free Grammars

Within the context of bioinformatics applications, Stochastic Context-Free Grammars (SCFGs) are employed in RNA structural analysis. SCFGs form the foundation model for modeling the patterns in RNA families within the RFAM database (Washington University, 2003). SCFGs have been applied within comparative genomics to identify RNA genes across two different but related organisms. A comparative analysis of the potential homologs in RNA secondary structure indicates the presence of an RNA gene and a probable secondary structure. Models for RNA secondary structure prediction have also been proposed (Eddy and Eddy, 2000).

9.4.3 Probabilistic Boolean Networks

Probabilistic Boolean Networks extend the properties of Boolean networks to determine gene-gene interactions. The advantage of Boolean networks stems from their ability to qualitatively model genetic interactions. As an example, the interactions that govern the activity of the Rb protein (Shmulevich et al., 2002) are shown in Fig. 9.14.

In Fig. 9.14, arrows represent activation lines while bars indicate inhibitions. The right side of the figure shows the logic modeling of this scenario with four inputs and one output. The cell cycle that explains the regulation consists of a series of states modeled with ON/OFF Boolean semantics, as can be seen in Fig. 9.14. The modeling of cellular interactions accommodates the actual states the cell transits through during its life cycle.

In reality, interactions are not as simple as shown in Fig. 9.14. A more flexible method is needed, as more than one pathway may contribute to gene regulation. To account for such flexibility, a probabilistic approach called Probabilistic Boolean Networks was developed (Shmulevich et al., 2002). This was implemented by extending the Boolean Networks to include more than one function per node. The basic component of such a network is shown in Fig. 9.15.

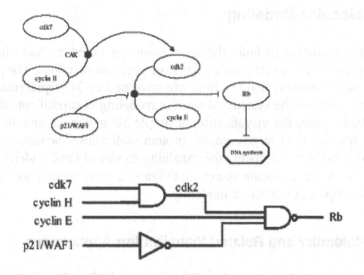

Fig. 9.14. Boolean cell regulation representation (Shmulevich et al., 2002)

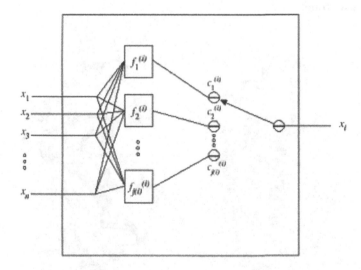

Fig. 9.15. Basic unit of Probabilistic Boolean Networks (Shmulevich et al., 2002)

Figure 9.15 shows the alternative functions ("predictors") that share common inputs $x1$ through xn to produce outputs of which one is selected. An entire probabilistic Boolean network would consist of n such units. The flexibility introduced by this probabilistic enhancement allows probabilistic Boolean networks to be used as a tool for modeling gene regulatory networks.

9.5 Molecular Modeling

Molecular modeling includes the set of computer-based methods that construct, present, and modify molecular structures and reactions. The properties of such structures and reactions are governed by 3D representation of the participants in the system. Molecular modeling is carried out on many scales that include the visualization of simple 3D molecules and the analysis and simulation of large complex protein molecules. The outcome from molecular modeling is mainly the capability to identify and understand the properties of the molecule under investigation. This section will discuss the major topics in molecular modeling.

9.5.1 Molecular and Related Visualization Applications

Molecular visualization is considered a valuable technique that aids the interpretation and understanding of experimental results. Presented in this chapter are current visualization techniques, and their implications, to assist the researcher.

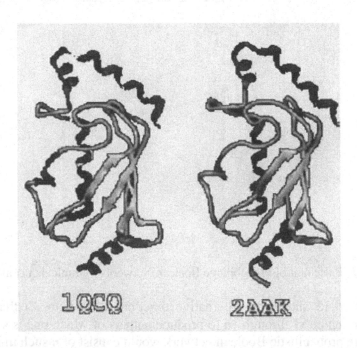

Fig. 9.16. Homologous Enzymes 1QCQ (Arabidopsis Thaliana) and 2AAK (Baker's Yeast) (Ravichandran, November 2003)

Homology studies are enhanced through the use of visualization techniques where domains can be visualized and the differential properties of the proteins can be discovered. In techniques like comparative modeling, discussed earlier, visualization can indicate resultant 3D differences between the target and template sequences. Figure 9.16 show two homologous enzymes of family Ubiquitin conjugating enzymes showing structural differences owing to their 43% sequence identity.

This technique is a powerful tool in the modeling of enzyme-substrate interactions. The active enzyme site is routinely modeled to determine chemical interactions with the substrate, providing process knowledge to the investigator. The active site of the enzyme representing the functional center can be investigated through molecular modeling to determine its composition and properties (Varfolomeev et al., 2002).

Visualization techniques are applied to drug design by modeling the drug targets, thereby enabling synthetic construction of the drug in a process called structure-based drug design. Such approaches focus on identifying molecules capable of disrupting the detrimental effects of the target molecule. A case study involves the search for deactivating HIV protease. The first step in such a process involves modeling the target molecule, in this case HIV protease. With the structure generated from processes like X-ray crystallography, the molecular model can be studied to locate a compound "inhibitor", either in a chemical library or via synthesis, to block the active site of the enzymes. The structure-based drug design approach has significant benefits over traditional drug development methods. When a structure is modeled visually, the design of drugs is a logical next step, whereas trial-and-error modifications of pre-existing drugs are carried out in the traditional manner. This approach promises more rapid drug discovery than traditional techniques. For instance, using HIV protease inhibitors, three drugs were developed in eight years, whereas using the traditional method, 10 to 15 costly years were spent in development (Zapp, 2002).

Much interest and research has been done and will continue to be done on the use of expression arrays to determine levels of gene expression under disease or other defined conditions. The capture and accurate representation of the massive amount of data from such studies has led to the development of the following visualization techniques:

1. Scatter plots
2. Heat maps
3. Multidimensional scaling (principal components analysis) and
4. Anatomical mapping

Scatter plots are used to show the level of gene expression from resultant microarray data. A related scenario would see diseased sequences labeled Cy5 (red) and non-diseased sequences labeled Cy3 (green). Once processed, the resultant data can be represented by a scatter plot, as seen in Fig. 9.17. Genes falling outside the x2 difference in expression levels are selected for analysis.

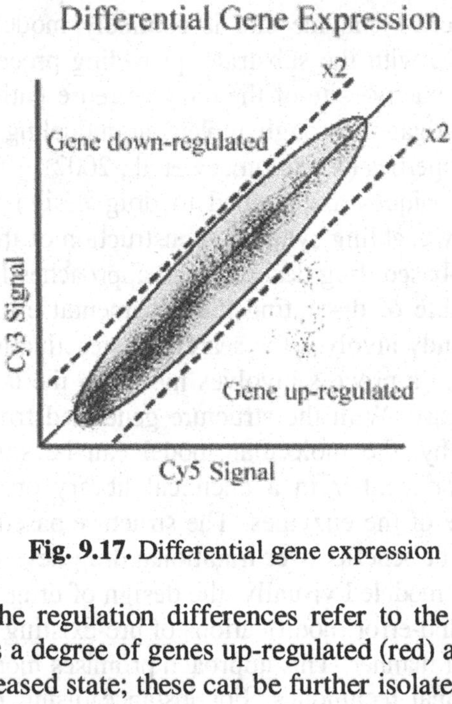

Fig. 9.17. Differential gene expression

In Fig. 9.17, the regulation differences refer to the disease state. The scatter plot shows a degree of genes up-regulated (red) and down-regulated (green) in the diseased state; these can be further isolated and their interactions more closely investigated.

Heat maps are a visual representation, of gene expression allowing for two-dimensional analysis. In Fig. 9.18, columns represent the different treatments while rows represent expression profiles. In this manner, genes can be clustered according to their expressions. The technique is useful for gauging the effect of drugs on gene products.

As seen earlier in the scatter plot, the color indicates the level of expression, with gene groupings showing similar expression profiles.

Multidimensional scaling (Principal Components Analysis) is a statistical multivariate technique for the identification of key variables within a multidimensional dataset. The goal of such an approach is to reduce dimensionality while filtering noise to produce data in a form consistent with visualization techniques.

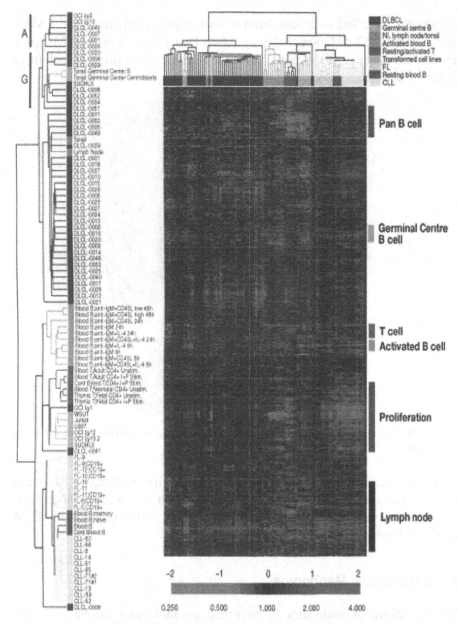

Fig. 9.18. Heat Map (Hunter February 2004)

Anatomical mapping represents a visualization technique that arise from tissue-specific gene expression data. Methodologies such as the Serial Analysis of Gene Expression (SAGE, Velculescu et al., 1995) exist to profile tissue-specific gene expressions. Databases that contain expression profiles for human tissues, such as GeneNote http://genecards.weizmann. ac.il/cgi-bin/genenote/home_page.pl; Shmueli et al., 2003) and other such databases, have led to a visualization technique called Anatomical Mapping, as termed by Hunter (February 2004). Using the Anatomical Mapping technique, specific tissue gene expression data can be mapped to human anatomical models, as shown in Fig. 9.19.

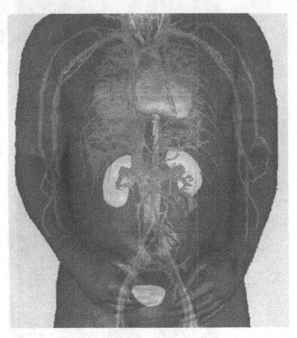

Fig. 9.19. Human anatomical model with gene expression overlay (Hunter February, 2004)

In this chapter, a subset of current visualization techniques has been briefly discussed. The major goal of visualization in molecular and resultant higher level methods is to aid understanding and interpretation of the target under analysis.

9.5.2 Molecular Mechanics

The modeling of molecules is governed by molecular mechanics. This process involves mathematical modeling of molecular geometries, energies, and other characteristics through adjusting bond lengths, bond angles, and torsion angles to equilibrium values determined by atomic hybridization and bonding schemes. Geometry is calculated as a function of steric energy using the laws of Newtonian physics and experimentally derived values (Richon, 2001). These processes help define and, consequently, refine molecular models.

9.5.3 Modern Computer Programs for Molecular Modeling

Many software tools exist to aid molecular modeling. Three major Web-based applications (Protein Explorer, Chime, and Deep View Swiss-Pdb Viewer) are presented in brief to highlight the scope of possible modeling.

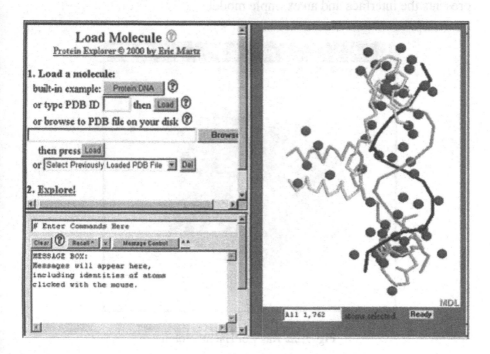

Fig. 9.20. Protein Explorer Interface

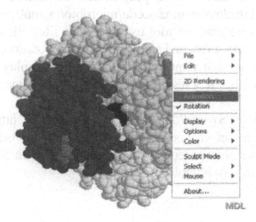

Fig. 9.21. Chime Haemoglobin

"Protein Explorer", available at http://www.proteinexplorer.org, is a free online utility to visualize 3D structures including proteins and nucleic acids showing ligand, inhibitor, and drug interactions. The target users for this software are university students and researchers, basically anyone who needs to view a 3D structure and its functional implications. Figure 9.20 presents the interface and an example model.

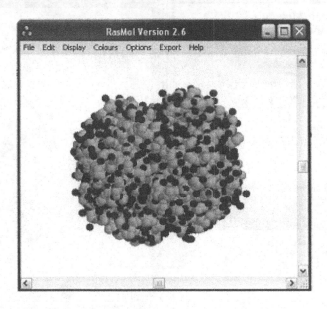

Fig. 9.22. RasMol Haemoglobin

Chime, located at http://www.umass.edu/microbio/chime/, is a 3D molecule visualization browser plug-in derived from the standalone RaMol application (http://www.umass.edu/microbio/rasmol/getras.htm). Chime, therefore, is a presentation tool used by Web sites allowing users to view 3D molecular structures, and supporting mouse rotation. RasMol is an offline visualization tool requiring PDB files for display. Protein Explorer employs Chime to view resultant 3D structures. Chime and RasMol interfaces are shown in Figures 9.21 and 9.22.

"Deep View Swiss-Pdb Viewer", located at http://us.expasy.org/-spdbv/, is a protein analysis tool downloadable for offline/online usage. This tool allows simultaneous sequence analysis with SWISS-Model integration, allowing for homology studies.

References

Baker, D., Sali, A. (2001) Protein Structure Prediction and Structural Genomics. Science 294:93-96.

Baldi, P., Chauvin, Y., Hunkapiller, T., McClure, M. (1994) Hidden Markov models of biological primary sequence information. In: Proc. Natl. Acad. Sci. USA 91:1059-1063.

Bates, P.A., Sternberg, M.J.E. (1999) Model building by comparison at CASP3: using expert knowledge and computer automation, Proteins: Structure, Function and Genetics. Suppl 3:47-54.

Batzoglou, S., Pachter, L., Mesirov, J.P., Berger, B., Lander, E.S. (2000) Human and Mouse Gene Structure: Comparative Analysis and Application to Exon Prediction. Genome Research 10:950-958.

Berman, H.M., Westbrook,J. Feng,Z. Gilliland,G. Bhat,TN., Weissig, H., Shindyalov, I.N., Bourne, P.E. (2000) The Protein Data Bank, Nucleic Acids Research 28:235-242.

Contreras-Moreira, B., Bates, P.A. (2002) Domain Fishing : a first step in protein comparative modeling. Bioinformatics 18:1141-1142.

Friedman, N., Linial, M., Nachman, I., Pe'er, D. (2000) Using Bayesian Network to Analyze Expression Data. Journal of Computational Biology 7:601-620.

Havel, T.F. and Snow, M.E. (1991) A new method for building protein conformations from sequence alignments with homologues of known structure. J. Mol. Biol. 217:1-7

Hunter, L. (February 2004) Lecture 17: Computing with Expression Array Results. http://compbio.uchsc.edu/Hunter_lab/Hunter/bioi7711/lecture17.ppt.

Karchin, R. (1999) Hidden Markov Models and Protein Sequence Analysis. In: Proc. 7th International Conference on Intelligent Systems for Molecular Biology.

Kemp, G. (February 2004) Bioinformatics III Lecture: Comparative Modeling. http://www.cs.chalmers.se/~kemp/teaching/bioinformaticsIII/2004/lecture2.pdf.

Kent, W.J. and Zahler, A.M. (2000) Conservation, Regulation, Synteny, and Introns in a Large-scale C. briggsae-C. elegans Genomic Alignment. Genome Research 10:1115-1125.

Kolinski, A., Betancourt, M.R., Kihara, D., Rotkiewicz, P. and Skolnick, J. (2001) Generalized Comparative Modeling (GENECOMP): A combination of sequence comparison, threading, and lattice modeling for protein structure prediction and refinement. Proteins: Structure, Function and Genetics 44:133-149.

Krogh, A. (1998) An Introduction to Hidden Markov Models for Biological Sequences. In: Computational Methods in Molecular Biology, pp 45-63.

Levitt, M. (1992) Accurate Modeling of Protein Conformation by Automatic Segment Matching. J. Mol. Biol. 226:507-533.

Purdue, E. (2000) Comparative Genomics. http://www.biospace.com/articles/ genomics_comparative.cfm, July.

Ravichandran, S. (November 2003) Homology Modeling: Concepts and Protocols. http://ncisgi.ncifcrf.gov/~ravichas/HomMod/Dec03HomMod.htm.

Richon, A.B. (2001) An Introduction to Molecular Modeling. Mathematech 1:83.

Rivas, E., Eddy, S.R. (2000) Secondary structure alone is generally not statistically significant for the detection of noncoding RNAs. Bioinformatics 16:573-585.

Sali, A. and Blundell, T.L. (1993) Comparative protein modeling by satisfaction of spatial restraints. J. Mol. Biol. 234:779-815.

Shmueli, O., Horn-Saban, S., Chalifa-Caspi, V., Shmoish, M., Ophir, R., Benjamin-Rodrig, H., Safran, M., Domany, E. and Lancet, D. (2003) GeneNote: whole genome expression profiles in normal human tissues. Comptes Rendus Biologies 326:1067-1072.

Shmulevich, I., Dougherty, E.R., Kim, S., Zhang, W. (2002) Probabilistic Boolean networks: a rule-based uncertainty model for gene regulatory networks. Bioinformatics 18:261-274.

Sjolander, K., Karplus, K., Brown, M., Hughey, R., Krogh, A., Mian, S.I. and Haussler, D. (1996) Dirichlet mixtures: a method for improved detection of weak but significant protein sequence homology. Computer Applications in the Biosciences 12:327-345.

Suter-Crazzolara, C. and Kurapkat, G, (2001) Comparative Genomics for the Mining of Data. Genetic Engineering News 21 11:34-35.

Tatusov, R.L., Koonin, E.V. and Lipman, D.J. (1997) A Genomic Perspective on Protein Families. Science 278:631-637.

UCSC, Computational Biology Group (February 2004) Sequence Alignment and Modeling System. http://www.cse.ucsc.edu/research/compbio/sam.html

Varfolomeev, S.D., Uporov, I.V. and Fedorov, E.V. (2002) Bioinformatics and Molecular Modeling in Chemical Enzymology. Active Sites of Hydrolases. Biochemistry (Moscow) 67:1099-1108.

Velculescu, V.E., Zhang, L., Vogelstein B, Kinzler KW (1995) Serial Analysis of Gene Expression. Science 270:484-487.

Washington University (December 2003) The Rfam database of RNA alignments and CMs. http://rfam.wustl.edu/

Westhead, D.R. (February 2004) Structural Bioinformatics. http://bbsrc-bioinf.leeds.ac.uk/b/structure/lecture2.ppt.

Zapp, M.A. (2002) The Structures of Life. National Institute of General Medical Sciences, http://www.nigms.nih.gov/news/science_ed/structlife.pdf.

10 Pattern Matching for Motifs

Brendan Tse[1,2], David Hume[1,2], Yi-Ping Phoebe Chen[3,4]

[1] CRC for Chronic Inflammatory Diseases
[2] Institute for Molecular Bioscience,
   University of Queensland, Brisbane, Australia
[3] School of Information Technology
   Faculty of Science and Technology
   Deakin University, 221 Burwood Highway, VIC3125, Australia
[4] ARC Centre in Bioinformatics

10.1 Introduction

Everybody is interested in getting all the possibly useful information in biological data. How do we get it? We cannot go into the details of each and every sequence.

A portion of a sequence, called subsequence, may occur repeatedly and have distinctive feature. This portion is known as motif, and will act as the starting point for any analysis of biological data. The motif may recur often in a set of protein sequences, with some variations. Generally, it has some important functional role. For example, it may contain information preserved by the evolutionary process.

The pattern is generally used to represent anything that occurs repeatedly. It is used in all walks of life. From a statistical point of view, it is a repeated occurrence of sequential data. There are sequence and structure patterns that can be used to characterize proteins. Motifs are short patterns. A motif may represent biological information like the tertiary structure of the protein. On the other hand, a pattern in statistical rather than biological. A pattern can be defined as a motif if it is conserved strongly within a given set of sequences. All motifs are patterns, but not vice versa.

Once the motif is found, we can look for its repetition. This can be done using different pattern matching techniques. However, this is not an easy task, evident from the fact that genomic data available from different databases across the world is so voluminous.

The complexity of eukaryotic organisms is not proportional to the number of protein/encoding genes in the genome. The extent to which complexity and gene number are unrelated became evident from the initial draft of the human genome. The current annotation of the human genome suggests there are not much more than 30,000 protein coding loci, only 30% more than *C. elegans* (worm) and five times greater than *S. cerevesiae* and (yeast). Analysis of the mouse transcriptome (Kawai et al., 2001, Okazaki et al., 2002) reveals that some additional complexity arises from the presence of many additional transcripts that do not encode proteins, and from the potential of alternative splicing to generate many different protein products from the same genomic locus. However, the final level of additional complexity arises from the control systems. Only a small proportion of the genome is transcribed into mature mRNAs that may, or may not, encode proteins, yet, very substantial segments of the genome within, and between, transcribed regions are highly conserved at least across mammalian species (see: http://ecrbrowser.dcode.org/). These conserved regions contain the instructions that determine when and where transcription occurs. In large measure, the complexity of higher eukaryotes arises from their ability to control transcription in space and time, so that a much larger number of possible combinations of gene products (that essentially equate with cell types and tissues) can be generated, and their functions coordinated and regulated.

The genomic code that determines when and where transcription occurs is written in the DNA sequence upstream and downstream of the transcription start site. Nuclear proteins that bind to these sequence elements in a sequence-specific manner determine the transcriptional activity of the locus. In general, our knowledge of transcription control of any particular gene has been determined empirically. At one time, experimenters cloned individual cDNAs, and used them as probes to measure levels of mRNA one at a time. More recently, the availability of cDNA microarrays has permitted complete transcriptome profiling of individual tissues or cell types responding to a stimulus. However, if we could read the transcriptional code, such experiments would become at least partly redundant. We would be able to predict from genomic DNA sequence that a particular gene will be transcribed in a certain location, and in association with genes, that might contribute to the same pathway or biological function. This is not yet possible, but through the use of pattern recognition algorithms, researchers can already identify statistically significant patterns that are shared by the control regions of co-expressed genes, and that may be used to identify more genes in the same set. These patterns may also constitute the binding sites for candidate transcriptional regulatory proteins that can be experimentally validated.

In this chapter, we will go through essentials of the relevant biology, and the problems and the challenges in the analysis of transcriptional control elements. We will discuss briefly the nature of transcription control, the basics of the major computational approaches, and the current limitations in this field.

10.2 Gene Regulation

The process of transcription is initiated by the binding of RNA polymerase and associated proteins of the preinitiation complex to the transcription start point (TSP). Binding and initiation are controlled by transcription factors bound to elements within the vicinity of the TSP. Although transcriptional output is commonly measured experimentally as if transcription were an analog process, it is actually digital. In a higher eukaryote, each diploid cell has two copies of each strand of DNA, packaged in a nucleoprotein complex called chromatin and visible as a chromosome. At the level of a single gene on one chromosome, there are two forms of regulation that are, essentially, all or nothing. Firstly, the locus can be in active or inactive chromatin. As a cell commits to a particular cell lineage, it switches off transcription of genes that will not be required for differentiated functions, and these genes are commonly methylated on CG dinucleotides, and assembled into heterochromatin, which is transcriptionally silent. Aside from silent genes, within a given cell there are many other genes that are not actively transcribed at any particular time, and may be acutely and reversibly induced. They are in an active chromatin state, but signals from the environment determine whether mRNA is produced. There is a great deal of evidence that this is also a digital phenomenon at the level of individual DNA templates in single cells (Hume, 2000). Since transcription is a digital process, the transcriptional code, and the binding of specific DNA binding proteins, work by determining the probability that a gene is available for transcription, and whether, subsequently, it is actually transcribed at any particular time. The actual level of mRNA in cells is also regulated at other levels; the rate of transcriptional elongation, splicing and processing, nuclear export and translation into protein; but that is not our concern here.

Transcription factors (TFs) are DNA-binding proteins that bind to DNA on specific cis-acting regulatory elements to increase or decrease the probability of transcription (Hume, 2000, Rombauts et al., and 2003). While genes of simpler eukaryotes contain relatively small numbers of binding sites for specific transcription factors, and these are usually found in a small window of 200-400bp 5' of the transcription start point (the so-called promoters), mammalian genes are more complex. Enhancer and silencer regions that, respectively activate or repress transcription, may be found tens of kilobases upstream of the TSP, within the introns of the gene, or tens of kb 3'. For example, the CSF-1 receptor contains regulatory elements in the first intron (Tagoh et al., 2002). Many of these enhancer, and silencer regions, like those of the CSF-1R gene, are highly conserved across mammalian species.

10.2.1 Promoter Organization

Although promoters, enhancers, and silencers have many sequence elements in common, promoters must have one unique function, the ability to specify the TSP. The start points of many mammalian genes are fixed for an AT-rich sequence, the TATA/Box, or a separate sequence, the initiator. The start point is located in about 30 bp upstream of TSP and has a consensus pattern of TATAAA. The initiator has a consensus pattern of YYANTAYY (Lemon and Tjian 2000); see Table 1. When these are absent, some genes that are expressed in many different cell types (so-called house-keeping genes) commonly have GC-rich sequences, and some genes expressed in cells of the immune system, such as macrophages, have purine-rich sequences. The latter classes tend not to initiate transcription at a precise point, but rather have multiple TSPs over a 50-100 bp window. In any case, each promoter type must provide the signal to recruit the basal transcriptional machinery, including the TATA-binding protein, TATA-associated proteins (TAFs), and RNA polymerase II (Lemon and Tjian 2000). In the absence of experimental data specifying the 5' end of mRNA, the sequence features of promoters are not adequate for providing computational identification. In mammals, the situation is complicated by the fact that many genes have multiple promoters that determine initiation in different tissues. The tartrate-resistant acid phosphatase gene, for example, has separate TATA-containing and TATA-less promoters directing high-level expression in osteoclasts and low-level housekeeping expression in other tissues (Walsh et al., 2003).

A partial exception to the problem of a priori promoter identification is found in CG-rich promoters. Broadly speaking, in mammals there are two classes of promoters – CpG-poor and CpG-rich promoters. The CpG island is a useful structure for predicting mammalian proximal promoters. The CpG dinucleotide is suppressed in frequency in mammalian genomes because of selective mutation, so clusters of high CG content (CpG islands) are a discernible landmark. CpG dinucleotides are often associated with methylation on cytosine, which, as mentioned above, is associated with gene inactivation and heterochromatin. In a vertebrate genome, about 60%-90% of all CpGs are methylated, but CpG clusters associated with active genes are generally unmethylated. They are usually few hundred to few thousand base pairs in length, and located near active regions around the promoters. Around 60% of the human and mouse genes contain CpG islands. (Antequera, 2003; Durbin et al., 1998; and Rombauts et al., 2003). However, it is not possible to determine the precise TSP within or around a CpG island, and many genes have several such islands.

Outside of the TSP region, promoters, enhancers, and silencers bind the same sets of DNA binding proteins. Any one transcriptional control region can span from as as little 50 to more than 1,000 bp. Binding sites for individual transcription factors are generally in the range from 5-20 bp, and within an enhancer or promoter there may be tandem repeats of sites for single factors, or for combinations of any number of factors. Sites can be overlapping and/or compound, for more than one factor binding cooperatively. A single gene with a promoter and multiple enhancers can readily have 50/100 identifiable transcriptional regulator sites. The combined effects of these sites determine the transcriptional regulation of the gene. No two genes have precisely the same set of motifs, present at the same location relative to the TSP. The challenge is to identify those motifs within the vicinity of a gene that are likely to be of functional significance, and to determine a pattern that can be compared to other genes to assess similarity and the likelihood of a common transcriptional output.

10.3 Motif Recognition

DNA binding proteins commonly contact multiple bases within their target sequence, and will tolerate single or even multiple base changes, albeit with reduced affinity. Sometimes, reduced affinity can be compensated for by cooperative binding by another factor to an adjacent site. The recognition site for any one factor is therefore recognized not as a single sequence, but as a family of motifs to which the factor can bind. The goal of pattern recognition in this context is to identify subsequences in your query sequence that are likely to bind a particular factor. The query sequence in this context can be a gene sequence or a selected genomic sequence where you want to match your pattern or motif. Generally, motif detection scans the query sequence by a given window size, and evaluates the subsequence in the current window to the selected motif definition. The window size is set to the length of the motif, and slides across the sequence one base at a time until it reach the end of the query sequence. A match occurs if the subsequence in the current window matches the motif definition under the preset user condition (Fig. 10.1c). Motifs are derived from sampling a collection of binding site sequences for a selected TFs usually determined experimentally and available in a number of public databases such as Trans-Fac.

The success and significance of matching through such a search depends upon the definition of a motif, which must maximize the true positive rate, as opposed to the false positive derived from random occurrence of the sequence in DNA. There are two ways of representing a motif, either by a consensus pattern or by a probability matrix. A consensus pattern is a string of letters, that defines your query sequence, which can match to at a given position (Fig. 10.1a). As described above, the approach uses a window with the size of the motif to scan the query sequence. As it scans through each subsequences the window, it attempts to match the sub-string to the consensus pattern (Fig. 10.1c). Normally, the user assigns a mismatch limit to allow a hit to have mismatches within the subsequence. A higher mismatch limit will allow matches to more degenerate motifs and a low limit will yield only stringent matches. The advantage of this approach is that matches are easily defined and interpreted, as either all or nothing; its disadvantage is that mismatches, if permitted, are given equal weighting, but a particular mismatch might be completely non-functional as a binding site. So, the false positive rate tends to be fairly high.

The matrix approach uses probabilities to define the motif. A matrix representation assigns a probability of a particular base occurring at a certain position in the motif. This approach takes account of the fact that certain contact residues in a motif may be absolutely required for significant binding, others may tolerate two or three alternatives, while others yet may be non-contact spacers tolerant of any base. In this approach, the query sequence is again scanned from one end to the other. The subsequence yield from each window slide generates a probability score. Here, a match was when the probability score is better then a defined threshold (Fig. 10.1b). In general, a probability value (p-value) is calculated; this value rates the probability the subsequence matched the motif of being randomly (Fig. 10.1d). Hence, the lower the p-value, the more significant is the match. If the score of the sequence within the current window is lower than any so far competed, it is the p-value cutoff and is considered a match. The advantage of this approach is that the user can define the threshold, providing a much greater control in filtering the matches. It provides a statistically meaningful way for describing the motif, generating a meaningful probability score, just identifying a match. The statistic - based approach offers solutions to cases where the contents of regions in the query sequence are biased toward the motif composition. With such an approach, one can correct the probability for a background; for example, a specific GC-rich sequence, such as a binding site for the factor Sp1, would require a higher level of match to reach significance if it occurred within a CpG island. Each its motif requires own probability cutoff, based on the background and the biological context of different query sequences. This requires more complex information, to be collected for each of the motifs.

Regardless of whether one takes a simple consensus or a matrix as the basis for searching, mammalian genes have search windows that are just too large. Given the size and degeneracy of transcription factor binding sites, all sites occur randomly in genomic DNA with significant frequency, and when one is dealing with control regions extending over tens of kilobases, an attempt to identify the functional elements in any single gene is futile. For this reason, the search has to be focused on narrower regions, or the significance has to be reinforced by searching a larger set of examples of genes that share regulation to identify patterns in common.

10.4 Motif Detection Strategies

There have been two major approaches to increasing the statistical power of pattern recognition motif searching algorithms, the "Multi-genes, single species" and the "Single gene, multi-species" and (Pennacchio and Rubin 2001, Wang and Stormo, 2003). The "Multi-genes, single species" approach relies on the conservation of the regulatory mechanism between clusters of co-regulated genes. We infer, for example, that the large set of genes induced by lipopolysaccharide in macrophages (Wells et al., 2003) will have common elements that are recognized by LPS-inducible transcription factors, such as the nuclear factor/kB. The "single gene, multi-species" approach is based upon the assumption that the core regulatory mechanism will be conserved across groups of evolutionarily related species, and that the motifs involved will approximately be in the same place or have approximately the same relative abundance. Neither approach is entirely adequate. The logical extension is to combine the two into "Multi-genes, multi-species" (Wang and Stormo, 2003).

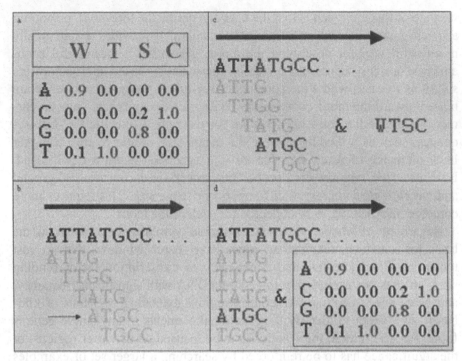

Fig. 10.1. Motif Detection. (a) An example of a consensus pattern at the top and an example of a probability weight matrix at the bottom. (b) An example of using a window size of four to scan across the query sequence and retrieve the subsequences within each window. (c) Here, a match is show when using a consensus pattern to scan the query sequence to obtain a match (in blue). (d) Use of an equivalent matrix to scan the query sequence to obtain the same match

10.4.1 Multi-genes, Single Species Approach

The transcriptional output of a cell in response to any signal involves coordinated expression of many different genes. The advent of cDNA microarray transcriptional profiling permits precise clustering of co-regulated genes. Even in simpler organisms such as yeast, a simple stimulus such as nutrient deprivation can induce hundreds of target genes. A large amount of experimental data supports the view that many clusters of co-regulated genes represent transcriptional targets of a small number of transcription factors, and that their promoters correspondingly contain recognition sites for those factors, albeit in subtly different contexts (DeRisi et al., 1997, and Lee et al., 2002).

The "multi-genes, single species" approach to identification of transcription factor motifs and more global transcriptional codes relies on searching the regulatory domains of as many co-regulated genes as possible in parallel. The main advantage of this approach is that it increases the significance value for prediction of motifs above the random background. For example, if a query sequence contains only one degenerate copy of the target motif, then prediction based upon that query sequence alone will not yield a statistically significant value to provide a confident match. On the other hand, if the same target motif occurs once or more often in each member of a cluster of 50 co-regulated genes, even a fairly degenerate motif that is common to the cluster might be identified with confidence.

Even with this statistical power, the performances of the predictions are influenced by the degeneracy of the motif and the size of the chosen search window in each gene, which is generally arbitrary. If the target motif has a degeneracy of approximately 30% or more, then the predictions becomes very unreliable (Wang and Stormo, 2003). The impact of degeneracy is in part dependent upon the random background frequency, which can, for example, be a function of base composition as well as length of the motif.

The assumption that co-regulated genes necessarily have common regulatory mechanisms is also not always correct. A large group of genes induced by a particular stimulus might be divided into sub-groupings based on their spatial and temporal profiles. Individual signals commonly initiate multiple parallel signaling pathways, which may target a subset of genes regulated by distinct sets of transcription factors. An example is the response of macrophages to lipopolysaccharide (Sweet and Hume, 1996).

10.5 Single Gene, Multi-species Approach

This concept is based upon the view that genuinely orthologous genes that have the same regulatory pattern in different species are likely also to share the basic features of transcriptional control. This approach is sometimes called phylogenetic profiling. The presumption is that the motifs that control transcription will be conserved. If we focus a motif search only on regions that are conserved between species, the search window can be greatly reduced, with a consequent increase in the probability of identifying functional elements. There are two provisos to such an analysis. Firstly, the species chosen must be sufficiently related that the gene complement is similar, but sufficiently divergent so that the functional elements have been conserved against a background of sequence divergence. In practice, for mammals the comparison between mouse and human is frequently informative, highlighting blocks of evolutionary conserved sequences among stretches of completely divergent sequences (see the Website cited above). The conservation of control sequences in blocks is likely to reflect the fact that motifs can only function if they are accessible within the chromatin structure, and chromatin remodeling generally occurs over larger domains coincident in part with supercoiling of the DNA in nucleosomes. By contrast, a comparison between humans and apes, or between rats and mice, would contribute much less to reduction of the search window. The comparison becomes more powerful more species are available, and the rapid sequencing of other mammals will undoubtedly increase the confidence of this approach.

In general, there are two ways to perform these analyses. The first approach is to extract the block of conserved non-coding sequences shared with orthologous genes, and focus the motif search solely on that region. The alternative is to carry out the motif search on each of the orthologs, and identify those elements that are present in all orthologs. The latter approach has the advantage of not assuming that the function motifs occur within blocks, and of not being dependent upon the accuracy of alignments. Alignments are not always straightforward, because insertions of repeats, such as line elements, can alter the spacing between enhancers and promoters. For example, in the urokinase plasminogen activator gene, there are three highly/conserved regions that function as enhancers, up to 8.2 kb upstream of the TSP, but their relative positions differ between species due to repeat element insertions (Stacey et al., 1995).

The predictive value of this method depends upon the accuracy of orthology relationships. This is particularly complex within multigene families, where evolutionary change can occur by gene duplication and deletion. In such circumstances, there may be no true ortholog. This was highlighted recently in a analysis of the S100 gene cluster, which has different numbers of genes in mouse and human (Ravasi et al.). When a cDNA of interest generates multiple hits on a genomic sequence, it is not necessarily the best hit that is the ortholog. Apart from the existence of multiple related functional protein/coding genes, one can encounter processed and unprocessed pseudogenes. In such circumstances, there may be no choice but to combine from the information literature on expression and function, evidence of synteny (gene order on the chromosomes of the two species), and any other available evidence before deciding upon orthology. Conversely, the presence of large regions of a conserved non-coding sequence can of itself support the view that two genes from different species are likely orthologs.

Some of the phenotypic differences between species arise precisely because they regulate transcription in distinct ways, even when the protein product has the same basic function. For example, the toll-like receptor 2 gene (TLR2) is functionally orthologous in mouse and human, but is regulated very differently and has little promoter conservation (Rehli, 2002). To some extent, this problem can now be obviated by comparing microarray expression profiles across species, and eliminating from consideration putative orthologs that are clearly not regulated in the same manner.

10.6 Multi-genes, Multi-species Approach

This approach inherits the strengths and weaknesses of both the above approaches. In general, the "single gene multi-species" approach is less computationally intensive, since one is typically dealing with only a small number of species, and is usually carried out first. For each member of a cluster of co-regulated genes, we assemble the conserved non-coding region and carry out an analysis to identify conserved motifs or motifs that fit the predetermined matrices discussed above. The predictions are then merged to determine which motifs are over-expressed in the cluster. The analysis can potentially be sufficiently large that false positives become unimportant. In fact, one can decide to include all putative orthologs for any gene within the cluster, and examine them individually in retrospect to decide which of them contain motifs common to the co-regulated set.

10.7 Summary

As noted in the introduction, any mammalian gene may have 50/100, or more, binding sites for transcription factors scattered among promoters and enhancers. Typically, there are multiple sites bound by any single transcription factor. As noted above, genuine transcriptional regulatory elements tend to be clustered within conserved non-coding regions. There are many transcription factors that bind or act cooperatively, for example, the Ets and AP1 families (Stacey et al., 1995), so that their respective recognition motifs commonly occur side-by-side if they are functional. Regardless of the method used above, one can achieve an additional constraint on analysis and greater confidence in predictions by searching for clusters of predicted elements using programs such as Cluster Bluster (Frith et al., 2003). If the same clusters occur in genes with similar regulatory patterns, or across species, the analysis can have an additional predictive power. When one includes multiple genes, the order and location of sites becomes irrelevant, and the output one seeks is the incidence of a particular site within a cluster, and its frequency when it is present. This constraint, in addition to those above, can help overcome the problem of transcription factor binding site degeneracy, and take us to a position in which it may be possible to design machine learning approaches that can distinguish classes of genes and likely transcriptional outputs based upon genomic sequence information alone.

References

Antequera, F. (2003) Structure, function and evolution of CpG island promoters. *Cellular and Molecular Life Sciences* 60: 1647-1658.

DeRisi, J.L., Iyer, V.R. and Brown, P.O. (1997) Exploring the Metabolic and Genetic Control of Gene Expression on a Genomic Scale. *Science* 278: 680-686.

Durbin, R., Eddy, S.R., Krogh, A. and Mitchison, G. (1998) *Biological sequence analysis : probabalistic models of proteins and nucleic acids.* Cambridge University Press, New York.

Frith, M.C., Li, M.C. and Weng, Z. (2003). Cluster-Buster: finding dense clusters of motifs in DNA sequences. *Nucl. Acids. Res.* 31: 3666-3668.

Hume, D.A. (2000) Probability in transcriptional regulation and its implications for leukocyte differentiation and inducible gene expression. *Blood* 96: 2323-2328.

Kawai, J., Shinagawa, A., Shibata, K., Yoshino, M., Itoh, M., Ishii, Y., Arakawa, T., Hara, A., Fukunishi, Y., Konno, H., Adachi, J., Fukuda, S., Aizawa, K., Izawa, M., Nishi, K., Kiyosawa, H., Kondo, S., Yamanaka, I., Saito, T., Okazaki, Y., Gojobori, T., Bono, H., Kasukawa, T., Saito, R., Kadota, K., Matsuda, H., Ashburner, M., Batalov, S., Casavant, T., Fleischmann, W., Gaasterland, T., Gissi, C., King, B., Kochiwa, H., Kuehl, P., Lewis, S., Matsuo, Y., Nikaido, I., Pesole, G., Quackenbush, J., Schriml, L. M., Staubli, F., Suzuki, R., Tomita, M., Wagner, L., Washio, T., Sakai, K., Okido, T., Furuno, M., Aono, H., Baldarelli, R., Barsh, G., Blake, J., Boffelli, D., Bojunga, N., Carninci, P., de Bonaldo, M.F., Brownstein, M.J., Bult, C., Fletcher, C., Fujita, M., Gariboldi, M., Gustincich, S., Hill, D., Hofmann, M., Hume, D.A., Kamiya, M., Lee, N.H., Lyons, P., Marchionni, L., Mashima, J., Mazzarelli, J., Mombaerts, P., Nordone, P., Ring, B., Ringwald, M., Rodriguez, I., Sakamoto, N., Sasaki, H., Sato, K., Schonbach, C., Seya, T., Shibata, Y., Storch, K.F., Suzuki, H., Toyo-oka, K., Wang, K.H., Weitz, C., Whittaker, C., Wilming, L., Wynshaw-Boris, A., Yoshida, K., Hasegawa, Y., Kawaji, H., Kohtsuki, S., and Hayashizaki, Y. (2001) Functional annotation of a full length mouse cDNA collection. *Nature* 409: 685-690.

Lee, T.I., Rinaldi, N.J., Robert, F., Odom, D.T., Bar-Joseph, Z., Gerber, G.K., Hannett, N.M., Harbison, C.T., Thompson, C.M., Simon, I., Zeitlinger, J., Jennings, E.G., Murray, H.L., Gordon, D.B., Ren, B., Wyrick, J.J., Tagne, J.B., Volkert, T.L., Fraenkel, E., Gifford, D.K. and Young, R.A. (2002) Transcriptional Regulatory Networks in Saccharomyces cerevisiae. *Science* 298: 799-804.

Lemon, B. and Tjian, R. (2000) Orchestrated response: a symphony of transcription factors for gene control. *Genes Dev.* 14: 2551-2569.

Okazaki, Y., Furuno, M., Kasukawa, T., Adachi, J., Bono, H., Kondo, S., Nikaido, I., Osato, N., Saito, R., Suzuki, H., Yamanaka, I., Kiyosawa, H., Yagi, K., Tomaru, Y., Hasegawa, Y., Nogami, A., Schonbach, C., Gojobori, T., Baldarelli, R., Hill, D.P., Bult, C., Hume, D.A., Quackenbush, J., Schriml, L.M., Kanapin, A., Matsuda, H., Batalov, S., Beisel, K.W., Blake, J.A., Bradt, D., Brusic, V., Chothia, C., Corbani, L.E., Cousins, S., Dalla, E., Dragani, T.A., Fletcher, C.F., Forrest, A., Frazer, K.S., Gaasterland, T., Gariboldi, M., Gissi, C., Godzik, A., Gough, J., Grimmond, S., Gustincich, S., Hirokawa, N., Jackson, I.J., Jarvis, E.D., Kanai, A., Kawaji, H., Kawasawa, Y., Kedzierski, R.M., King, B.L., Konagaya, A., Kurochkin, I.V., Lee, Y., Lenhard, B., Lyons, P.A., Maglott, D.R., Maltais, L., Marchionni, L., McKenzie, L., Miki, H., Nagashima, T., Numata, K., Okido, T., Pavan, W.J., Pertea, G., Pesole, G., Petrovsky, N., Pillai, R., Pontius, J.U., Qi, D., Ramachandran, S., Ravasi, T., Reed, J.C., Reed, DJ., Reid, J., Ring, B.Z., Ringwald, M., Sandelin, A., Schneider, C., Semple, C.A.M., Setou, M., Shimada, K., Sultana, R., Takenaka, Y., Taylor, M.S., Teasdale, R.D., Tomita, M., Verardo, R., Wagner, L., Wahlestedt, C, Wang, Y., Watanabe, Y., Wells, C., Wilming,L.G., Wynshaw-Boris, A., Yanagisawa, M., et al. 2002. Analysis of the mouse transcriptome based on functional annotation of 60,770 full length cDNAs. *Nature* 420: 563-573.

Pennacchio, L.A. and Rubin, E.M. (2001) Genomic strategies to identify mammalian regulatory sequences. *Nature Reviews Genetics* 2: 100-109.

Ravasi, T., Hsu, K., Goyette, J., Schroder, K., Yang, Z., Rahimi, F., Miranda, L.P., Alewood, P.F., Hume, D.A. and C. Geczy. PROBING THE S100 PROTEIN FAMILY THROUGH GENOMIC AND FUNCTIONAL ANALYSIS. Genomics.

Rehli, M. (2002) Of mice and men: species variations of Toll-like receptor expression. *Trends in Immunology* 23: 375-378.

Rombauts, S., Florquin, K., Lescot, M., Marchal, K., Rouze, P. and Van de Peer, Y. (2003) Computational Approaches to Identify Promoters and cis-Regulatory Elements in Plant Genomes. *Plant Physiology* 132: 1162-1176.

Stacey, K., Fowles, L., Colman, M., Ostrowski, M. and Hume, D. (1995) Regulation of urokinase-type plasminogen activator gene transcription by macrophage colony-stimulating factor. *Mol. Cell. Biol.* 15: 3430-3441.

Sweet, M.J. and Hume, D.A. (1996) Endotoxin signal transduction in macrophages. *Journal of Leukocyte Biology* 60: 8-26.

Tagoh, H., Himes, R., Clarke, D., Leenen, P.J.M., Riggs, A.D., Hume, D. and Bonifer, C. (2002) Transcription factor complex formation and chromatin fine structure alterations at the murine c-fms (CSF-1 receptor) locus during maturation of myeloid precursor cells. *Genes Dev.* 16: 1721-1737.

Walsh, N.C., Cahill, M., Carninci, P., Kawai, J., Okazaki, Y., Hayashizaki, Y., Hume, D.A., Cassady, A.I. (2003) Multiple tissue-specific promoters control expression of the murine tartrate-resistant acid phosphatase gene. *Gene* 307: 111-123.

Wang, T. and Stormo, G.D. (2003) Combining phylogenetic data with co-regulated genes to identify regulatory motifs. *Bioinformatics* 19: 2369-2380.

Wells, C., Ravasi, T., Faulkner, G., Carinci, P., Okazaki, Y., Hayashizaki, Y., Sweet, M.J., Wainwright, B.J., Hume, D.A. (2003) Genetic control of the innate immune response. *BMC Immunology* 4.

11 Visualization and Fractal Analysis of Biological Sequences

Zu-Guo Yu[1,2], Vo Anh1 and Yi-Ping Phoebe Chen[3,4]

[1] Program in Statistics and Operations Research,
Queensland University of Technology, GPO Box 2434, Brisbane,
QLD 4001, Australia.
[2] School of Mathematics and Computing Science,
Xiangtan University,
Hunan 411105, China.
[3] School of Information Technology,
Faculty of Science and Technology, Deakin University,
Burwood, VIC 3125, Australia.
[4] ARC Centre in Bioinformatics

11.1 Introduction

Biological sequences can be treated as either deoxyribonucleic acid (DNA) sequences or *amino acid sequences* (also known as *protein sequences*).

In the past two decades, there has been tremendous interest in trying to unravel the mysteries of DNA. The hereditary information of organisms (except for RNA/viruses) is encoded in their DNA sequences. These sequences are one-dimensional linear polymers that are produced from four different monomers (nucleotides), namely, adenine (*a*), cytosine (*c*), guanine (*g*), and thymine (*t*). A large amount of information concerning origin of life, evolution of species, development of individuals, and expression and regulation of genes exists in these sequences (Luo et al., 1998). As far as encoded information is concerned, we can ignore the fact that DNA exists as a double helix of two "conjugated" strands and treat it as a one-dimensional symbolic sequence made out of the four letters from the *alphabet* {*a*, *c*, *g*, *t*}. A DNA sequence identifies a given species and distinguishes it from all other species, even those having the same nucleotide composition. The nucleotide sequence is called the *primary structure* since it is the most basic level of a structure, and also defines the higher levels of the structure (secondary, tertiary, etc.). The most basic step in the study of DNA is to determine its nucleotide sequence. After a DNA is sequenced, the next step is to find different functional regions in it. How to gain more bio-information from these DNA sequences is a challenging problem. The nucleotide sequences stored in GenBank have exceeded hundreds of billions of base pairs, and they increase ten-folds/every five years. It has become essential to improve on new theoretical methods to perform DNA sequence analyses. In the theory of molecular biology, there is an important law called the *central dogma*, shown in Fig. 11.1. The relationship DNA and the biological functions can be understood from this figure.

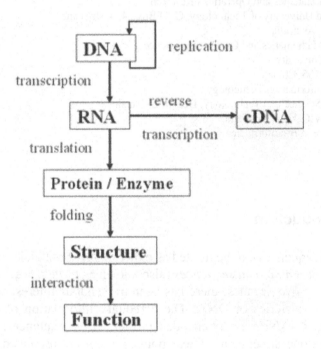

Fig. 11.1. The central dogma in showing how DNA controls the biological functions

Finding the three-dimensional structure of proteins is a complex physical and mathematical problem of prime importance in molecular biology, medicine, and pharmacology (Chothia, 1992, and Shih, 2000). A protein is composed of one or more chains that are covalently joined. The chains of amino acids are called *polypeptides*. Twenty different kinds of amino acids are found in proteins. So a protein sequence is commonly formed by twenty different kinds of amino acids, namely, Alanine (*A*), Arginine (*R*),

Asparagine (*N*), Aspartic acid (*D*), Cysteine (*C*), Glutamic acid (*E*), Glutamine (*Q*), Glycine (*G*), Histidine (*H*), Isoleucine (*I*), Leucine (*L*), Lysine (*K*), Methionine (*M*), Phenylalanine (*F*), Proline (*P*), Serine (*S*), Threonine (*T*), Tryptophan (*W*), Tyrosine (*Y*), and Valine (*V*) (Brown, 1998, p. 109). The one-letter and three-letter abbreviations, the molecular weight, and the polarity of the R group of these amino acids are shown in Table 11.1. The coding of DNA sequences can be translated into amino acid sequences as stipulated in the *genetic code* shown in Table 11.2.

Table 11.1. Twenty kinds of amino acids

Amino acid	Abbreviation		Molecular weight	Polarity of R group
	3-letter	1-letter		
Alanine	ala	A	89.1	Non-polar
Arginine	arg	R	174.2	Positive polar
Asparagine	asn	N	132.1	Uncharged polar
Aspartic acid	asp	D	133.1	Nagative polar
Cysteine	cys	C	121.2	Uncharged polar
Glutamic acid	glu	E	147.1	Negative polar
Glutamine	gln	Q	146.2	Uncharged polar
Glycine	gly	G	75.1	Uncharged polar
Histidine	his	H	155.2	Positive polar
Isoleucine	ile	I	131.2	Non-polar
Leucine	leu	L	131.2	Non-polar
Lysine	lys	K	146.2	Positive polar
Methionine	met	M	149.2	Non-polar
Phenylalanine	phe	F	165.2	Non-polar
Proline	pro	P	115.1	Non-polar
Serine	ser	S	105.1	Uncharged polar
Threonine	thr	T	119.1	Uncharged polar
Tryptophan	trp	W	204.2	Non-polar
Tyrosine	tyr	Y	181.2	Uncharged polar
Valine	val	V	117.2	Non-polar

The standard abbreviation that is used most frequently is the 3-letter one. The 1-letter abbreviation should only be used to save space when listing the amino acid sequence of a polypeptide. The above table is taken from page 109 of Brown (1998).

It is believed that the dynamical folding process and stable structure, or native conformation, of a protein are determined by its primary structure, namely, its amino acid sequence (Anfinsen, 1973, and Shih, et al., 2002). The 20 amino acids in natural polypeptides can occur in any number and any order. Because the number of amino acids in a polypeptide molecule usually ranges from 100 to 1,000, the number of different protein molecules possible is enormous. Once an amino acid sequence is known, the number of foldable spatial structures possible is also enormous. Prediction of the high level structures, such as secondary and spatial structures from the amino acid sequence, is a challenging problem, particularly for large proteins. A number of coarse-grained models have been proposed to provide insight into these very complicated issues (Shih et al., 2002).

Table 11.2. Genetic code

UUU	phe	UCU	ser	UAU	tyr	UGU	cys
UUC	phe	UCC	ser	UAC	tyr	UGC	cys
UUA	leu	UCA	ser	UAA	stop	UGA	stop
UUG	leu	UCG	ser	UAG	stop	UGG	trp
CUU	leu	CCU	pro	CAU	his	CGU	arg
CUC	leu	CCC	pro	CAC	his	CGC	arg
CUA	leu	CCA	pro	CAA	gln	CGA	arg
CUG	leu	CCG	pro	CAG	gln	CGG	arg
AUU	ile	ACU	thr	AAU	asn	AGU	ser
AUC	ile	ACC	thr	AAC	asn	AGC	ser
AUA	ile	ACA	thr	AAA	lys	AGA	arg
AUG	met	ACG	thr	AAG	lys	AGG	arg
GUU	val	GCU	ala	GAU	asp	GGU	gly
GUC	val	GCC	ala	GAC	asp	GGC	gly
GUA	val	GCA	ala	GAA	glu	GGA	gly
GUG	val	GCG	ala	GAG	glu	GGG	gly

The content of this table is taken from Brown (1998), p. 120.

A well known model in this class is the HP model proposed by Dill (1985). In this model, 20 kinds of amino acids are divided into two types, namely, hydrophobic (**H**) (or non-polar) and polar (**P**) (or hydrophilic). In the past decade, the HP model has been extensively studied by several groups (e.g. Shih et al., 2000; Li et al., 1996; Wang and Yu, 2000). From studying the model on lattices, a small number of structures are found with exceptionally high designability that a large number of protein sequences possess as their ground states (Li et al., 1996). These highly designable structures are found to have protein-like secondary structures (Shih et al., 2000; Li et al., 1996; Micheletti et al., 1998). But the HP model may be too simple and lack sufficient information on the heterogeneity and complexity of the natural set of residues (Wang and Wang, 2000). According to Brown (1998), in the HP model, one can divide the polar class into three subclasses: positive polar, uncharged polar and negative polar, (see Table 11.1). So 20 different kinds of amino acids can be divided into four classes: non-polar, negative polar, uncharged polar, and positive polar. In this model, one considers more details than in the HP model. We call this model a *detailed HP model*.

In summary, we note some important problems in DNA and protein sequence analyses:

- Distinguishing the functional regions in a DNA sequence; in particular, distinguishing coding sequences from noncoding sequences, something that is helpful in finding new genes;
- Finding patterns in DNA and protein sequences;
- Studying the classification and evolution of organisms; and
- Predicting the native structure of a protein from its amino acid sequence.

This chapter will present some tools built on the theory of fractal geometry, which may play a useful role in approaching the above problems. Fractal geometry provides a mathematical formalism for describing complex spatial and dynamical structures (Mandelbrot, 1982, and Feder, 1988). The fractal method has been successfully used to study many problems in Physics, Mathematics, Engineering, and Biology over the past two decades. Multifractal analysis is a useful way to characterize the spatial heterogeneity of both theoretical and experimental fractal patterns (Grassberger and Procaccia, 1983). Multifractal analysis was initially proposed to treat turbulence data. In recent years it has been applied successfully in many different fields, including time series analysis and financial modeling (Yu et al., 2001). In this chapter, we detail some geometrical representations of DNA and protein sequences, and apply the techniques to perform their fractal/multifractal analyses.

11.2 Fractal Analysis

11.2.1 What Is a Fractal?

The word "fractal" was coined by Mandelbrot from the Latin *fractus*, meaning broken, to describe objects that are too irregular to fit into a traditional geometrical setting (Falconer, 1990). Any fractal has a fine structure, i.e., details at all scales. Many fractals have some degree of self-similarity: they are made up of parts that resemble the whole in some way. Sometimes the resemblance may be weaker than strict geometrical similarity; for example, the self-similarity may be approximate or statistical. Falconer (1990) suggested that it seems best to regard a *fractal* as a set F that has the following properties:

1. F has a fine structure, i.e., details on arbitrarily small scales;
2. F is too irregular to be described in traditional geometrical language, both locally and globally;
3. Often, F has some form of self-similarity, perhaps approximate or statistical;
4. Usually, the "fractal dimension" of F (defined in some way) is greater than its topological dimension; and
5. In most cases of interest, F is defined in a very simple way, perhaps recursively (e.g., Cantor set).

The concept of "dimension" plays a central role in the study of fractals. Fundamental to most definitions of dimension is the idea of "measurement at scale δ". For each δ, we measure a set in a way that ignores irregularities of size less than δ, and we want to see how these measurements behave as $\delta \to 0$. If we denote by $M_\delta(F)$ the measurement, a dimension of F is then determined by a power law (if any) obeyed by $M_\delta(F)$ as $\delta \to 0$. If

$$M_\delta(F) \propto c\delta^{-s}$$

for some constants c and s, we might say that F has "dimension" s, with c regarded as the "s-dimensional measure" of F. Taking logarithms,

$$\ln M_\delta(F) \approx \ln c - s \ln \delta$$

in the sense that the difference of the two sides tends to 0 with δ, and

$$s = \lim_{\delta \to 0} \frac{\ln M_\delta(F)}{-\ln \delta}.$$

These formulae are appealing for computational and experimental purposes, since s can be estimated as the gradient of a log-log graph plotted over a suitable range of δ (Falconer, 1990). Box counting or box dimension is one of the most widely used dimensions.

11.2.2 Recurrent Iterated Function System Model

Barnsley and Demko (1985) originally named a system of contractive maps $w = \{w_1, w_2, ..., w_N\}$ an iterated function system (IFS). Let E_0 be a compact set in a compact metric space, and define $E_{\sigma_1\sigma_2...\sigma_n} = w_{\sigma_1} \circ w_{\sigma_2} \circ ... \circ w_{\sigma_n}(E_0)$ and

$$E_n = \bigcup_{\sigma_1,\sigma_2,...,\sigma_n \in \{1,2,...,N\}} E_{\sigma_1\sigma_2...\sigma_n}$$

Then $E = \bigcap_{n=1}^{\infty} E_n$ is called the *attractor* of the IFS. The attractor is usually a fractal and the IFS is a relatively general model to generate many well known fractal sets such as the Cantor set and the Koch curve. Given a set of probabilities $p_i > 0, \sum_{i=1}^{N} p_i = 1$, pick an $x_0 \in E$ and define the iteration sequence

$$x_{n+1} = w_{\sigma_n}(x_n) \qquad\qquad n = 0,1,2,3,..., \quad (11.1)$$

where the indices σ_n are chosen randomly and independently from the set $\{1,2,...,N\}$ with probabilities $\Pr(s_n = i) = p_i$. Then every orbit $\{x_n\}$ is dense in the attractor E (Barnsley and Demko, 1985, Vrscay, 1991). For n large enough, we can view the orbit $\{x_0, x_1, ..., x_n\}$ as an approximation of E. This process is called *chaos game*.

Given a system of contractive maps $w = \{w_1, w_2, ..., w_N\}$ on a compact metric space E^*, we associate with these maps a matrix of probabilities $P = (p_{ij})$ which is row stochastic, i.e., $\sum_j p_{ij} = 1$, $i = 1,2,...,N$. Consider a random chaos game sequence generated by

$$x_{n+1} = w_{\sigma_n}(x_n) \qquad\qquad n = 0,1,2,3,...,$$

where x_0 is any starting point, but now the indices σ_n are chosen with a probability that depends on the previous index σ_{n-1},

$$\Pr(s_{n+1} = i) = p_{s_n,i}$$

which is the fundamental difference between this process and the usual chaos game Equation (11.1). Then (E^*, w, P) is called a *recurrent iterated function system* (RIFS).

Let μ be the invariant measure on the attractor E of an IFS or RIFS, χ_B the characteristic function of the Borel subset $B \subset E$, then, from the ergodic theorem for IFS or RIFS (Barnsley and Demko, 1985),

$$\mu(B) = \lim_{n \to \infty} \left[\frac{1}{n+1} \sum_{k=0}^{n} \chi_B(x_k) \right].$$

In other words, $\mu(B)$ is the relative visitation frequency of B during the chaos game. A histogram approximation of the invariant measure may then be obtained by counting the number of visits made to each pixel on the computer screen.

11.2.3 Moment Method to Estimate the Parameters of the IFS (RIFS) Model

The coefficients in the contractive maps and the probabilities in the RIFS model are parameters we want to estimate from an observed measure for its representation or simulation. A moment method can be used to estimate these parameters (Vrscay, 1991). If μ is the invariant measure and A the attractor of an RIFS in R, the moments of μ are given by

$$g_i = \int_A x^i d\mu, \quad g_0 = \int_A d\mu = 1. \tag{11.2}$$

If $w_i(x) = c_i x + d_i$, $i = 1,...,N$, the following well known recursion relations hold for the IFS model:

$$[1 - \sum_{i=1}^{N} p_i c_i^n] g_n = \sum_{j=1}^{n} \binom{n}{j} g_{n-j} (\sum_{i=1}^{N} p_i c_i^{n-j} d_i^j). \tag{11.3}$$

Thus, setting $g_0 = 1$, the moments $g_n, n \geq 1$, may be computed recursively from the knowledge of $g_0, g_1,..., g_{n-1}$ (Vrscay, 1991).

For the RIFS model, we have

$$g_n = \sum_{j=1}^{N} g_n^{(j)}, \tag{11.4}$$

where $g_n^{(j)}, j = 1,2,...,N$, are given by the solution of the following system of linear equations:

$$\sum_{j=1}^{N}(p_{ji}c_i^n - \delta_{ij})g_n^{(j)} = -\sum_{k=0}^{n-1}\binom{n}{k}\left(\sum_{j=1}^{N}c_i^k d_i^{n-k} p_{ji}g_k^{(j)}\right),$$

(11.5)

$$i=1,...,N,\ n\geq 1$$

For $n=0$, we set $g_0^{(i)} = m_i$, where m_i are given by the solution of the linear equations

$$\sum_{j=1}^{N}p_{ji}m_j = m_i,\quad i=1,2,...,N,\ \text{and}\ g_0 = \sum_{i=1}^{N}m_i = 1.$$

(11.6)

If we denote by G_k the moments obtained directly from the observed measure using Equation (11.2), and by g_k the formal expression of moments obtained from Equations (11.3-11.6), then through solving the optimal problem

$$\underset{c_i,d_i,p_{ij}\ or\ P_i}{}\sum_{k=1}^{n}(g_k - G_k)^2, \text{ for some chosen } n,$$

(11.7)

we obtain the estimated values of the parameters in the IFS or RIFS model.

To our knowledge (Anh et al., 2001), it is much harder to simulate a measure than to fit its multifractal spectrum (because different measures may have the same multifractal spectrum). We found that the RIFS model can be used to simulate the measure representation of complete genomes, while the IFS model is useful for the simulation of the measure representation of protein sequences. In our study, the estimated parameters of an RIFS or IFS model are used to discuss the classification and evolutionary tree of living organisms and the structural classification of large proteins.

11.2.4 Multifractal Analysis

The most common numerical implementation of multifractal analysis is via the so-called *fixed-size box counting algorithms* (Halsy et al., 1986). In the one-dimensional case, for a given measure μ with support $E \subset R$, we consider the *partition sum*

$$Z_\varepsilon(q) = \sum_{\mu(B)\neq 0}[\mu(B)]^q$$

(11.8)

$q \in R$, where the sum runs over all different nonempty boxes B of a given side ε in a grid covering of the support E, that is,

$$B = [k\varepsilon, (k+1)\varepsilon] \tag{11.9}$$

The scaling exponent $\tau(q)$ is defined as

$$\tau(q) = \lim_{\varepsilon \to 0} \frac{\ln Z_\varepsilon(q)}{\ln \varepsilon} \tag{11.10}$$

and the generalized fractal dimensions of the measure are defined as

$$D_q = \tau(q)/(q-1) \qquad \text{for } q \neq 1 \tag{11.11}$$

and

$$D_q = \lim_{\varepsilon \to 0} \frac{Z_{1,\varepsilon}}{\ln \varepsilon}, \qquad \text{for } q = 1 \tag{11.12}$$

where $Z_{1,\varepsilon} = \sum_{\mu(B) \neq 0} \mu(B) \ln \mu(B)$. The generalized fractal dimensions are numerically estimated through a linear regression of

$$\frac{1}{q-1} \ln Z_\varepsilon(q)$$

against $\ln \varepsilon$ for $q \neq 1$, and similarly through a linear regression of $Z_{1,\varepsilon}$ against $\ln \varepsilon$ for $q = 1$. D_1 is called the information dimension and D_2 the correlation dimension. The D_1 corresponding to positive values of q give relevance to the regions where the measure is large. The D_q corresponding to negative values of q deal with the structure and the properties of the most rarefied regions of the measure.

By following the thermodynamic formulation of multifractal measures, Canessa (2000) derived an expression for the "analogous" specific heat as

$$C_q \equiv -\frac{\partial^2 \tau(q)}{\partial q^2} \approx 2\tau(q) - \tau(q+1) - \tau(q-1) \tag{11.13}$$

He showed that the form of C_q resembles a classical phase transition at a critical point for a financial time series. In the following we calculate the "analogous" specific heat of many kinds of measures we define for biological sequences. The types of phase transition are useful in the classification of bacteria.

11.3 DNA Walk Models

11.3.1 One-Dimensional DNA Walk

A significant contribution in the study of DNA sequences is the investigation of the long-range correlation. One-dimensional DNA walk was firstly proposed by Peng et al., (1992). They define that the walk is "up," $u(i) = +1$, when a pyrimidine (c or t) occurs at position i along the DNA chain, while the walk is "down," $u(i) = -1$, if a purine (a or g) occurs at position i. The question they want to answer is

Would such a walk display only short-range correlation or only long-range correlation (i.e., scale-free "fractal" phenomenon)?

Define

$$y(l) = \sum_{i=1}^{l} u(i).$$

The root mean-square fluctuation $F(l)$ is defined by

$$F(l) = \left[\overline{\Delta y(l,l_0) - \overline{\Delta y(l,l_0)}} \right]^{2 \; 1/2}$$

where

$$\Delta y(l,l_0) = y(l_0 + l) - y(l_0).$$

The average (denoted by a bar) is taken over all positions l_0 in the sequence. Using the root mean-square fluctuation, we can characterize the following cases:

Case 1 Random or local correlation: $F(l) \propto l^{1/2}$.

Case 2 Long-range correlation: $F(l) \propto l^{\alpha}$ with $1/2 < a < 1$.

Having calculated the exponents α for all DNA sequences available in GenBank at that time, they found:

1. For coding sequences, the exponents are close to 0.5, indicating random walks or local correlation.
2. For noncoding sequences, $\alpha \approx 0.67$, indicating that the walks display long-range correlation.

But their results have been disputed by some other researchers because they did not distinguish a between g in purines and c between t in pyrimidines in their DNA walk model. Buldyrev et al., (1994, 1998) and gave some explanations and improvements. By undertaking a more detailed analysis, Larhammar and Chatzidimitriou-Dreismann (1993) concluded that both coding and noncoding sequences exhibit long-range correlation. A subsequent work by Prabhu and Claverie (1992) also substantially corroborates these results.

11.3.2 Two-Dimensional DNA Walk

Luo et al., (1988, 1998) defined two- or three-dimensional DNA walk models which distinguish c from t in pyrimidines, and a from g in purines. Define

$$\vec{u}(i) = \begin{cases} +\vec{X} & if \quad s_i = a, \\ -\vec{X} & if \quad s_i = t, \\ +\vec{Y} & if \quad s_i = c, \\ -\vec{Y} & if \quad s_i = g. \end{cases}$$

For a sequence consisting of N_0 bases, define

$$< R^2{}_{i,i+N} >_{N_0} = \sum_{j=0}^{N-1}\sum_{k=0}^{N-1} < \vec{u}(i+j) \bullet \vec{u}(i+k) >,$$

$$< R^2{}_N > = \frac{1}{N_0 - N + 1} \sum_{i=1}^{N_0 - N + 1} < R^2{}_{i,i+N} >_{N_0} .$$

Then the local fractal dimension is defined by

$$D_{N_0} = \ln(\frac{N+1}{N}) / \ln(\frac{< R^2{}_{N+1} >_{N_o}}{< R^2{}_N >_{N_0}})^{1/2} .$$

The local fractal dimension $D_{N_0}(N)$ changes smoothly only for $N \le N_0$. So we define

$$
D_f = \begin{cases} \dfrac{2}{N_0} \sum_{N=1}^{N_0/2} D_{N_0}(N) & \text{for} \quad N_0 \quad \text{even,} \\[3mm] \dfrac{2}{N_0+1} \sum_{N=1}^{(N_0+1)/2} D_{N_0}(N) & \text{for} \quad N_0 \quad \text{odd.} \end{cases}
$$

D_f is called the *average fractal dimension*. When N is large enough, $D_{N_0}(N) = 2$ for a random walk. Luo et al., (1988, 1998) found that

1. Almost all D_f of DNA sequences are different from 2; hence DNA sequences exhibit long-range correlation.
2. D_f of exons is larger than that of introns.

11.3.3 Higher-Dimensional DNA Walk

Berthelsen et al., (1992) considered the global fractal dimension of human DNA sequences treated as pseudorandom walks. Because this pseudorandom walk model is rather complicated to detail here, we refer the interested reader to the original paper. They considered the fractal dimension of this kind of representation of long DNA sequences and found

1. The global fractal dimensions of coding sequences are different from those of noncoding sequences.
2. The DNA sequences used are not random sequences.

11.4 Chaos Game Representation of Biological Sequences

11.4.1 Chaos Game Representation of DNA Sequences

Based on a technique from chaotic dynamics, Jeffrey (1990) proposed a chaos game representation (CGR) of DNA sequences by using the four vertices of a square in the plane to represent a, c, g, and t. The first point of the plot is placed half-way between the center of the square and the vertex corresponding to the first letter, the ith point of the plot is placed half-way between the $(i-1)$th point and the vertex corresponding to the ith letter in the DNA sequence. The method produces a plot of a DNA sequence that displays both local and global patterns. Self-similarity or fractal structures were found in these plots. Some open questions from the biological point of view based on the CGR were proposed (Jeffrey, 1990).

11.4.2 Chaos Game Representation of Protein Sequences

The idea of CGR of DNA sequences proposed by Jeffrey (1990) was generalized and applied for visualizing and analysing protein databases by Fiser et al., (1994). Generalization of CGR of DNA may take place in several ways. In the simplest case, the square in CGR of DNA is replaced by an n-sided regular polygon (n-gon), where n is the number of different elements in the sequence to be represented. As proteins consist of 20 kinds of amino acids, a 20-sided regular polygon (regular 20-gon) is the most adequate for protein sequence representation. A few thousand points result in an "attractor" that allows visualization of the rare or frequent residues and sequence motifs.

A new method was proposed for the chaos game representation of different families of proteins (Basu et al., 1998). Using concatenated amino acid sequences of proteins belonging to a particular family and a 12-sided regular polygon, each vertex of which represents a group of amino acid residues leading to conservative substitutions, the method generates the CGR of the family and allows pictorial representation of the pattern characterizing the family. The CGRs of different protein families are found to exhibit distinct visually identifiable patterns (Basu et al., 1998). This implies that different functional classes of proteins follow specific statistical biases in the distribution of different mono-, di-, tri-, or higher order peptides along their primary sequences.

11.4.3 Chaos Game Representation of Protein Structures

The chaos game representation can also be used to study 3D structures of proteins (Fiser et al., 1994). Protein conformations can be characterized by a sequence of dihedral angles (ϕ, ψ) of the single bonds of C_α atoms in the polypeptide chain. Due to steric restrictions that stem from high energy atomic overlap, there are only 16 areas on the (ϕ, ψ) map the Ramachandran plot available for low energy structures. The conformation of a polypeptide chain can be characterized by the sequence of these low energy areas along the polypeptide chain. Thus protein structures can be visualized in a way analogous to that put forward for sequences by using 16-gons instead of 20-gons.

In most cases, a less detailed structure description, with reference to helix, sheer, turn, and "random coil" structures, is used for characterizing the polypeptide structure (Fiser et al., 1994). When one deals with exactly four kinds of elements, the original CGR was suggested (Jeffrey, 1990) for DNA can be used by replacing the four nucleotides with the four secondary structure elements at the vertices of the square. However, one of the four structural elements, the random coil, is not a regular one, so it is not as important as the other three. Therefore, instead of a square, one of the regular structure elements (helix, sheet, or turn) can be selected and placed at the vertices of a regular triangle, while the random coil structure is represented by the center of this triangle (Fiser et al., 1994). If the distribution of the secondary structure elements were random, it would have a Sierpinski-like triangle, but as the central point is also used a reference point, a new Sierpinski triangle appears without overlapping the original one.

11.4.4 Chaos Game Representation of Amino Acid Sequences Based on the Detailed HP Model

In the detailed HP model, the 20 kinds of amino acids are divided into four classes: non-polar, negative polar, uncharged polar, and positive polar. The eight residues designating the non-polar class are ALA, ILE, LEU, MET, PHE, PRO, TRP, and VAL; the two residues designating the negative polar class are ASP, GLU; the seven residues designating the uncharged polar class are ASN, CYS, GLN, GLY, SER, THR, and TYR; and the remaining three residues ARG, HIS, and LYS, designate the positive polar class.

For a given protein sequence with length L, $s = s_1 s_2 ... s_L$, where $s_i, i = 1, 2, ..., L$, is one of the 20 kinds of amino acids. We define

$$a_i = \begin{cases} 0, & if \quad s_i \in \quad\quad non-polar, \\ 1, & if \quad s_i \in \quad negative-polar, \\ 2, & if \quad s_i \in \quad uncharged-polar, \\ 3, & if \quad s_i \in \quad positive-polar. \end{cases} \quad (11.14)$$

We then obtain a sequence $X(s) = a_1 a_2 ... a_L$, where a_i is a letter in the alphabet {0, 1, 2, 3}. We next define the chaos game representation for a sequence $X(s)$ in the square $[0,1] \times [0,1]$ in a similar way to that of DNA sequences (Jeffrey 1990), where the four vertices correspond to the four letters 0, 1, 2, 3: The first point of the plot is placed half-way between the center of the square and the vertex corresponding to the first letter of the sequence $X(s)$; the ith point of the plot is then placed half-way between the $(i-1)$th point and the vertex corresponding to the ith letter. We then call the obtained plot the *chaos game representation* of the protein sequence s based on the detailed HP model.

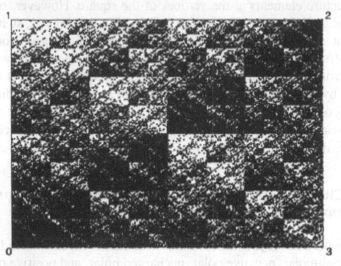

Fig. 11.2. The chaos game representation for the linked protein sequence from the genome of *Buchnera* sp. APS (185,827 amino acids)

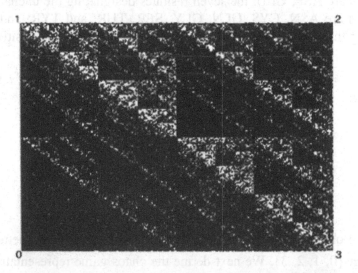

Fig. 11.3. The chaos game representation for the linked protein sequence from the genome of *Methanobacterium thermoautotrophicum* deltaH, (528,191 amino acids)

Each coding sequence in the complete genome of an organism can be translated into a protein sequence using the genetic code (Brown, 1998, p. 122). We next link all translated protein sequences from a complete genome to form a long protein sequence according to the order of the coding sequence in the complete genome. As a result, we obtain a linked protein sequence for each organism. In this Subsection, we consider only this kind of linked protein sequence for the organisms and view them as symbolic sequences. Then the CGR defined above of the linked protein sequence of an organism is called the CGR of the organism. For example, the CGR of Buchnera sp. APS is given in Fig. 11.2 and that of *Methanobacterium thermoautotrophicum* deltaH is given in Fig. 11.3. Fractal patterns are apparent in these CGRs.

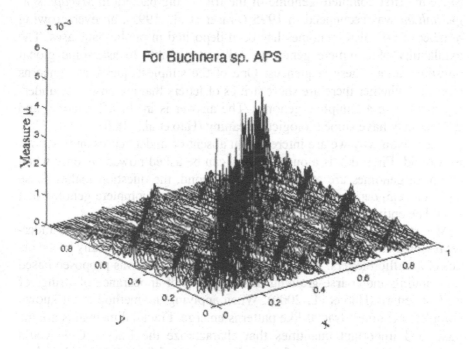

Fig. 11.4. The histogram of μ based on a 64×64 mesh of *Buchnera* sp. APS

Considering the points in a CGR of an organism, we can define a measure μ by $\mu(B) = \#(B) / N_1$, where $\#(B)$ is the number of points lying in the subset B of the CGR and N_1 is the length of the sequence. We can divide the square $[0,1] \times [0,1]$ into meshes of size 64×64, 128×128, 512×512 or 1024×1024. This results in a measure for each mesh. The measure μ based on a 64×64 mesh of *Buchnera* sp. APS is given in Fig.

11.4 as an example. We then can obtain a 64×64, 128×128, 512×512 or 1024×1024 matrix A, where each element is the measure value on the corresponding mesh. We call A the *measure matrix* of the organism. Multi-fractal analysis of these measures can be performed based on the CGR representation (see Yu et al., 2003). Because the linked protein sequences of Eukaryotes are too long, the CGR method described in this Subsection does not seem suitable for their analysis.

11.5 Two-Dimensional Portrait Representation of DNA Sequences

Since the first complete genome of the free-living bacterium *Mycoplasma genitalium* was sequenced in 1995 (Fraser et al., 1995), an ever growing number of complete genomes has been deposited in public databases. The availability of complete genomes makes it possible to ask some global questions about these sequences. One of the simplest questions concerns checking whether there are short strings of letters that are absent or under-represented in a complete genome. The answer is in the affirmative, and the fact may have some biological meaning (Hao et al., 2000).

The reason why we are interested in absent or under-represented strings is twofold. First, this is a question that can be asked nowadays only when complete genomes are at our disposal. Second, the question makes sense since one can derive a *factorizable* language from a complete genome that would be entirely defined by the set of forbidden words.

We start by considering how to visualize the avoided and under-represented strings in a bacterial genome whose length is usually in the order of a million letters. A simple visualization method was proposed based on counting and coarse-graining the frequency of appearance of strings of a given length (Hao et al., 2000). When applying the method to all known complete genomes, fractal-like patterns emerge. Fractal dimensions are the basic and important quantities that characterize the fractal. One would naturally ask: what are the fractal dimensions of fractals related to languages defined by tagged strings? In this Subsection we will answer the question.

11.5.1 Graphical Representation of Counters

We call any string made of K letters from the set $\{g, c, a, t\}$ a K-string. For a given K, there are in total 4^K different K-strings. In order to count the number of each kind of K-strings in a given DNA sequence 4^K counters are needed. These counters may be arranged as a $2^K \times 2^K$ square, as shown in Fig. 11.5 for $K = 1,2,3$.

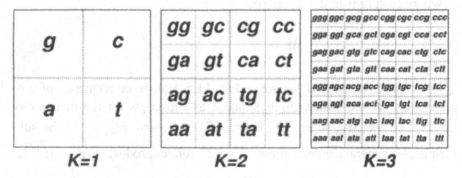

Fig. 11.5. The arrangement of string counters for $K=1$ to 3 in squares of the same size

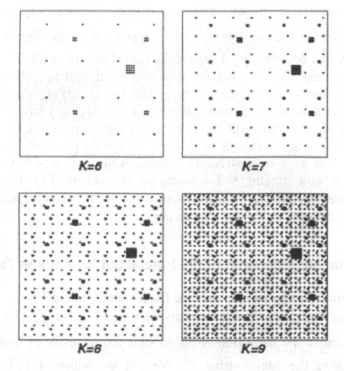

Fig. 11.6. *ctag*-tagged strings in $K=6$ to 9 frames

In fact, for a given K the corresponding square may be represented as a direct product of K copies of identical matrices:

$$M^{(K)} = M \otimes M \otimes ... \otimes M ,$$

where each M is a 2×2 matrix

$$M = \begin{bmatrix} g & c \\ a & t \end{bmatrix},$$

that represents the $K=1$ square in Fig. 11.5. For the convenience of programming, we use binary digits 0 and 1 as subscripts for the matrix elements, i.e., let $M_{00} = g$, $M_{01} = c$, $M_{10} = a$, and $M_{11} = t$. The subscripts of a general element of the $2^K \times 2^K$ direct product matrix $M^{(K)}$,

$$M^{(K)}_{I,J} = M_{i_1 j_1} M_{i_2 j_2} ... M_{i_K j_K},$$

are given by $I = i_1 i_2 .. i_K$ and $J = j_1 j_2 ... j_K$. These may be easily calculated from an input DNA K-string $s = s_1 s_2 ... s_K$, where $s_i \in \{g,c,a,t\}$. We call this $2^K \times 2^K$ square a K-frame. Put in a frame of fixed K and described by a color code biased toward small counts, each bacterial genome shows a distinctive pattern which indicates absent or under-represented strings of certain types (Hao et al., 2000). For example, many bacteria avoid strings containing the string $ctag$. Any string that contains $ctag$ as a substring will be called a $ctag$-tagged string. If we mark all $ctag$-tagged strings in frames of different K, we get pictures as shown in Fig. 11.6. The large-scale structure of these pictures persists, but more details appear with growing K. Excluding the area occupied by these tagged strings, one gets a fractal F in the limit $K \to \infty$. It is natural to ask what the fractal dimension of F for a given tag is.

11.5.2 Fractal Dimension of the Fractal Set for a Given Tag

Problem: How do we calculate the fractal dimension of F?

In formal language theory, we start with the alphabet $\Sigma = \{a,c,g,t\}$. Let Σ^* denote the collection of all possible strings made of letters from Σ, including the empty string ε. We call any subset $L \subset \Sigma^*$ a *language* over the alphabet Σ. Any string over Σ is called a *word*. If we denote the given tag as w_0, for our case,

$$L = \{\text{words do not contain } w_0 \text{ as factor}\}.$$

F is then called the fractal related to language *L*.

In using the box dimension, we can consider a more general case, i.e. the case of more than one tag. We denote the set of tags as *B*, and assume that there is element that is a factor of any other element in *B*. We define

$$L_1 = \{\text{words that do not contain any of the elements of } B \text{ as a factor}\}.$$

Now, let a_K be the number of all strings of length *K* that belong to language L_1. As the linear size δ_K in the *K*-frame is $1/2^K$, the box dimension of *F* may be calculated as

$$\dim_B(F) = \lim_{K \to \infty} \frac{\ln a_K}{-\ln \delta_K} = \lim_{K \to \infty} \frac{\ln a_K^{1/K}}{\ln 2} \tag{11.15}$$

We next define the generating function of a_K as

$$f(s) = \sum_{K=0}^{\infty} a_K s^K,$$

where *s* is a complex variable.

First, L_1 is a dynamic language. From Theorem 2.5.2 of Xie (1996), we have

$$\lim_{K \to \infty} a_K^{1/K} \text{ exists,} \tag{11.16}$$

which we denote as *l*. From Equation (11.15), we have

$$\dim_B(F) = \frac{\ln l}{\ln 2}. \tag{11.17}$$

For any word $w = w_1 w_2 ... w_n$, $w_i \in \Sigma$ for $i = 1, 2, ..., n$, we denote

$$Head(w) = \{w_1, w_1 w_2, w_1 w_2 w_3, ..., w_1 w_2 ... w_{n-1}\},$$

$$Tail(w) = \{w_n, w_{n-1} w_n, w_{n-2} w_{n-1} w_n, ..., w_2 w_3 ... w_n\}.$$

For any two given words *u* and *v*, we denote $overlap(u, v) = Tail(u) \cap Head(v)$. If $x \in Head(v)$, then we can write $v = xx'$. We denote $x' = v/x$ and define

$$u : v = \sum_{x \in overlap\,(u,v)} s^{|v/x|},$$

where $|v/x|$ is the length of word v/x. From the Golden-Jackson cluster method (Noonan and Zeilberger 1999), we know that

$$f(s) = \frac{1}{1 - 4s - weight(C)},$$

where $weight(C) = \sum_{v \in B} weight(C[v])$ and $weight(C[v])$ $(v \in B)$ are solutions of the linear equations

$$weight(C[v]) = -s^{|v|} - (v : v)weight(C[v]) - \sum_{u \in B, u \neq v}(u : v)weight(C[u]) \cdot$$

It is easy to see that $f(s)$ is a rational function. Its maximal analytic disc at center 0 has radius $|s_0|$, where s_0 is the minimal module zero point of $1/f(s)$. On the other hand, according to the Cauchy criterion of convergence, we have $1/l$ as the radius of convergence of the series expansion of $f(s)$. Hence $|s_0| = 1/l$. From Equation (11.17), we obtain the following result.

Table 11.3. Generating function and dimension for some single tags

Tag	$f(s)$	$\dim_B(F)$	Tag	$f(s)$	$\dim_B(F)$
g	$\dfrac{1}{1-3s}$	$\dfrac{\ln 3}{\ln 2}$	ggg	$\dfrac{1+s+s^2}{1-3s-3s^2-3s^3}$	1.98235
gc	$\dfrac{1}{1-4s+s^2}$	1.89997	$ctag$	$\dfrac{1}{1-4s+s^4}$	1.99429
gct	$\dfrac{1}{1-4s+s^3}$	1.97652	$gcgc$	$\dfrac{1+s^2}{1-4s+s^2-4s^3+s}$	1.99463

Conclusion: The box dimension of F is

$$\dim_B(F) = -\ln|s_0|/\ln 2,$$

where s_0 is the minimal module zero point of $1/f(s)$ and $f(s)$ is the generating function of language L_1.

In particular, the case of a single tag, i.e., B contains only one word, is easily treated, and some of the results are shown in Table 11.3.

The fractal dimension of the limit set of portraits was discussed in Yu et al., 2000; Hao et al., 2001. We give only the result regarding the box dimension. The connection between Hao's scheme and the chaos game representation is established through the multifractal property (Tino, 2002).

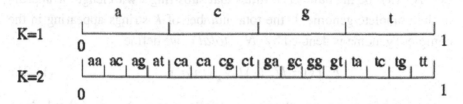

Fig. 11.7. The subintervals of [0,1[which are used to represent K-strings for $K=1$ and $K=2$

11.6 One-Dimensional Measure Representation of Biological Sequences

11.6.1 Measure Representation of Complete Genomes

Measure representation

The measure representation of complete genomes can be used to carry out their multifractal analysis (Yu et al., 2001). We divide the interval [0,1] into 4^K disjoint subintervals, and use each subinterval to represent a counter. The order of these intervals corresponds to the dictionary order of these K-strings.

Letting $s = s_1 s_2 ... s_K$, where $s_i \in \{g, c, a, t\}$, $i = 1, 2, ..., K$, be a substring with length K, we define

$$x_{left}(s) = \sum_{i=1}^{K} \frac{x_i}{4^i}, \tag{11.18}$$

where

$$x_i = \begin{cases} 0, & \text{if } s_i = a, \\ 1, & \text{if } s_i = c, \\ 2, & \text{if } s_i = g, \\ 3, & \text{if } s_i = t, \end{cases} \tag{11.19}$$

and

$$x_{right}(s) = x_{left}(s) + \frac{1}{4^K}. \tag{11.20}$$

We then use the subinterval $[x_{left}(s), x_{right}(s)]$ to represent substring s. Let $N_K(s)$ be the number of times that substring s with length K appears in the complete genome. If the total number of K-strings appearing in the complete genome is denoted by $N_K(total)$, we define

$$F_K(s) = N_K(s)/N_K(total) \tag{11.21}$$

to be the frequency of substring s. It follows that $\sum_{\{s\}} F_K(s) = 1$. Now we can define a measure μ_K on $[0,1]$ by $d\mu_K(x) = Y_K(x)dx$, where

$$Y_K(x) = 4^K F_K(s), \quad \text{when } x \in [x_{left}(s), x_{right}(s)] \tag{11.22}$$

It is easy to see $\int_0^1 d\mu_K(x) = 1$ and $\mu_K([x_{left}(s), x_{right}(s)]) = F_K(s)$. We call μ_K the *measure representation* of the organism corresponding to the given K. As an example, the histogram of substrings in the genome of *M. genitalium* for $K = 3$ and 6 are given in Fig. 11.8. Self-similarity is apparent in these measures.

For simplicity of notation, the index K is dropped in $F_K(s)$, etc., from now on, where its meaning is clear.

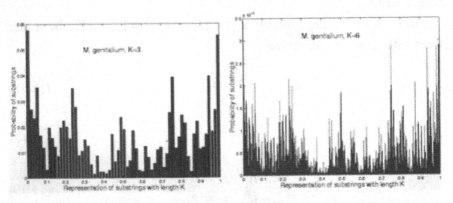

Fig 11.8. Histograms of substrings with lengths K=3 and K=6 in the complete genome of *M. genitalium*

Remark: The ordering of a, c, g, t in Equation (11.19) will give the natural dictionary ordering of K-strings in the one-dimensional space. A different ordering of K-strings would change the nature of the correlations. When we want to compare different organisms using the measure representation, once the ordering of a, c, g, t in Equation (11.19) is given, it is fixed for all organisms.

Multifractal analysis

Multifractal analysis was performed on the measure representations of a large number of complete genomes (Yu et al., 2001). As examples, the D_q and C_q curves of some organisms are shown in Figures 11.9 and 11.10 respectively.

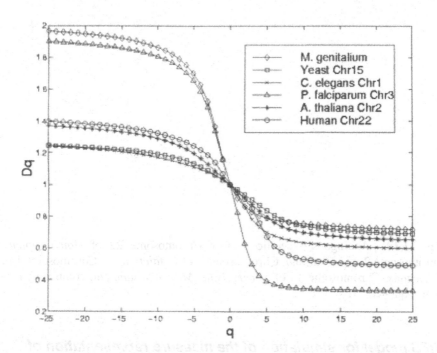

Fig. 11.9. Dimension spectra of Chromosome 22 of *Homo sapiens*, Chromosome 2 of *A. thaliana*, Chromosome 3 of *P. falciparum*, Chromosome 1 of *C. elegans*, and Chromosome 15 of *S. cerevisiae* and *M. genitalium*

From the measure representations and the values of the D_q spectra and related C_q curves, it was concluded that these complete genomes are not random sequences. For substrings with length $K = 8$, the D_q spectra of all organisms studied are multifractal-like and sufficiently smooth for the C_q

curves to be meaningful. With the decreasing value of K, the multifractality lessens. The C_q curves of all bacteria resemble a classical phase transition at a critical point. But the "analogous" phase transitions of chromosomes of non-bacteria organisms are different. Apart from Chromosome 1 of *C. elegans*, they exhibit the shape of the double peaked specific heat function.

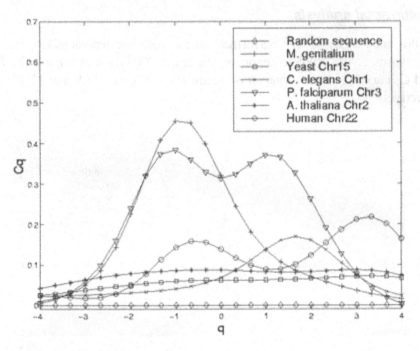

Fig. 11.10. "Analogous" specific heat of Chromosome 22 of *Homo sapiens*, Chromosome 2 of *A. thaliana*, Chromosome 3 of *P. falciparum*, Chromosome 1 of *C. elegans*, Chromosome 15 of *S. cerevisiae*, *M. genitalium*, and completely random sequence

RIFS model for simulation of the measure representation of complete genome

From the measure representation of a complete genome, we see that it is natural to choose $N=4$ and

$$w_1(x) = x/4, w_2(x) = x/4+1/4, w_3(x) = x/4+1/2, w_4(x) = x/4+3/4$$

in the RIFS model. For a given measure representation of the complete genome of an organism, we obtain the estimated values of the matrix of probabilities by solving the optimal problem. For example, when $K=8$, the estimated values of the matrix of probabilities of *Buchnera sp. APS* is

$$\begin{pmatrix} 0.423483 & 0.207054 & 0.099711 & 0.269753 \\ 0.354290 & 0.187515 & 0.129088 & 0.329107 \\ 0.299749 & 0.167843 & 0.148956 & 0.383452 \\ 0.290126 & 0.100192 & 0.179554 & 0.430129 \end{pmatrix}.$$

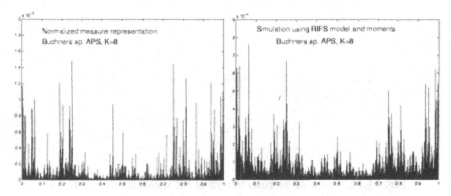

Fig. 11.11. The measure representation (left) and the RIFS simulation (right) of the complete genome of *Buchnera* sp. APS when $K=8$

Based on the above matrix, the histogram approximation of the generated measure of *Buchnera sp. APS* using the RIFS model is shown on the right in Fig. 11.11. This is quite similar to the figure on the left Fig. 11.11. In order to clarify how close the simulation measure is to the original measure representation, we convert the measure to its walk representation. If $t_j, j=1,2,...,4^K$ is the histogram of a measure and t_{ave} is its average, then we define $T_j = \sum_{i=1}^{j}(t_i - t_{ave}), j=1,2,...,4^K$ as the walk representation of the measure. In Fig. 11.12, we show the walk representations of the measures in Fig. 11.11. From Fig. 11.12, it is seen that the difference between the two walk representations is very small. We simulated the measure representations of the complete genomes of many organisms using the RIFS model (Anh et al., 2002). We found that RIFS is a good model to simulate the measure representation of organisms. From above, once the matrix of probabilities is determined, the RIFS model is obtained. Hence the matrix of probabilities obtained from the RIFS model can be used to represent the measure of the complete genome of an organism. Different organisms can be compared using their matrices of probabilities obtained from the RIFS model.

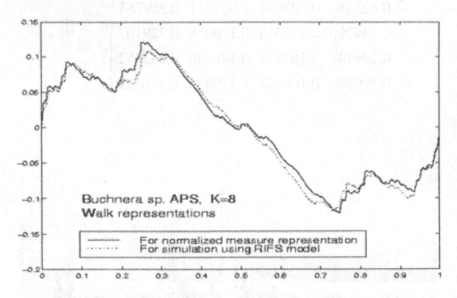

Fig. 11.12. The walk representations of the measures in Fig. 11.11

11.6.2 Measure Representation of Linked Protein Sequences

Measure representation

The concept of linked protein sequences was given in Subsection 11.4.3. We call any string made of K letters from the alphabet {A, C, D, E, F, G, H, I, K, L, M, N, P, Q, R, S, T, V, W, Y} that corresponds to twenty kinds of amino acids a K-string. For a given K, there are in total 20^K different K-strings. In order to count the number of each kind of K-strings in a given protein sequence, 20^K counters are needed. We divide the interval [0,1] into 20^K disjoint subintervals, and use each subinterval to represent a counter. Letting $s = s_1 s_2 ... s_K$, where $s_i \in$ {A, C, D, E, F, G, H, I, K, L, M, N, P, Q, R, S, T, V, W, Y}, $i = 1, 2, ..., K$ be a substring with length K, we define

$$x_{left}(s) = \sum_{i=1}^{K} \frac{x_i}{20^i}, \tag{11.23}$$

where x_i is one of the integer value from 0 to 19 corresponding to $s_i =$ A, C, D, E, F, G, H, I, K, L, M, N, P, Q, R, S, T, V, W, Y respectively (similar to Equation (11.19)), and

$$x_{right}(s) = x_{left}(s) + \frac{1}{20^K} \tag{11.24}$$

We then use the subinterval $[x_{left}(s), x_{right}(s)]$ to represent the substring s. Let $N_K(s)$ be the number of times that a substring s with length K appears in the amino acid sequence. If the total number of K-strings appearing in the amino acid sequence is denoted by $N_K(total)$, we define

$$F_K(s) = N_K(s) / N_K(total) \tag{11.25}$$

to be the frequency of substring s. It follows that $\sum_{\{s\}} F_K(s) = 1$. Now we can define a measure μ_K on $[0,1]$ by $d\mu_K(x) = Y_K(x)dx$, where

$$Y_K(x) = 20^K F_K(s), \quad \text{where} \quad x \in [x_{left}(s), x_{right}(s)] \tag{11.26}$$

It is easy to see $\int_0^1 d\mu_K(x) = 1$ and $\mu_K([x_{left}(s), x_{right}(s)]) = F_K(s)$. We call μ_K the *measure representation* of an amino acid sequence or a protein corresponding to the given K.

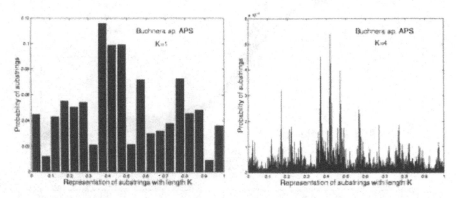

Fig. 11.13. Histograms of substrings with lengths $K=1$ and $K=4$ in the linked protein sequence from the complete genome of *Buchnera* sp. APS

If we consider linked protein sequences, we also call μ_K the *measure representation* of the linked protein sequence of the organism corresponding to the given K. As an example, the histogram of substrings in the linked protein sequence of *Buchnera* sp. APS for $K = 1$ and $K = 4$ are given in Fig. 11.13.

For simplicity of notation, the index K is dropped in $F_K(s)$, etc., from now on, where its meaning is clear. We can order all the $F(s)$ in the increasing order of $x_l(s)$. We then obtain a sequence of real numbers consisting of 20^K elements, which we denote as $F(t)$, $t = 1, 2, ..., 20^K$.

Remark: The ordering of 20 letters in the definition of the measure follows the natural dictionary ordering of K-strings in the one-dimensional space. Different orderings of 20 letters give almost the same multifractal spectrum and D_q curve when the absolute value of q is relatively small (refer to the measure representation of the DNA sequence given above). Hence our results based on multifractal analysis are considered independent of the ordering. In a comparison of different organisms using this measure representation, once the ordering is given, it is fixed for all organisms.

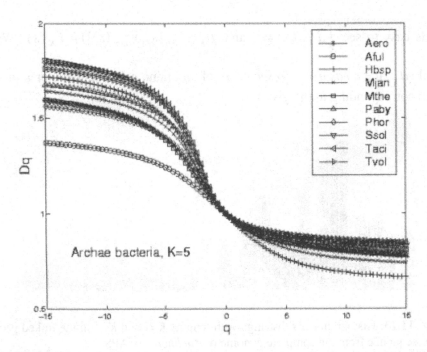

Fig. 11.14. Dimension spectra of measure representation μ of protein sequences of some Archae bacteria

Multifractal analysis

In Yu et al., *PRE* (2003), multifractal analysis was performed on the measure representations of the linked protein sequences of a large number of complete genomes. From the values of the D_q (generalized dimensions) spectra and related C_q (analogous specific heat) curves, it is concluded that these protein sequences are not completely random sequences. For substrings with length $K = 5$, the D_q spectra of all organisms studied are multifractal-like and sufficiently smooth for the C_q curves to be meaningful. The C_q curves of all bacteria resemble a classical phase transition at a critical point. But the "analogous" phase transitions of higher organisms studied exhibit the shape of the double peaked specific heat function.

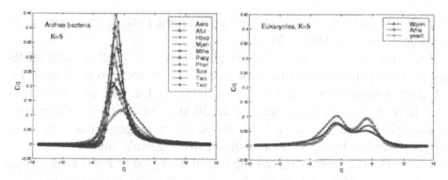

Fig. 11.15. "Analogous" specific heat of measure representation μ of protein sequences of some organisms

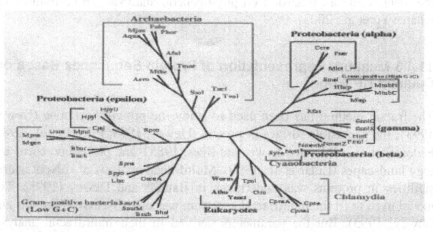

Fig. 11.16. The neighbor-joining phylogenetic tree based on the correlation distance using $F^d(s)$ with $K = 5$

Correlation distance and phylogenetic tree

If s' is one of the 20 letters, we denote by $P(s')$ the frequency of letter s' in the linked protein sequence. Then for any K-substring $s = s_1 s_2 ... s_K$, where $s_i \in \{A, C, D, E, F, G, H, I, K, L, M, N, P, Q, R, S, T, V, W, Y\}, i = 1, 2, ..., K,$
we define

$$F'(s) = P(s_1)P(s_2)...P(s_K).$$

We next define

$$F^d(s) = F(s) - F'(s). \tag{11.27}$$

For all 20^K different K-strings, we can also order the $F^d(s)$ sequence according to the dictionary order of s.

From the point of view of Qi et al., (2004), we need to subtract the background structure from the sequence $\{F(s)\}$ in order to get a more satisfactory evolutionary tree. Qi et al., (2004) used a Markov model to do this. Here we use the frequencies of the 20 kinds of amino acids appearing in the linked protein sequence. By the nature of its generation, this probability measure behaves as a multiplicative cascade and displays long memory. Hence, subtracting out the fractal background $F'(s)$ as described above has the effect of reducing long memory in the measure representation. Then, we can use the correlation distance based on the sequence $\{F^d(s)\}$ to construct a phylogenetic tree of organisms (see Fig. 11.16). Further details and a discussion on phylogenetic analysis can be found elsewhere (Yu et al., 2003).

11.6.3 Measure Representation of Protein Sequences Based on Detailed HP Model

The fractal method has been used to study the protein backbone (Dewey 1993}, the accessible surface of protein (Dewey, 1993; Pfiefer et al., 1985; Fedorov et al., 1993; and Lewis and Rees, 1985) and protein potential energy landscapes (Lidar et al., 1999). Multifractal analysis of solvent accessibilities in proteins was undertaken in Balafas and Dewey (1995). The model used to fit the multifractal spectrum was also discussed (Balafas and Dewey, 1995). But the parameters derived in their multifractal analysis cannot be used to predict the structural classification of a protein from its amino acid sequence.

Based on the idea of DNA walk model and different mappings, a decoded walk model was proposed to study the correlation property of protein sequences (Pande et al., 1994) using "Bridge analysis" and Straint and Dewey (1995) using multifractal analysis. Deviations of the decoded walk from random behavior provide evidence of memory.

Inspired by the idea of measure representation of DNA sequences (Yu et al., 2001a), we proposed a visual representation, i.e., a measure representation, of protein sequences based on the detailed HP model (Yu et al., 2004).

Through the map defined by Eq. 11.6 based on the detailed HP model, we can transform a protein sequence to a number sequence $X(s) = a_1 a_2 ... a_L$, where a_i is a letter in the alphabet $\{0,1,2,3\}$. Using the same idea as that for DNA sequences in the previous Subsection, we can define the measure representation μ_K of K-strings in the sequence $X(s) = a_1 a_2 ... a_L$. (We call μ_K the *measure representation* of the given protein sequence based on the detailed HP model. As an example, the original measure representation based on the detailed HP model of protein 1DAB (Protein Data Bank ID) is shown in the left figure of Fig. 11.17.

IFS model to simulate the measure representation of protein sequences based on the detailed HP model

In order to simulate the measure representation based on the detailed HP model of a protein sequence using IFS or RIFS model, we see that it is natural to choose $N = 4$ and

$$w_1(x) = x/4, w_2(x) = x/4 + 1/4, w_3(x) = x/4 + 1/2, w_4(x) = x/4 + 3/4$$

in the IFS model. For a given measure representation of a protein sequence, we obtain the estimated values of the probabilities p_1, p_2, p_3, p_4 in the IFS model by solving the optimization problem. Based on the estimated values of the probabilities, we can use the chaos game to generate a histogram approximation of the invariant measure of the IFS which we can compare with the real measure representation of the protein sequence. An IFS simulation of protein *P.69 Pertactin* (Protein Data Bank ID: 1DAB) is shown in the right figure of Fig. 11.17. In order to clarify how close the simulation measure is to the original measure representation, we convert the measure to its walk representation. If t_j, $j = 1,2,...,4^K$ is the histogram of a measure and t_{ave} is its average, then we define

$T_j = \sum_{i=1}^{j} (t_i - t_{ave}), j = 1,2,...,4^K$ as the walk representation of the meas-

ure. In Fig. 11.18, we show the walk representations of the measures in Fig. 11.17. From Fig. 11.18, it is seen that the difference between the two walk representations is very small.

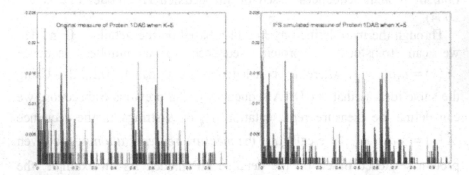

Fig. 11.17. The measure representation (left) and the IFS simulation (right) of protein *P.69 Pertactin* (PDB ID: 1DAB)

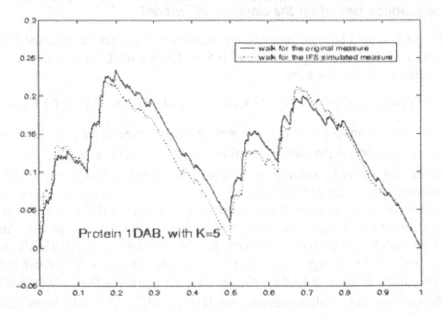

Fig. 11.18. The walk representations of the measures in Fig. 11.17

Table 11.4. The estimated parameters in the IFS model of all 32 proteins selected.

Class	PDB ID	p_1	p_2	p_3	p_4
α	1AVC	0.433053	0.057476	0.360621	0.148850
	1B89	0.434701	0.090537	0.355757	0.119005
	1BJ5	0.395675	0.171289	0.263892	0.169145
	1HO8	0.425220	0.116664	0.324997	0.133119
	1IAL	0.454049	0.145905	0.279686	0.120360
	1QSA	0.429905	0.095604	0.366038	0.108453
	2BCT	0.479382	0.051937	0.343780	0.124902
	5EAS	0.438919	0.079522	0.386794	0.094765
β	1B9S	0.374272	0.055143	0.447158	0.123429
	1DAB	0.443784	0.082010	0.399380	0.074825
	1EUT	0.404940	0.086955	0.409295	0.098810
	1FNF	0.392416	0.124496	0.393389	0.089700
	1JX5	0.418789	0.121671	0.364252	0.095288
	1MAL	0.369149	0.074231	0.483407	0.073214
$\alpha + \beta$	1B90	0.412281	0.069013	0.413590	0.105117
	1BBU	0.408854	0.203032	0.238907	0.149207
	1BYT	0.419483	0.124814	0.313159	0.142543
	1CLC	0.411955	0.089417	0.393040	0.105588
	1E7U	0.407123	0.186941	0.242776	0.163161
α / β	1A8I	0.435450	0.100694	0.329504	0.134352
	1ACJ	0.437285	0.087811	0.359227	0.115677
	1AOV	0.378102	0.092808	0.390054	0.139036
	1BFD	0.503850	0.103505	0.303115	0.089530
	1CRL	0.445648	0.061138	0.432773	0.060441
Others	1DPI	0.434653	0.174507	0.229232	0.161609
	1EFG	0.463732	0.090136	0.318268	0.127863
	1EPS	0.455629	0.080760	0.366760	0.096850
	1F1O	0.438389	0.119861	0.290525	0.151225
	1KVP	0.409277	0.105865	0.364443	0.120415
	1PMD	0.384736	0.133984	0.386281	0.094999
	1TPT	0.462826	0.143851	0.272910	0.120413
	4ACE	0.437279	0.087855	0.359186	0.115681

It is well known that statistical methods and nonlinear scale methods require large data samples. The methods introduced in this Subsection can only be used on long protein sequences (corresponding to large proteins). The amino acid sequence of 32 large proteins is selected from the RCSB Protein Data Bank (PDB). These 32 proteins belong to five structure classes (Russell, 2000) according to their secondary structures: α, β, $\alpha + \beta$ (α, β alternate), α / β (α, β segregate), and other (no α and no β) proteins.

First, we convert the amino acid sequences of these proteins into their measure representations with $K = 5$. If K is too small, there are not enough combinations of letters from the set $\{0, 1, 2, 3\}$, yielding no statistical sense. But if K is too large, the frequencies of most substrings are zero, yielding no biological information from the measure representation. Considering the length of the selected proteins, which range from 350 to 1,000, we have found it is suitable to choose $K = 5$.

We simulated the measure representations of 32 proteins using the IFS and RIFS models (Yu et al., 2004). We found that IFS is a good model to simulate the measure representation based on the detailed HP model of protein. We also found that the IFS model is better than the RIFS model in simulating the measure representation of protein sequences. The estimated parameters in the IFS model of 32 proteins are given in Table 11.4.

Once the probabilities are determined, the IFS model can be used for the measure representation of the protein sequence. From Table 11.4, we find the probability p_3 (which corresponds to the uncharged polar property) can be used to distinguish proteins from classes α and β (the values of p_3 of proteins in class α are less than those of proteins in class β), and the probability p_1 (which corresponds to the non-polar property) can be used to distinguish proteins from classes $\alpha + \beta$ and α / β (the values of p_1 for proteins in class α / β are less than those of proteins in class $\alpha + \beta$). Hence we believe that the non-polar residues and uncharged residues play a more important role than other kinds of residues in the protein folding process. This information is useful for the prediction of protein structure.

References

Anfinsen, C. (1973) Principles that govern the folding of protein chains. Science 181: 223-230.

Anh, V.V., Lau, K.S. and Yu, Z.G. (2001) Multifractal characterization of complete genomes. J. Phys. A: Math. Gene. 34: 7127-7139.

Anh, V.V., Lau, K.S. and Yu, Z.G., (2002) Recognition of an organism from fragments of its complete genome, Phys. Rev. E 66: 031910.

Balafas, J.S. and Dewey, T.G. (1995) Multifractal analysis of solvent accessibilities in proteins. Phys. Rev. E. 52: 880-887.

Barnsley, M.F. and Demko, S. (1985) Iterated function systems and the global construction of Fractals. Proc. R. Soc. Lond. A 399: 243-275.

Basu, S., Pan, A., Dutta, C. and Das, J. (1998) Chaos game representation of proteins. J. Mol. Graphics and Modeling 15: 279-289.

Berthelsen, C.L., Glazier, J.A. and Skolnick, M.H. (1992) Global fractal dimension of human DNA sequences treated as pseudorandom walks. Phys. Rev. A 45: 8902-8913.

Brown, T.A. (1998) Genetics (3rd Edition). CHAPMAN & HALL, London

Buldyrev, S.V., Dokholyan, N.V., Goldberger, A.L., Havlin, S., Peng, C.K., Stanley, H.E. and Visvanathan, G.M. (1998) Analysis of DNA sequences using method of statistical physics. Physica A 249 : 430-438.

Buldyrev, S.V., Goldgerger, A.I., Havlin, S., Peng, C.K. and Stanley, H.E. (1994) in: *Fractals in Science*, Edited by A. Bunde and S. Havlin, Springer-verlag Berlin Heidelberg, Page 49-87.

Canessa, E. (2000) Multifractality in time series. J. Phys. A: Math. Gene. 33: 3637-3651.

Chothia, C. (1992) One thousand families for the molecular biologists. Nature (London) 357: 543-544.

Dewey, T.G. (1993) Protein structure and polymer collapse. J. Chem. Phys. 98: 2250-2257.

Dill, K.A. (1985) Theory for the folding and stability of globular proteins, Biochemistry 24: 1501-1509.

Falconer, K.J. (1990) Fractal geometry: Mathematical foundations and applications. John wiley & sons LTD.

Feder, J. (1988) Fractals. Plenum Press, New York, London..

Fedorov, B.A., Fedorov, B.B. and Schmidt, P.W. (1993) An analysis of the fractal properties of the surfaces of globular proteins, J. Chem. Phys. 99: 4076-4083.

Fiser, A., Tusnady, G.E., Simon, I. (1994) Chaos game representation of protein structures. J. Mol. Graphics 12:302-304.

Fraser, C.M. et al. (1995) The minimal gene complement of Mycoplasma genitalium. Science 270: 397-404.

Grassberger, P. and Procaccia, I. (1983) Characterization of strange attractors. Phys. Rev. Lett. 50: 346-349.

Halsy, T., Jensen, M., Kadanoff, L., Procaccia, I. and Schraiman, B. (1986) Fractal measures and their singularities: the characterization of strange sets. Phys. Rev. A 33: 1141-1151.

Hao, B.L., Lee, H.C. and Zhang, S.Y. (2000) Fractals related to long DNA sequences and complete genomes. Chaos, Solitons and Fractals 11(6): 825-836.

Hao, B.L., Xie, H.M., Yu, Z.G. and Chen, G.Y. (2001) Factorizable language: from dynamics to bacterial complete genomes. Physica A 288: 10-20.

Jeffrey, H.J. (1990) Chaos game representation of gene structure. Nucleic Acids Research 18(8): 2163-2170.

Larhammar, D. and Chatzidimitriou-Dreismann, C.A. (1993) Biological origins of long-range correlations and compositional variations in DNA. Nucl. Acids Res. 21:5167-5170.

Lewis, M., Rees, D.C. (1985) Fractal Surface of Proteins. Science 230: 1163-1165.

Li, H., Helling, R., Tang, C. and Wingreen, N.S. (1996) Emergence of Preferred Structures in a Simple Model of Protein Folding, Science 273: 666-669.

Li, W.H. and Graur, D. (1991) Fundamental of Molecular Evolution. Sinauer Associates, Inc. Sunderland, Massachusetts.

Lidar, D.A., Thirumalai, D., Elber, R. and Gerber, R.B. (1999) Fractal analysis of protein potential energy landscapes. Phys. Rev. E 59: 2231-2243.

Luo, L., Lee, W., Jia, L., Ji, F. and Lu, T. (1998) Statistical correlation of nucleotides in a DNA sequence. Phy. Rev. E 58(1): 861-871.

Luo, L. and Tsai, L. (1988) Fractal analysis of DNA walk. Chin. Phys. Lett. 5: 421-424.

Mandelbrot, B.B. (1982) The Fractal Geometry of Nature. W. H. Freeman, New York.

Micheletti, C., Banavar, J.R., Maritan, A. and Seno, F. (1998) Steric Constraints in Model Proteins, Phys. Rev. Lett. 80: 5683-5686.

Noonan, J. and Zeilberger, D. (1999) The Goulden-Jackson cluster method: extensions, applications and implementations, J. Difference Eq. Appl. 5, 355-377, http://www.math.rutgers.edu/~zeilberg/papers1.html.

Pande, V.S., Grosberg, A.Y. and Tanaka, T. (1994) Nonrandomness in Protein Sequences: Evidence for a Physically Driven Stage of Evolution? Proc. Natl. Acad. Sci. USA 91: 12972-12975

Peng, C.K., Buldyrev, S., Goldberg, A.L., Havlin, S., Sciortino, F., Simons, M. and Stanley, H.E. (1992) Long-range correlations in nucleotide sequences. Nature 356: 168-170.

Pfiefer, P., Welz, U. and Wipperman, H. (1985) Fractal surface dimension of proteins: Lysozyme. Chem. Phys. Lett. 113: 535-540

Prabhu, V.V. and Claverie, J.M. (1992) Correlations in intronless DNA. Nature 359: 782-782.

Qi, J., Wang, B. and Hao, B.L. (2004) Prokaryote phylogeny based on complete genomes--tree construction without sequence alignment. J. Mol. Evol. 58:1-11.

Russell, R.B. (2000) Classification of Protein Folds, in *Protein structure prediction: Methods and Protocls*, Eds, D. Webster, Humana Press Inc., Totowa, NJ.

Shih, C.T., Su, Z.Y., Gwan, J.F., Hao, B.L., Hsieh, C.H. and Lee, H.C. (2000) Mean-Field HP Model, Designability and Alpha-Helices in Protein Structures, Phys. Rev. Lett. 84(2): 386-389.

Shih, C.T., Su, Z.Y., Gwan, J.F., Hao, B.L., Hsieh, C.H., Lee, H.C. (2002) Geometric and statistical properties of the mean-field HP model, the LS model and real protein sequences. Phys. Rev. E 65: 041923.

Strait, B.J. and Dewey, T.G. (1995) Multifractals and decoded walks: Applications to protein sequence correlations, Phys. Rev. E. 52: 6588-6592.

Tino, P. (2001) Multifractal properties of Hao's geometric representation of DNA sequences, Physica A 304: 480-494.

Vrscay, E.R. (1991) Iterated function systems: theory, applications and the inverse problem, in Fractal *Geometry and analysis*, Eds, J. Belair, NATO ASI series, Kluwer Academic Publishers.

Wang, B. and Yu, Z.G. (2000) One way to characterize the compact structures of lattice protein model. J. Chem. Phys. 112(13): 6084-6088

Wang, J. and Wang, W. (2000) Modeling study on the validity of a possibly simplified representation of proteins. Phys. Rev. E 61: 6981-6986.

Xie, H.M. (1996) Grammatical Complexity and One-Dimensional Dynamical Systems. World Scientific, Singapore.

Yu, Z.G., Anh, V.V. and Lau, K.S. (2001) Measure representation and multifractal analysis of complete genome. Phys. Rev. E 64: 031903.

Yu, Z.G., Anh, V.V. and Lau, K.S. (2003) Multifractal and correlation analysis of protein sequences from complete genome. Phys. Rev. E 68:021913.

Yu, Z.G., Anh, V.V. and Lau, K.S. (2004) Fractal analysis of large proteins based on the Detailed HP model. Physica A (in press).

Yu, Z.G., Hao, B.L., Xie, H.M. and Chen, G.Y. (2000) Dimension of fractals related to language defined by tagged strings in complete genome. Chaos, Solitons and Fractals 11(14): 2215-2222.

12 Microarray Data Analysis

Alan W.-C. Liew[1], Hong Yan[1,2], Mengsu Yang[3] and Y.-P. Phoebe Chen[4]

[1] Department of Computer Engineering and Information Technology
City University of Hong Kong, Tat Chee Avenue, Kowloon, Hong Kong
[2] School of Electrical and Information Engineering
University of Sydney, NSW 2006, Australia
[3] Department of Biology and Chemistry
City University of Hong Kong, Tat Chee Avenue, Kowloon, Hong Kong
[4] School of Information Technology
Deakin University, Australia

12.1 Introduction

Microarray deals with DNA samples. It is a device that cotains an array of microscopic glass slides coated with DNA molecules. Of late, it has evolved into hign density DNA chip. Using this microarray, expressions of genes are measured using the laser spectroscopic technique. We will not go into the details of the microarrray technology. Rather, we will go into details of analysis of measured data for gene expression.

What do we get out of this analysis of minute DNA samples? How reliable is the information extracted from this analysis? These are the puzzling questions that concern everyone involved in biology and bioinformatics.

In this chapter, we will discuss several analytical techniques and tools used in image analysis of microarray for data extraction and data analysis for pattern discovery.

Image analysis is very crucial to analysis of measured data as it gives details of particular elements of the array. Several techniques and tools are available for analysis of measued data to gain insight into any pattern that emerges. The most popular among them are the cluster analysis, temporal expression profile analysis, and gene regulatory analysis. We will discusss about them in detail.

12.2 Microarray Technology for Genome Expression Study

Important insights into gene function can be gained by gene expression profiling. Gene expression profiling is the process of determining when and where particular genes are expressed. For example, some genes are turned on (expressed) or turned off (repressed) when there is a change in external conditions or stimuli. In multicellular organisms, gene expressions in different cell types are different during different developmental stages in life. Even within the same cell type, gene expressions are dependent on the cell cycle. DNA mutation may alter the expressions of certain genes, which causes illnesses such as abnormal tumor growths or cancers. Furthermore, the expression of one gene is often regulated by the expression of another gene. A detailed analysis of all this information will provide an understanding the networking of different genes and their functional roles.

Traditional techniques of gene expression study are laborious and slow (Sambrook and Russell, 2001). In the past, genes and their expression profiles were studied one at a time. Although some of these techniques have very good sensitivity and serve certain applications, they are inadequate for the holistic study of the complete genome of an organism since the expressions of different genes are generally interdependent.

Microarray technology, which allows massively parallel, high throughput profiling of gene expression in a single hybridization experiment, has recently emerged as a powerful tool for genetic research (Schena et al.,1995; Moore, 2001; and Lockhart and Winzeler, 2000). The technique allows the simultaneous study of tens of thousands (for example, standard high density arrays currently have around 30,000 to 40,000 cDNAs spotted on each array) of different DNA nucleotide sequences on a single microscopic glass slide. Besides the enormous scientific potential of cDNA microarrays in the fundamental study of gene expressions, gene regulations, and interactions, they also have very important applications in pharmaceutical and clinical research. For example, by comparing gene expressions in normal and diseased cells, microarrays can be used to identify disease genes for therapeutic drugs or for assessing the effect of a treatment.

In a microarray experiment, two samples of cRNA are reverse transcribed from mRNA purified from cellular contents are labeled with different fluorescent dyes (usually Cy3 and Cy5, which have different emission wavelengths) to constitute the cDNA targets. The two cDNA targets are then hybridized onto a cDNA microarray. The microarray holds hundreds or thousands of spots, each of which contains a known different DNA sequence called probe. These spots are printed onto a glass slide by a robotic arrayer. The DNA in the spots is bonded to the glass to keep it from washing off during the hybridization reaction. If a target contains a cDNA whose sequence is complementary to the DNA probe on a given spot, that cDNA will hybridize to the spot, where it will be detectable by its fluorescence. Spots with more bound targets will have more fluorescent dyes, and will therefore fluoresce more intensely.

Once the cDNA targets have been hybridized to the array and any loose target has been washed off, the array is scanned by a laser scanner to determine how much of each target is bound to each spot. The hybridized microarray is scanned for the red wavelength (at approximately 635 nm for the cyanine5, on Cy5 dye) and the green wavelength (at approximately 530 nm for the cyanine3, on Cy3 dye); this produces two sets of images typically in 16 bits Tiff format. The ratio of the two fluorescence intensities at each spot indicates the relative abundance of the corresponding DNA sequence in the two cDNA samples that are hybridized to the DNA sequence on the spot. By examining the expression ratio of each spot in the Cy3 and Cy5 images, gene expression study can be studied. Fig. 12.1 shows a schematic of the cDNA microarray technique and Fig. 12.2 outlines the steps for performing a cDNA microarray experiment.

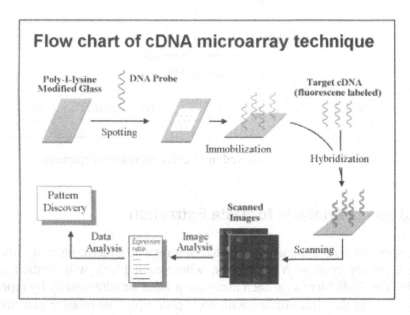

Fig. 12.1. A schematic of the cDNA microarray technique

The large amount of data in the microarray images necessitates the use of computer analysis. In general, analysis of microarray data can be categorized into two parts: image analysis for data extraction and data analysis on the gene expression ratio (Liew et al., 2003b). The ultimate goal in image analysis is to automatically quantify each spot giving information about the relative extent of hybridization of the two cDNA samples, a process known as quantitation. However, automatic and reliable analysis of microarray images has proved to be difficult due to the poor contrast between spots and background, and the many contaminations/artifacts arising from the hybridization procedures, such as irregular spot shape and size, dust on the slide, large intensity variation within the spots and the background, and nonspecific hybridization.

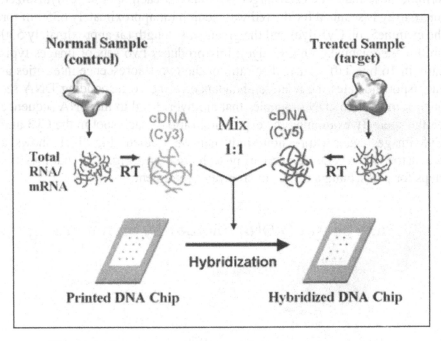

Fig. 12.2. The steps involved in a cDNA microarray experiment

12.3 Image Analysis for Data Extraction

The spots on a microarray are printed in a regular pattern: an array image will typically contain NxM blocks, where each block will contain pxq spots. The NxM blocks on each array are printed simultaneously by repeatedly spotting the slide surface with NxM print tips. The relative placement of adjacent blocks is therefore determined by the spacing between adjacent print tips. Adjacent spots inside each block are separated during printing by slightly offsetting the print tips after each spotting. These spots must be individually segmented from the background to compute the expression ratio.

Although precise robotic arrayers are used to ensure precise positioning during printing, variations in spot positions cannot be totally avoided. The positional variations become significant when very high density printing is carried out, since the size of each spot is in the μm range. Differences in the size of the transferred drops on the print tips also cause variations in spot size and shape. The hybridization process further introduces variability, such as different labeling efficiencies for different DNA sequences, and specific and non-specific hybridization on the spots and background. The post-hybridized slide treatments, such as the washing off of the unbounded cDNA targets with solvents and slide dehydration, also create image artifacts. Finally, the imaging process could give rise to geometric distortion, blurring, intensity saturation, and poor contrast in the image. All these factors make the microarray image highly variable and complicate the spot segmentation task.

Many software packages, both free and commercial, have been developed for microarray image analysis, some of these software packages are *GenePix* (Axon, 2001), *ScanAlyze* (Eisen, 1999), *QuantArray* (Packard, Yale and Bohnert, 2001), *Dapple* (Buhler et al., 2000), *Spot* (Buckley, 2002), *DeArray* (Chen et al., 1997), *Matarray* (Wang et al., 2001), and *GeneIcon* (Liew et al., 2003a). A typical spot segmentation task usually involves the following steps: (1) preprocess the pair of microarray images, (2) identify the location of all blocks on the microarray image, (3) generate the grid within each block that subdivides the block into *pxq* subregions, each containing at most one spot, and (4) segment the spot, if any, in each subregion. We give a brief account of each of the steps in our image analysis algorithm (*GeneIcon*) below.

12.3.1 Image Preprocessing

The input microarray images consist of a pair of 16-bit images in TIFF format, laser scanned from a microarray slide, using two different wavelengths. For computational efficiency, a spot segmentation algorithm usually operates on a single image. Let X denotes the composite image obtained from R (Cy5) and G (Cy3); then, one possible way to compute X is

$$X = \left\lfloor 0.5 * \left(G' + \left(\frac{median(G')}{median(R')} \right) R' \right) \right\rfloor,$$

where $G' = \sqrt{G}$, $R' = \sqrt{R}$, and $\lfloor \ \rfloor$ denotes rounding to the nearest integer in the range [0, 255].

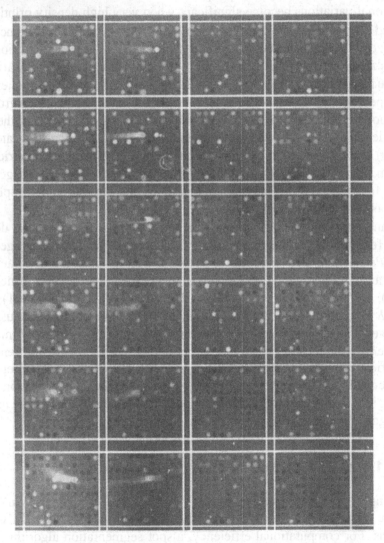

Fig. 12.3. Segmentation of a microarray image into blocks

12.3.2 Block Segmentation

The blocks in a microarray image are arranged in a very rigid pattern due to the printing process, and each block in a microarray image is surrounded by regions void of any spots. Hence, an effective way for block segmentation is through an analysis of the vertical and horizontal image projection profiles. In our image analysis algorithm, the projection profiles are obtained from an adaptively binarized image. By performing analysis on the projection profiles, accurate block segmentation can be achieved. Figure 12.3 shows an example of block segmentation of a microarray image.

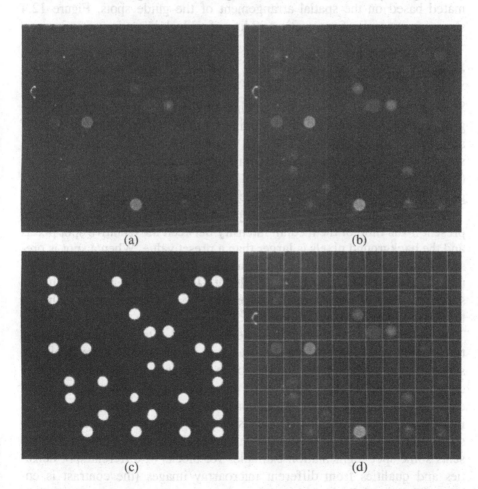

Fig. 12.4. (a) A block of spots from a microarray image shown as an RGB color image, where the green component is given by Cy3, the red component given by Cy5 and the blue component is set to zero. (b) The corresponding composite image. (c) The guide spots found. (d) Grid generated from the guide spot image

12.3.3 Automatic Gridding

Our gridding strategy consists of first locating the good quality spots (we called them guide spots), and then inferring the geometry of the grid from these spots. While gridding, we also correct for any global rotation, and remove any erroneous spots that do not fit the estimated grid geometry. In order to account for the variable background and spot intensity, a novel adaptive thresholding procedure and morphological processing are used to detect the guide spots. After the guide spots are found, global rotation in the image is compensated for, and the correct grid parameters are estimated based on the spatial arrangement of the guide spots. Figure 12.4 shows an example of automatic gridding of a block in a microarray image.

12.3.4 Spot Extraction

Spot segmentation is performed in each of the subregions defined by the grid. The segmentation involves finding a circle that separates the spot, if any, from the background. The spot segmentation task consists of three steps: (1) background equalization for intensity variation in the subregion, (2) statistical intensity modeling and optimum thresholding of the subregion, and (3) finding the best-fit circle that segments the spot.

If a guide spot is present, a spot is present. Otherwise, a spot is assumed present if the ratio of the median intensity between the tentative spot pixels and the background pixels is larger than a preset value. When a spot is present, the intensity distribution of the pixels within the subregion is modeled using a 2-class Gaussian Mixture Model. The pixel intensity within the subregion may be transformed if necessary, i.e., log transformed if the intensity is lognormally distributed, prior to the Gaussian Mixture modeling. The optimum threshold can then be computed. Once the subregion is thresholded and segmented, a best-fit circle is computed for the final spot segmentation. Although the actual spot shape usually deviates from strictly circular, we constrain the spot shape to be circular to ensure that the spot extraction procedure is robust to poor quality segmentation while providing a reasonable fit to good quality spots. Nevertheless, for good quality spots, adaptive shape segmentation can be easily adopted. Figure 12.5 presents some spot segmentation examples for blocks of different spot densities and qualities from different microarray images (the contrast is enhanced for visual display).

12.3.5 Background Correction, Data Normalization and Filtering, and Missing Value Estimation

Once the spots in a microarray image are extracted, the intensity value of each spot can be obtained and the log ratio, i.e., $M = \log_2 R/G$, which indicates the differential expression of the two DNA samples (the red and the green dyes), can be computed. However, due to contaminations and experimental errors, some preprocessing of the raw intensity value is needed before the expression data can be subjected to further analysis. The preprocessing steps usually involve (i) background correction, (ii) data normalization, (iii) data filtering, and/or (iv) missing values estimation.

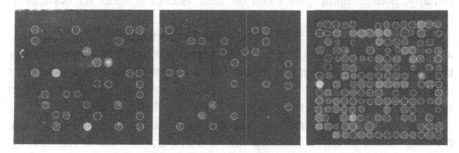

Fig. 12.5. cDNA Microarray spot segmentation results

The motivation for background correction is the belief that a spot's measured intensity includes a contribution not due to the specific hybridization of the target to the probe. This could arise from non-specific hybridization and stray fluorescence emitted from other chemicals on the glass slide. Such a contribution should be removed from the spot's measured intensity to obtain a more accurate quantification of hybridization. Different approaches, ranging from simple subtraction of local background intensity (Eisen, 1999 and Axon, 2001) to sophisticated statistical correction have been proposed (Kooperberg et al., 2002).

The purpose of normalization is to adjust for any bias that arises from variation in the microarray process rather than from biological differences between the RNA samples. Position variation on a slide may arise due to differences between the print tips on the arrayer, variation over the course of the print run, or nonuniformity in the hybridization. Differences between slides may arise from differences in ambient conditions when the slides were prepared. Another common variation is the red-green bias due to the differences between the labeling efficiencies, the scanning properties of the two fluors, and the scanner settings. It is necessary to normalize the spot intensities before any subsequent analysis is carried out.

The most widely used within-slide normalization method assumes that the red-green bias is constant on the log scale across the slide. The log ratios are corrected by subtracting a constant c to get the normalized values $M_{norm} = \log_2(R/G) - c$. The global constant c is usually estimated from the mean or the median log-ratios value over a subset of the genes assumed to be not differentially expressed (Chen et al., 1997 and Wolfinger et al., 2001). However, the imbalance in the red and green intensities is usually not constant across the spots within and between slides, and can vary according to overall spot intensity, location on the slide, slide origin, and, possibly, other variables. Other more sophisticated normalization methods are available to account for these dependencies (Yang et al., 2002). Additionally, housekeeping genes can be used as control spots for normalization.

Not all data extracted from a microarray experiment are useful. For example, some temporal expression data might have missing values at many time points. Some expression ratios might be unreliable due to the poor quality of the spots. Thus, the expression data are usually filtered prior to subsequent data analysis stage (Eisen, 1999, and Axon, 2001).

Gene expression microarray experiments usually suffered from the missing values problem. Missing values occur due to various reasons, including artifacts on the microarray image, insufficient resolution, image corruption, etc. The unreliable spots on the microarray image are usually manually flagged and excluded from subsequent analysis, resulting in the missing of data at those locations. The existence of missing values has important implications for subsequent data analysis. For example, the inability of many clustering algorithms to process the missing values means that profiles containing missing values are often discarded. However, instead of ignoring gene expression profiles containing missing values (thus throwing away useful information), such missing values can often be estimated based on available knowledge and assumptions about the data.

Reliable estimation of missing values is important. If an erroneous missing value imputation is performed, gene expressions containing a high number of missing values can be assigned to the wrong cluster in subsequent cluster analysis. The most common methods to deal with missing values are simply replacements by zero or by the average of the expression profile. Such estimation techniques, however, make very crude use of the available knowledge within the data. Other more advanced techniques, such as the K-nearest neighbor method (*KNNimpute*) or the singular value decomposition method (*SVDimpute*), have recently been proposed (Troyanskaya et al., 2001).

Intuitively, if we can incorporate more available information about the missing values into their estimation, we can obtain better estimates. We have recently proposed a missing value imputation technique based on this idea (Gan et al., 2004). Let the gene expression data be tabulated as a matrix A of size MxN, where M denotes the M genes being studied and N denotes the N arrays produced under N different experimental conditions. If we perform a singular value decomposition on matrix A, we get

$$A_{M \times N} = U_{M \times M} \Sigma_{M \times N} V_{N \times N}^{T}$$

Let $L = \min\{M, N\}$, matrix V^T now contains L eigengenes, and matrix U contain L eigenarrays. Unlike *SVDimpute,* our method makes use of information in both the eigengenes and eigenarrays for missing value imputation. Moreover, we allow uncertainties in the estimated values by modeling them as convex sets, and use the projection onto convex sets (POCS) algorithm to iteratively refine the estimated values. Using the new algorithm, we were able to obtain a normalized root mean squared error reduction of between 16% and 20% more than *KNNimpute* and *SVDimpute* on the gene expression datasets of the yeast cell/cycle from Spellman et al. (http://cellcycle-www.stanford.edu; Spellman et al., 1998).

12.4 Data Analysis for Pattern Discovery

Once expression data isobtained from the microarray images, the information embedded in the data needs to be discovered and analyzed. In gene expression study, the data is arranged in matrix form, where the rows correspond to genes and the columns correspond to the genes' responses under different experimental conditions. One can examine the expression profiles of different genes by comparing rows in the expression matrix, or study the responses of genes to different experimental conditions by examining the columns of the expression matrix.

12.4.1 Cluster Analysis

A standard tool in gene expression data analysis is cluster analysis. Cluster analysis is a fundamental technique in exploratory data analysis and pattern discovery. It aims at finding groups in a given dataset such that objects in the same group are similar to each other while objects in different groups are dissimilar. Since genes with related functions are expected to have similar expression patterns, clustering of genes may suggest possible roles for genes with unknown functions based on the known functions of some other genes that are placed in the same cluster. Many clustering algorithms, for example, K-means, Self-Organizing Maps (SOMs), Hierarchical clustering, Self-Organizing Tree Algorithm, principal components analysis (PCA), and Multidimensional Scaling, have been applied to the study of high-dimensional gene expression data (Brazma and Vilo, 2000; Alon et al, 1999; Perou et al., 1999; White et al., 1999; Yeung and Ruzzo, 2001; Tang et al., 2002; Eisen, 1998; Tamayo et al., 1999; and Duda, 2001). Clustering of gene expression data has been applied to the study of temporal expression of yeast genes in sporulation (Chu et al., 1998), the identification of gene regulatory networks (Chen and Filkov et al., 1999), and the study of cancer (Golub et al., 1999).

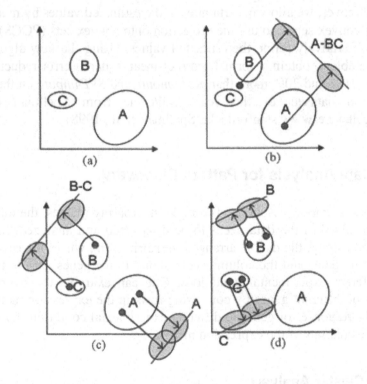

Fig. 12.6. The binary hierarchical clustering framework. (a) Original gene expression data treated as one class. (b) The class split into two clusters, A and BC. (c) Cluster A cannot be split further, but cluster BC is split into two clusters, B and C. (d) Both cluster B and C cannot be split any more, and we have three clusters A, B, and C (See Clausi, 2002)

Traditional clustering techniques can generally be classified into two categories, hierarchical and partitional. Hierarchical clustering transforms a pairwise dissimilarity matrix of patterns into a sequence of nested partitions, such as a dendrogram. Partitional clustering, on the other hand, performs a partitions of patterns into K clusters, such that other patterns in a cluster are more similar to each other than to patterns in the clusters. Both categories of clustering algorithms have their merits and weaknesses and both have been used extensively in gene expression data study (see, for example, the cluster analysis packages of Stanford Microarray Database: http://genome-www5.stanford.edu/MicroArray/SMD/restech.html).

BHC Clustering

We recently proposed a novel hierarchical partitioning framework that combines the features of both categories of algorithms, what we called the binary hierarchical clustering (BHC) (Szeto et al., 2003). In essence, our algorithm performs a successive binary subdivision of the data into interestingly smaller partitions in a hierarchical manner, until any further splitting of a partition into two smaller partitions is insignificant. The hierarchical structure is manifested in the binary tree structure of the clustering result, where a parent node gives rise to two children nodes if the projection onto the optimal fisher discriminant axis satisfies a certain threshold. The partitioning behavior of our algorithm is incorporated in the cluster splitting process, where the fuzzy C-means clustering algorithm is used to split a parent cluster into two children clusters. The basic idea and major steps of our algorithm are illustrated in Figures 12.6 and 12.7.

At each stage of the binary partitioning module of Fig. 12.7, the BHC algorithm uses the fuzzy C-means algorithm and the average linkage hierarchical clustering algorithm to split the data into two classes, and then refines and verifies the validity of the split by using the Fisher discriminant analysis. The main advantages of the BHC clustering algorithm are (Clausi, 2002): (1) the number of clusters can be estimated from the data directly, using a binary hierarchical framework and a mathematically well defined index; (2) no constraint about the number of samples in each cluster is required; and (3) no prior assumption about the class distribution is needed.

The binary hierarchical framework leads to a tree structure representation. The tree is constructed in such a way that adjacent clusters are more similar in terms of the Mahalanobis distance than non-adjacent clusters. By visualizing the clustering results using a tree structure, the relationships between clusters, the adjacency between clusters, and the variations within clusters can be observed easily. The tree structure visualization allows visual interpretation of the clustering result using additional biological knowledge, in a manner similar to that of hierarchical clustering. Figures

12.8 and 12.9 show some clustering results using the cell cycle expression data of yeast from Spellman et al. (http://cellcycle-www.stanford.edu; Spellman et al., 1998). The dataset contains expression profiles for 6,220 genes under different experimental conditions. Genes with similar expression profiles are seen to cluster successfully into the same group.

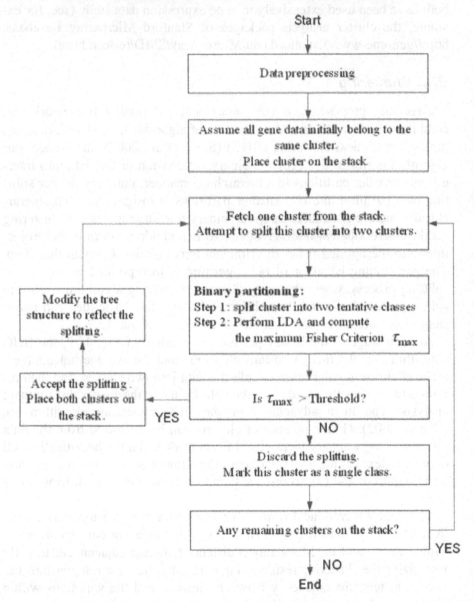

Fig. 12.7. Data flow diagram of the BHC clustering algorithm

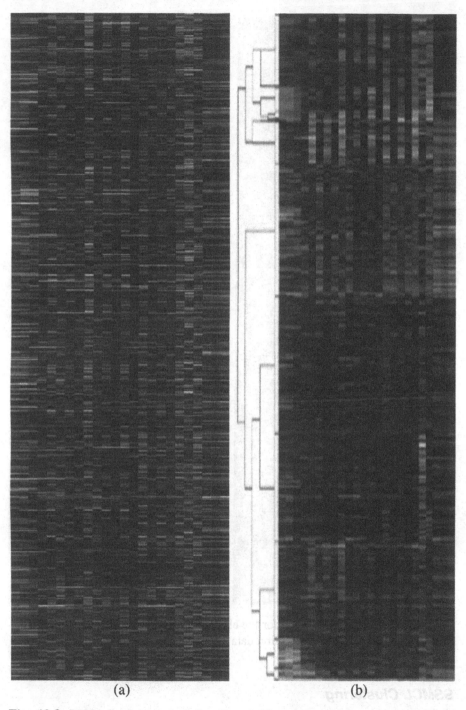

Fig. 12.8. BHC clustering result for the cdc15 experiment dataset. (a) Original gene expression data; (b) Expression data after BHC clustering

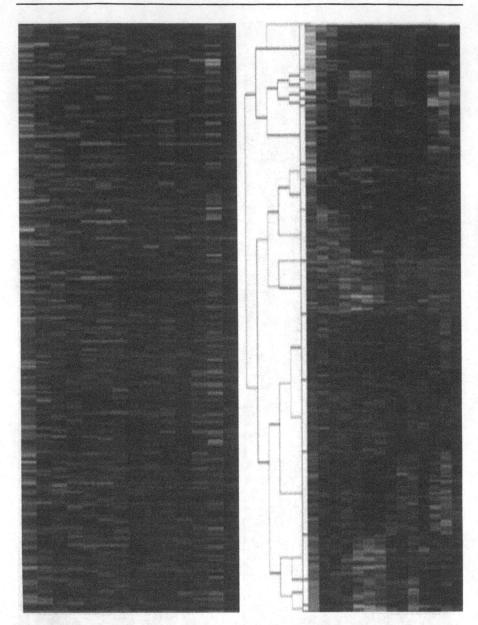

Fig. 12.9. BHC clustering result for the elutriation experiment dataset. (a) Original gene expression data; (b) Expression data after BHC clustering

SSMCL Clustering

In conventional clustering algorithms, if the number of prototypes is less than that of the natural clusters in the dataset, there must be at least one prototype that wins patterns from more than two clusters, and this behavior is called one-prototype-take-multiple-clusters (OPTMC) (see Fig. 12.10a). The implications of not finding natural clusters are: (i) a natural cluster might be erroneously divided into two or more classes, or worse still, (ii) several natural clusters, or parts of them are erroneously grouped into one class. Such behaviors would lead to wrong inferences about the data.

In view of the above shortcomings, we recently proposed a new partitional clustering framework called Self-Splitting and Merging Competitive Learning Clustering (SSMCL) (Wu et al., 2004). The new algorithm is able to identify the natural clusters through the adoption of a new competitive learning paradigm called the one-prototype-take-one-clusters (OPTOC) (Zhang and Liu, 2002). The OPTOC learning paradigm allows a cluster prototype to focus on just one natural cluster, while minimizing the competitions from other natural clusters (see Fig. 12.10b). The OPTOC behavior of a cluster prototype is achieved through the use of a dynamic neighborhood, which causes the prototype to eventually settle at the center of a natural cluster while ignoring competition from other clusters.

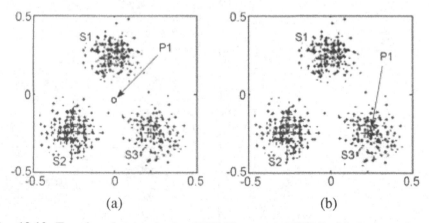

(a)   (b)

Fig. 12.10. Two learning methods: OPTMC versus OPTOC. (a) One prototype takes the center of three clusters (OPTMC). (b) One prototype takes one cluster (OPTOC) and ignores the other two clusters, (See Zhang and Liu, 2002)

Since it is very difficult to estimate reliably the correct number of natural clusters in a complex high dimensional dataset, an over-clustering and merging strategy was used to estimate the number of *distinct clusters* in the dataset. The over-clustering and merging strategy can be viewed as a top-down (divisive clustering), followed by a bottom-up (agglomerative clustering), process. In the top-down step, loose clusters (as measured by their variances) are successively split into two clusters until a pre-specified

370   Alan W.-C. Liew et al.

number of clusters, set to be larger than the true number of clusters in the data, is obtained. The over-clustering minimizes the chance of missing some natural clusters in the data. The merging step then attempts to merge similar clusters together, until finally all remaining clusters are distinct from each other. The merging scheme is based on the observation that a natural cluster should be expected to have a unimodal distribution. When two clusters are close to each other to the extent that their joint probability density function (pdf) is unimodal, these two clusters are merged into one. Together with the OPTOC framework, the over-clustering and merging framework allow a systematic estimation of the correct number of natural clusters in the dataset.

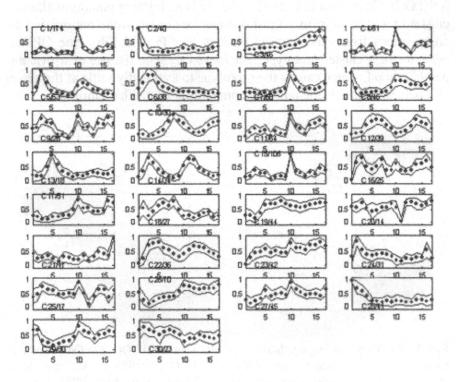

Fig. 12.11. The clustering results for the yeast cell cycle data. The number of clusters is set to 30

The SSMCL algorithm was used to cluster the yeast cell cycle data downloaded from http://genomics.stanford.edu (Spellman et al., 1998). The data was first over-clustered into 30 clusters (see Fig. 12.11). Cluster merging is then performed on the result until finally 22 clusters are obtained (see Fig. 12.12). Whereas similar clusters can be seen in Fig. 12.11, the 22 clusters in Fig. 12.12 are all visually distinct from each other.

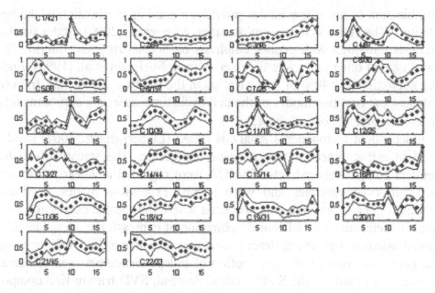

Fig. 12.12. The final clustering results for the yeast cell cycle data after cluster merging. 22 distinct clusters are obtained

12.4.2 Temporal Expression Profile Analysis and Gene Regulation

Time series of whole genome expression data are a particularly valuable sources of information because they can describe dynamic biological processes such as the cell cycles or metabolic processes (DeRisi et al, 1997, and Spellman et al., 1998). They allow the determination of causal relationships between the expressions of different genes. Such causal relationships allow the extraction of gene regulatory information, and ultimately lead to a better understanding of the complicated gene networking process within a cell.

Several methods were proposed to extract the significant modes of variation from the large array of time series expression data. Holter et al., (2000) used Singular Value Decomposition (SVD) to extract the "characteristic modes" of gene expression in the sporulation dataset (Chu et al., 1998), a yeast cell cycle dataset (cdc15) (Spellman et al., 1998), and a serum-treated human fibroblasts dataset (Iyer et al., 1999). They found that the first two modes capture 62%, 69%, and 72% of the variation for the cdc15, fibroblast, and sporulation datasets, respectively. They showed that the behavior of the widely disparate gene systems analyzed in their work is dominated by a small subset of the characteristic modes and that a linear combination of just a few modes provides a good approximation of the behavior of the entire system in most cases. Alter et al. (2000) used a similar analysis (although with greater emphasis on normalizing and filtering the data) on two other cell cycle time series from Spellman et al. (1998), finding approximately 40% of the variation in the top two eigengenes. In both datasets, the first two modes of the cell cycle time series are approximately sinusoidal and 90° out of phase.

Independent Components Analysis (ICA) (Liebermeister, 2002) can be used to extract linear modes of gene expression. The statistically independent components extracted by ICA were regarded as linear influences of unobserved variables and were termed expression modes. A linear model of gene expression was proposed where the sample expression profiles are determined by a linear combination of expression modes. The ICA model assumes that the different modes exert *independent influences* on the genes. In contrast, the assumption of independence between principal modes is not made in the SVD method. Instead, SVD tries to find components that maximally explain the variation in the data. Both temporal expression data (Yeast cell cycle data from Spellman at al., 1998) and non-temporal B-cell Lymphoma data (Alizadeh et al., 2000) were analyzed by Liebermeister.

The temporal nature of time series gene expression data was explicitly modeled by Dewey and Galas (2001) using a dynamic model. They modeled the entire set of time series gene expression data using a first order Markov model, which is equivalent to a first order autoregressive (AR) model. SVD was used to solve for the Markov transition matrix (which specifies the transition of the data from one time step to another time step) in the resulting matrix equation. By incorporating additional terms into the first order equation, they showed that some nonlinearity can be included into the linear dynamic model. The expression profiles for the diauxic shift (DeRisi et al., 1997) and for the cell cycle data (Spellman et al., 1998) were analyzed. The construction of a genetic network consisting of "dynamic classes" based on the transition matrix was also demonstrated.

All the methods mentioned above analyze the gene expression data as a whole, and attempt to summarize the dataset by a few dominant components. The characteristic of each gene is then obtained by projecting its expression profile onto the dominant components. The dominant components can be viewed as the "summary statistics" of the entire dataset. These methods can therefore be considered global in this sense.

Another class of algorithms attempt to perform pairwise comparison of gene expressions to identify pairs of genes from the set of gene expression profiles that have direct regulatory relationships. Such a comparison is local, in the sense that no "summary statistics" of the entire dataset is used in the comparison. Algorithms that perform such pairwise analysis for extracting regulatory information from time series; include microarray data of the simple correlation analysis method (Eisen et al., 1998), the edge detection method (Eisen M.B. et al., 1998), the event method (Kwon et al., 2003), and the spectral component correlation method (Yeung L.K. et al., 2004).

Among the various pairwise comparison approaches, the correlation-based method is perhaps the most popular one. This method determines whether or not two genes have a regulatory relationship by checking the global similarity between their expression profiles using the Pearson correlation measure. However, it does not take into account the fact that there is often a time delay before the regulator gene product can exert its influence on the target gene. Such a time delay can significantly degrade the performance of the method. The correlation method also strongly favors global similarity over more localized similarities arising from conditional regulatory relationships.

The edge detection method and the event-based method are designed specifically to overcome the shortcomings of the correlation-based analysis. The edge detection method scans through each gene expression curve to determine where major changes in expression levels (edges) occur. To produce a score, the edge detection method sums up the number of edges in two gene expression curves that share the same direction and are within reasonable distances of each other. Gene pairs that are likely to have an activation relationship would give high scores. Similar to the edge method, the event method also examines the slope of the expression profile at each time interval. Instead of deriving a similarity score directly from the slope, the event method associates an event with each slope. Depending on the slope value, the algorithm marks each event as either rising (R), constant (C), or falling (F), resulting in a string of events for each expression profile. A pairwise sequence alignment of the event strings is then performed to obtain a numerical score that reflects the regulatory relationship between two genes.

If the expression of gene A varies periodically at constant frequency, we expect the expression of gene B to more or less at the same frequency. This frequency of variation, however, may not be easily seen from the two time series expression profiles due to noise and other factors. In addition, if gene B is under the influence of both gene A and gene C ("two-regulating-one" situation), and the expression profiles of these influencing genes vary at different frequencies, then the relationship between gene A and gene B may not be easily seen from their time series profiles. This would cause problems for correlation-based similarity comparison, as well as the edge detection method and the event-based method.

A spectral component correlation approach (Yeung et al., 2003) is proposed to measure the correlation between time series expression data, and use the results to infer to potential regulatory relationships between genes. The technique summarizes the essential features of an expression pattern by means of a frequency spectrum estimated by autoregressive modeling (Marple, 1987). Specifically, the pattern is decomposed into a set of damped sinusoids of different frequencies so that each sinusoid can be considered separately during the analysis. We consider both types of transcriptional regulation, activation and inhibition. In the activation process, the product of gene A affects the transcription process of gene B such that the production rate for gene B increases. On the other hand, the inhibition process involves gene A's production decreasing the production of gene B.

The idea behind our technique is to decompose a time series expression profile $x[n]$ into a set of discrete time damped sinusoids of various frequencies. Hence we model the sequence as

$$x[n] = \sum_{i=1}^{M} x_i[n] = \sum_{i=1}^{M} \alpha_i \exp(\sigma_i n) \cos(\omega_i n + \phi_i).$$

The parameters in this model, α_i, σ_i, ω_i, and ϕ_i ($i = 1, 2, 3, \ldots M$), are the amplitude, damping factor, normalized frequency and phase angle of component i., respectively The correlation of $x[n]$ with another sequence $y[n]$ can then be reformulated as a sum of scaled componentwise correlations,

$$x[n] \circ y[n] = \sum_i \sum_j \sqrt{\frac{E_{x_i} E_{y_j}}{E_x E_y}} x_i[n] \circ y_j[n],$$

where $\circ$ denotes the correlation operation, and each term with the letter E represents either total energy of a sequence or energy of a particular component. This equation shows how a correlation of two sequences can be separated into a set of scaled componentwise correlations between each spectral component. Such componentwise correlations may provide more insights into the regulatory relationship. For instance, for the "two-regulating-one" situation, the correlation between the expression profiles of gene A and gene B may not be strong enough to suggest their relationship due to the presence of spectral components in gene B induced by gene C. However, the spectral components of gene B due to gene A would exhibit strong correlations to gene A's expression profile. Therefore, these scaled componentwise correlations can be used instead as a more reliable measurement for the relationship between these genes.

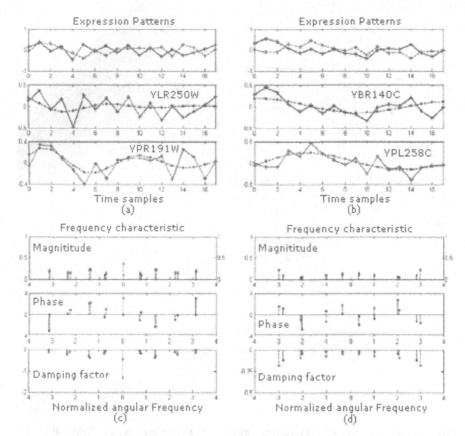

Fig. 12.13. (a) Known activation regulation involving genes YLR256W and YPR191W. (b) Known activation regulation involving genes YBR240C and YPL258C. In both (a) and (b), the top graphs show the gene expression profiles for the regulatory pairs, whilethe middle and bottom graphs show each of the expression profiles (with their corresponding lowest frequency components) individually. (c) Frequency characteristics obtained from the AR modeling technique for the expression profiles of genes YLR256W and YPR191W. (d) Frequency characteristics obtained from the AR modeling technique for the expression profiles of genes YBR240C and YPL258C. The top, middle, and bottom graphs in both (c) and (d) show the magnitudes, phases, and damping factors of the estimated frequency components for these expression profiles of these regulatory pairs, respectively

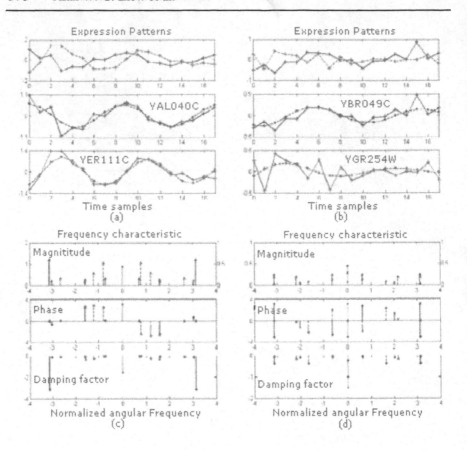

Fig. 12.14. (a) Known activation regulation involving genes YAL040C and YER111C. The dominant frequency components for these two genes are plotted in the middle and bottom graphs. Although they both strongly oscillate at a frequency of about 0.76 radians per second, the time lag, together with other unmatched components, makes them have the low correlation value of -0.3885. (b) Known inhibition regulation involving genes YBR049C and YGR254W with correlation coefficient -0.3226. The dominant frequency components for these gene pairs are plotted in the middle and bottom graphs. (c) Frequency characteristics for the regulatory gene pair YAL040C and YER111C. The dominant frequencies for these two profiles are 0.7248 radians per second and 0.8066 radians per second, respectively. (d) Frequency characteristics for the regulatory gene pair YBR049C and YGR254W. The dominant frequencies are 0.6395 radians per second for the first gene and 0.6271 radians per second for the second gene

We use the spectral component correlation algorithm to analyze the alpha-synchronized yeast cell cycle dataset from Spellman et al. (1998). We were able to detect many regulatory pairs that were missed by the traditional correlation method due to weak correlation. Figure 12.13 shows two known activation pairs. The first one involves genes YLR256W and

YPR191W, and the second one involves genes YBR240C and YPL258C. As can be seen, the two genes in each regulatory pair do not have similar expression patterns, and their correlation coefficients are -0.1491 and -0.1127 for the first and second pair, respectively. However, looking at the magnitude plots of the frequency components, we find that the time series profiles in each regulatory pair have very similar spectral characteristics. Their low correlation coefficients are due to phase differences between closely matched frequency components. Figures 12.13(a) and 12.14(b) plot for each pair the original expression patterns against their corresponding lowest frequency components. The low frequency components identify the general variations for the profiles, and the time lags between the activators and activatees are clearly revealed.

Table 12.1. Estimated frequency components for various expression profiles.

a	YAL040C				YER111C			
i	σi	ωi	αi	φi	σi	ωi	αi	φi
1	-1.5993	0.0000	0.8670	3.1416	-0.0203	0.8066	0.5167	-2.5294
2	-0.0047	0.7248	0.3177	-0.0226	-0.2575	1.2087	0.2854	-2.8483
3	-0.0729	1.5913	0.1697	-2.3890	-0.3592	1.5766	0.1318	-2.6949
4	-0.1313	3.0256	0.2068	0.6806	-0.0869	2.6468	0.1626	-0.0445
5	-3.1281	3.1416	1.1970	0.0000	-	-	-	-

b	YBR049C				YGR254W			
i	σi	ωi	αi	φi	σi	ωi	αi	φi
1	-1.0018	0.0000	0.4460	0.0000	-1.4952	0.0000	0.0740	3.1416
2	-0.0384	0.6395	0.2385	2.6440	0.1026	0.6271	0.1378	-1.9743
3	-0.0953	2.0240	0.0479	1.2530	-0.3656	1.6564	0.0821	2.2515
4	-0.0677	3.1416	0.2381	3.1416	-0.1718	2.1764	0.1833	0.2889
5	-0.3813	3.1416	0.0234	-3.1416	-0.0340	3.1416	0.1867	0.0000

(a) Components for genes YAL040C and YER111C. (b) Components for genes YBR049C and YGR254W. Components with strong correlation are highlighted.

For those regulations with strong oscillatory but time-shifted expression pairs, we can easily identify them by using only the spectral magnitude information, while ignoring the phase information. An example is given in Fig. 12.14(a), in which the expression profiles and spectrums for an activation pair involving genes YAL040C and YER111C are shown. These two patterns strongly oscillate at around 0.76 rad/s, but still have a relatively low correlation value of -0.3885 because of the time lag between them aother and unmatched components. The spectral magnitude plot (the top graph in Fig. 12.14(c)) shows that their dominant components are closely matched with each other. It should be noted that the component for gene YAL040C with frequency of 3.1416 rad/s is not considered dominant due to its large decaying factor (see the bottom graph in Fig. 12.14(c)). Another example, an inhibition regulation, is shown in Fig. 12.14(b). Careful examination of the phase angles of the dominant components in these examples suggests that the activatee has a phase lag between 0 and 180° relative to the activator's phase angle, whereas the inhibitee has a phase lead between 0 and 180° relative to the inhibitor's phase angle.

When comparing two expression patterns, it is often necessary to neglect certain irrelevant components that may otherwise corrupt the correlation between them. In fact, a large number of known regulations having weak correlations are caused by such irrelevant components. For example, the components at 0.7248 rad/s for gene YAL040C and 0.8066 rad/s for gene YER111C (see Table 12.6) clearly dominate over other components. The componentwise correlation with phase alignment using just this component is 0.7665. Compared to the original correlation value of -0.3885, the componentwise correlation strongly suggests similarity between the two patterns.

Table 12.2. Results for the two correlation methods applied to all 439 known regulatory pairs.

a	Traditional Correlation < 0.5	Traditional Correlation > 0.5	Total
Componentwise Correlation < 0.5	111	9	120
Componentwise Correlation > 0.5	196*	27	223
Total	307	36	343

b	Traditional Correlation < -0.5	Traditional Correlation > -0.5	Total
Componentwise Correlation < 0.5	1	40	41
Componentwise Correlation > 0.5	4	51*	55
Total	5	91	96

(a) Statistics for the 343 activation pairs. (b) Statistics for the 96 inhibition pairs.

When the componentwise correlation analysis is applied to all 439 known regulations, the results indicated that 223 of the 343 activations and 55 of the 96 inhibitions have their componentwise correlations score greater than 0.5 (see Table 12.1). We found that a large number of visually dissimilar expression pairs have very similar dominant frequency components. For example, among those 307 pairs having traditional correlation coefficients of less than 0.5, 196 of them have componentwise correlation coefficients greater than 0.5. Furthermore, 60 of the 196 pairs have their componentwise correlation coefficients greater than 0.9, and the expression patterns in each of these pairs strongly oscillate at almost identical frequencies. The spectral component correlation method allows the hidden componentwise relationships between two expression profiles, which are otherwise hidden in the traditional correlation method, to be revealed.

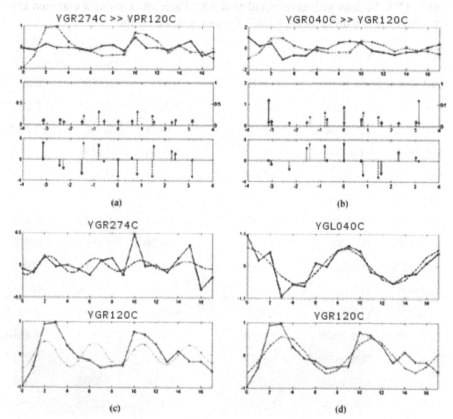

Fig. 12.15. Two activation regulations with gene YPR120C as an activatee. (a) Activation regulation with gene YGR274C as an activator. (b) Activation regulation with gene YAL040C as an activator. (c) Correlated frequency components for the first pair. (d) Correlated frequency components for the second pair

For those regulations involving a single gene being simultaneously regulated by two or more genes with different expression frequencies, it could be possible to identify them by checking for the existence of regulators' frequencies in the expression profile of the gene being regulated. Figure

12.15 shows two known activation regulations with a common gene, YPR120C, as an activatee. The figure reveals that the first regulation has its expression profiles correlated at a frequency of about 1.48 rad/s, whereas the second regulation has its profiles correlated at a frequency of about 0.76 rad/s. We have also found eight "n-regulating-one" activation sets having the following properties: i) each set contains a common activatee, and ii) the activatee has two different correlation frequencies for its regulators. These activation sets are summarized in Table 12.3.

Table 12.3. Various activation regulation sets. Each set contains a common activatee that has two different correlated frequency components.

Activator	Activatee	Traditional Correlation	Componentwise correlation	Activator Frequency	Activatee Frequency
YKL109W	YGL167C	0.2877	0.9237	0.6505	0.6842
YLR433C	YGL167C	0.1980	0.5287	1.3502	1.6359
YHR079C	YJL034W	-0.6594	0.9894	0.7063	0.7205
YPL085W	YJL034W	0.2717	0.6120	1.7581	1.9513
YKL109W	YLL041C	0.3792	0.9917	0.5339	0.5230
YBL021C	YLL041C	0.2586	0.9564	1.3748	1.3725
YGL237C	YLL041C	-0.4687	0.8484	0.6456	0.5230
YOR358W	YLL041C	0.3800	0.8008	1.2639	1.3725
YLR182W	YLR286C	-0.1208	0.8984	1.1082	1.0378
YLR071C	YLR286C	0.0349	0.6662	0.3324	0.4353
YLR131C	YLR286C	-0.2762	0.6535	0.5338	0.4353
YEL009C	YOR202W	0.0554	0.9276	1.2653	1.1670
YRL082C	YOR202W	0.6075	0.8912	0.3199	0.3517
YEL009C	YPR035W	-0.3737	0.9541	1.2653	1.2241
YFL021W	YPR035W	-0.2153	0.9002	0.4095	0.3662
YGR274C	YPR120C	0.4075	0.8541	1.5266	1.4566
YAL040C	YPR120C	-0.4331	0.7288	0.7248	0.8120
YLR256W	YPR191W	-0.1491	0.9173	0.7762	0.7295
YGL237C	YPR191W	-0.7333	0.8821	0.6456	0.7295
YBL021C	YPR191W	-0.2231	0.7569	1.3748	1.4294
YOR358W	YPR191W	0.0937	0.7209	0.6227	0.7295
YKL109W	YPR191W	0.2663	0.6254	0.5339	0.7295

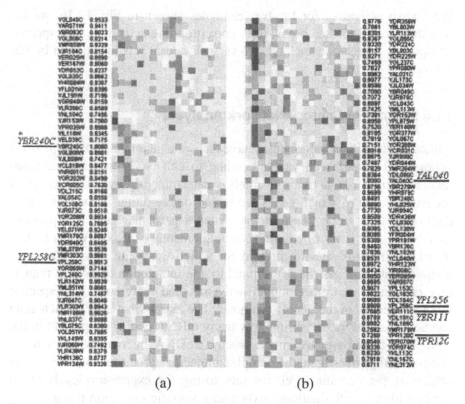

(a)   (b)

Fig. 12.16. Genes in the Filkov's dataset have their componentwise correlation coefficients, relative to gene (a) YBR240C and gene (b) YAL040C, greater than 0.7. The known activation regulations with genes YBR240C and YAL040C as activators are highlighted

To see how causal relationships can be inferred from the algorithm, we chose the genes YBR240C and YAL040C as references and foundall other genes in the Filkov's dataset (Filkov et al., 2002) which has a componentwise correlation coefficient greater than 0.7. There are 55 of the 288 genes for YBR240C and 59 of the 288 genes for YAL040C that satisfy this threshold. These two sets of genes with their scores are shown in Fig. 12.16, and their oscillatory properties are clearly revealed when they are arranged such that their phases are in descending order. Within these genes, one known activation regulation gene YBR240C is contained in the first set and three one known activation regulation for gene YAL040C are contained in the second set. Note that genes below the reference gene have their phases lag by $0°$ to $180°$ relative to the reference gene's phase, and they can be considered as potential activated candidates. On the other hand, genes above the reference gene have their phases lead by $0°$ to $180°$, and they can be considered as potential inhibited candidates. If we look at the known activatees for the two examples shown in Fig. 12.16, we see that they are all located below their corresponding activators. The spectral component correlation method allows such causal relationships to be observed.

12.4.3 Gene Regulatory Network Analysis

Although all cells in an organism have the same genomic data, the proteins synthesized in each cell vary according to cell type, time, and environmental factors. The activity of a cell is determined by which of its genes are expressed, i.e., which genes are turned on, resulting in the active production of their respective proteins. When a particular gene is expressed, its DNA is first transcribed into the complementary mRNA, which is then translated into the specific protein for which this gene codes. The transcription rate of a gene is determined by the interaction of diverse regulatory proteins, i.e., transcriptional activators and repressors, with specific DNA sequences in the gene's promoter. The expression level of each gene can be measured by measuring how many mRNA copies are present in the cell. High throughput techniques such as cDNA microarray allow us to systematically investigate the complex molecular processes and their interactions at the genome level. By monitoring the expression levels of all genes within a cell simultaneously under specific condition using cDNA microarray, we can determine which genes are up-regulated, down-regulated, or not expressed under a specific conditions, and detect any correlations between the levels of expression of different genes. Using such information, the logic of gene regulation in a cell can be deciphered (De-Risi et al., 1997).

Different models of gene regulation have been proposed. The simplest genetic regulatory network is the Boolean network first introduced by Kauffman in the late 1960s (Kauffman, 1969). The network is represented as a directed graph $G = (V, F)$, whose nodes V represent elements of the network, and F defines a topology of edges between the nodes and a set of Boolean functions. The Boolean network models each gene as being either ON or OFF, and the state of each gene at the next time step is determined by Boolean function of its input at the current time step. Despite its simplicity, Boolean networks are able to provide valuable insights in the behavior of gene interactions (Kauffman, 1993, and Wuensche, 1999) and have been applied in the analysis of real gene expression data for applications such as the identification of drug targets for cancer therapy (Szallasi and Liang, 1998, and Huang, 1999).

Although the Boolean network has proved useful in gene regulation studies, there are concerns about the biological plausibility of such a simple model. For one thing, gene expression data have not binary but continuous. Moreover, gene expression data is generally noisy and contain a high level of uncertainty. Such considerations have led to the proposal of various modifications on the basic Boolean network, such as the noisy Boolean network (Akutsu et al., 2000), the probabilistic Boolean network (Shmulevich et al., 2002a,b), and the hybrid Boolean network, where each gene has a continuously valued internal state and a Boolean external state (Glass, 1975, and Glass and Pasternack, 1978), or asynchronously updated logic with intermediate threshold values (Thomas 1991, and Thieffry and Thomas, 1998).

Other gene regulatory network models has also been proposed. The mRNA expression levels have been modeled (D'haeseleer et al., 1999, 2000) during Central Nervous System (CNS) development and injury by using a linear additive model, where the expression level of a gene is modeled as the weighted sum of the expression levels of other genes. Chen and He et al. (1999) proposed a number of linear differential equation models, which include both mRNA and protein levels, and showed how such models can be solved using linear algebra and Fourier transforms. Butte et al. (2000) introduced the concept of relevance network, where pairs of patterns are compared and groups of patterns higher than a specific threshold will aggregate to form relevance networks. Several groups have proposed the use of Bayesian networks for genetic regulatory network modeling (Friedman et al., 2000; Hartemink et al., 2002; and Imoto et al., 2002a,b). Bayesian networks are a type of graphical model for capturing complex relationships between a large amount of random variables by the directed acyclic graph encoding the Markov assumption. The modeling based on recurrent neural networks has also being shown to be potentially useful (Marnellos and Mjolsness, 1998; Marnellos et al., 2000; Vohradsky, 2001a,b; and Vu and Vohradsky 2002). In such a model, the regulatory process is considered as the combinatorial action of gene products on the rate of expression of a particular gene, and the action is modulated by a particular transfer function to generate the response curves. The accumulation of gene product, controlled by the regulators, is modified by degradation, usually modeled as a first order chemical reaction. In contrast with linear additive model, the recurrent neural network can model the nonlinearity in the genetic regulatory process due to the presence of a nonlinear transfer function in the model.

Genetic regulatory network modeling is an active area of research in functional genomics. Although complete modeling of the genetic regulatory process is currently unattainable, with the availability of more experimental data on the cellular and biochemical processes at the genome level, better understanding of the biology and chemistry of the transcription and translation processes, and better modeling techniques, one can be hopeful of unraveling complex genetic interactions and the mechanisms of cellular processes in the near future.

References

Akutsu, T., Miyano, S. and Kuhara, S. (2000) Inferring qualitative relations in genetic networks and metabolic pathways. Bioinformatics **16**: 727-734.

Alon, U., Barkai, N., Notterman, D.A., Gish, K., Ybarra, S., Mack, D. and Levine, A.J. (1999) Gene expression revealed by clustering analysis of tumor and normal colon tissues probed by oligonucleotide arrays. Proc. Nat. Acad. Sci. USA. **96**: 6745-6750.

Alter, O., Brown, P.O., Botstein, D. (2000) Singular value decomposition for genome-wide expression data processing and modeling. Proc. Nat. Acad. Sci. USA. **97**: 10101-10106.

Axon Instruments Inc. GenePix Pro 3.0, 2001.

Brazma,, A. and Vilo, J. (2000) Minireview: Gene expression data analysis. European Molecular Biology Laboratory, Outstation Hinxton – the European Bioinformatics institute, Cambridge CB10 ISD UK.

Buckley, M. (2002) The Spot User's Guide. CSIRO Mathematical and Information Sciences, Australia. http://www.cmis.csiro.au/iap/spot.htm.

Buhler, J., Ideker, T., Haynor, D. (2000) Dapple: Improved Techniques for Finding Spots on DNA Microarrays. Technical Report UWTR 2000-08-05, University of Washington.

Butte, A.J., Tamayo, P., Slonim, D., Golub, T.R., and Kohane, I.S. (2000). Discovering functional relationships between RNA expression and chemotherapeutic susceptibility using relevance networks. Proc. Nat. Acad. Sci. USA. **97**(22): 12182-12186.

Chen, T., He, H.L., Church, G.M. (1999) Modeling gene expression with differential equations. Pacific Symposium on Biocomputing **4**: 29-40.

Chen, T., Filkov, V. and Skiena, S.S. (1999) Identifying gene regulatory networks from experimental data. Proceedings of the Third Annual International Conference on Computational Molecular Biology RECOMB99, Lyon, France, March 1999, pp 94-103.

Chen, Y., Dougherty, E.R. and Bittner, M.L. (1997) Ratio-based decisions and the Quantitative Analysis of cDNA Microarray Images. J. Biomedical Optics. **2**: 364-374.

Chu, S., DeRisi, J., Eisen, M., Mulholland, J., Botstein, D., Brown, P.O. and Herskowitz, I. (1998) The transcriptional program of sporulation in budding yeast. Science **282** (5389): 699-705

Clausi, D.A. (2002). K-means Iterative Fisher (KIF) unsupervised clustering algorithm applied to image texture segmentation. Pattern Recognition **35**: 1959-1972.

D'Haeseleer, P., Wen, X., Fuhrman, S. and Somogyi, R. (1999) Linear modeling of mRNA expression levels during CNS development and injury. Pacific Symposium on Biocomputing **4**: 41-52.

D'Haeseleer, P., Liang and S., Somogyi, R. (2000) Genetic network inference: from co-expression clustering to reverse engineering. Bioinformatics **16**(8): 707-726.

DeRisi, J.L., Lyer, V.R. and Brown, P.O. (1997) Exploring the metabolic and genetic control of gene expression on a genomic scale. Science **278**: 680-686.

Duda, R.O., Hart, P.E. and Stork, D.G. (2001). Pattern Classification. Wiley-Interscience, NewYork.

Eisen, M. (1999) ScanAlyze User Manual. Stanford University. http://rana.lbl.gov/EisenSoftware.htm.

Eisen, M.B., Spellman, P.T., Brown, P.O. and Botstein, D. (1998) Cluster analysis and display of genome-wide expression patterns. Proc. Nat. Acad. Sci. USA. **95**: 14863-14868.

Filkov, V., Skiena, S. and Zhi, J. (2002) Analysis Techniques for microarray time series data. J. Comp. Biol. **9**(2): 317-330.

Friedman, N., Linial, M., Nachman, I. and Pe'er, D. (2000) Using Bayesian network to analyze expression data. J. Comp. Biol., **7**: 601-620.

Glass, L. (1975) Combinatorial and topological methods in nonlinear chemical kinetics. J. Chem. Phys. **63**(4): 1325-1335.

Glass, L. and Pasternack, J.S. (1978) Stable oscillations in mathematical models of biological control systems. J. Math. Biol. **6**: 207-223.

Golub, T.R., Slonim, D.K., Tamayo, P., Huard, C., Gaasenbeek, M., Mesirov, J.P., Coller, H., Loh, M.L., Downing, J.R., Caligiuri, M.A., Bloomfield, C.D. and Lander, E.S. (1999) Molecular classification of cancer: Class discovery and class prediction by gene expression monitoring. Science **286**: 531-537.

Hartemink, A.J., Gifford, D.K., Jaakkola, T.S. and Young, R.A. (2002) Combining location and expression data for principled discovery of genetic regulatory network models. Pacific Symposium on Biocomputing **7**: 437-449.

Imoto, S., Goto, T. and Miyano, S. (2002a) Estimation of genetic networks and functional structures between genes by using Bayesian networks and nonparametric regression. Pacific Symposium on Biocomputing **7**: 175-186.

Imoto, S., Kim, S., Goto, T., Aburatani, S., Tashiro, K., Kuhara, S. and Miyano, S. (2002b) Bayesian network and nonparametric heteroscedastic regression for nonlinear modeling of genetic network. Journal of Bioinformatics and Computational Biology, in press. (Preliminary version has appeared in Proc. 1st IEEE Computer Society Bioinformatics Conference, 219-227, 2002).

Holter, N.S., Mitra, M., Maritan, A., Cieplak, M., Banavar, J.R. and Fedoroff, N.V. (2000) Fundamental patterns underlying gene expression profiles: Simplicity from complexity. Proc. Nat. Acad. Sci. USA. **97**: 8409-8414.

Huang, S. (1999) Gene expression profiling, genetic networks, and cellular states: an integrating concept for tumorigenesis and drug discovery. J. Mol. Med. 77:469-480.

Iyer, V.R., Eisen, M.B., Ross, D.T., Schuler, G., Moore, T., Lee, J.C.F. and Trent, J.M., Staudt, L.M., Hudson, Jr. J., Boguski, M.S., Lashkari, D., Shalon, D., Botstein, D. and Brown, P.O. (1999) The transcriptional program in the response of human fibroblasts to serum. Science 283(5398): 83-97.

Kauffman, S.A. (1969) Metabolic stability and epigenesist in randomly connected nets. J. Theor. Biol. 22: 437-467.

Kauffman, S.A. (1993) The origin of order: Self-organization and selection in evolution. Oxford University Press, New York.

Kooperberg, C., Fazzio, T.G., Delrow, J.J. and Tsukiyama, T. (2002) Improved background correction for spotted DNA microarrays. J. Comp. Biol. 9(1): 55-66.

Kwon, A.T, Hoos, H.H. and Ng, R. (2003) Inference of transcriptional regulation relationships from gene expression data. Bioinformatics 19(8):905-912.

Liebermeister, W. (2002) Linear modes of gene expression determined by independent component analysis. Bioinformatics 18(1): 51-60.

Liew, A.W.C., Yan, H. and Yang, M. (2003a) Robust Adaptive Spot Segmentation of DNA Microarray Images. Pattern Recognition 36(5): 1251-1254.

Liew, A.W.C., Szeto, L.K., Tang, S.S. and Yan, H. (2003b) A computational approach to gene expression data extraction and analysis. To appear in special issue on "Genomic Signal Processing". J. VLSI Signal Processing-Systems for Signal, Image, and Video Technology.

Lockhart, D.J. and Winzeler, E.A. (2000) Genomics, gene expression and DNA arrays. Nature 405:827–846.

Marnellos, G., Mjolsness, E. (1998) A gene network approach to modeling early neurogenesis in Drosophila. Pacific Symposium on Biocomputing 3: 30-41.

Marnellos, G., Deblandre, G.A., Mjolsness, E. and Kintner, C. (2000) Delta-Notch lateral inhibitory patterning in the emergence of ciliated cells in Xenopus: experimental observations and a gene network model. Pacific Symposium on Biocomputing 5: 329-340.

Marple, S. (1987) Digital Spectral Analysis with Applications. Prentice Hall Inc., Englewood Cliffs, New Jersey.

Moore, S.K. (2001). Making Chips to probe genes. IEEE Spectrum, March 2001, pp.54-60.

Packard BioChip Technologies, LLC, QuantArray Microarray Analysis Software

Perou, C.M., Jeffrey, S.S., van de Rijn, M., Rees, C.A., Eisen, M.B., Ross, D.T., Pergamenschikov, A., Williams, C.F., Zhu, S.X., Lee, J.C.F., Lashkari, D., Shalon, D., Brown, P.O. and Botstein, D. (1999) Distinctive gene expression patterns in human mammary epithelial cells and breast cancers. Proc. Nat. Acad. Sci. USA. 96: 9212–9217.

Sambrook, J. and Russell, D.W. (2001) Molecular Cloning: A Laboratory Manual. 3rd Ed., Cold Spring Harbor Laboratory Press, New York.

Schena, M., Shalon, D., Davis, R.W. and Brown, P.O. (1995) Quantitative monitoring of gene expression patterns with a complementary DNA microarray. Science **270**:467-470.

Shmulevich, I., Dougherty, E.R. and Zhang, W. (2002a) From Boolean to probabilistic Boolean networks as models of genetic regulatory networks. Proc. IEEE **90**(11): 1778-1792.

Shmulevich, I., Dougherty, E.R., Kim, S. and Zhang, W. (2002b) Probablistic Boolean networks: a rule-based uncertainty model for gene regulatory networks. Bioinformatics **18**: 261-274.

Spellman, P.T., Sherlock, G., Zhang, M.Q., Iyer, V.R., Anders, K., Eisen, M.B., Brown, P.O., Botstein, D. and Futcher, B. (1998) Comprehensive Identification of Cell Cycle-regulated Genes of the Yeast Saccharomyces cerevisiae by Microarray Hybridization. Molecular Biology of the Cell **9**: 3273-3297.

Szallasi, Z. and Liang, S. (1998) Modeling the normal and neoplastic cell cycle with realistic Boolean genetic networks: their application for understanding carcinogenesis and assessing therapeutic strategies. Pacific Symposium on Biocomputing **3**: 66-76.

Szeto, L.K., Liew, A.W.C., Yan, H. and Tang, S.S. (2003) Gene expression data clustering and visualization based on a binary hierarchical clustering framework. J. Vis. Lang. Computing **14**: 341-362.

Tamayo, P., Slonim, D., Mesirov, J., Zhu, Q., Kitareewan, S., Dmitrovsky, E., Lander, E.S. and Golub, T.R. (1999) Interpreting patterns of gene expression with self-organizing maps: Methods and application to hematopoietic differentiation. Proc. Nat. Acad. Sci. USA. **96**: 2907–2912.

Tang, C., Zhang, L. and Zhang, A. (2002) Interactive visualization and analysis for gene expression data. IEEE Proceedings of the Hawaii International Conference on System Sciences. Big Island, HI. January 2002. **6**: 143-166.

Thieffry, D. and Thomas, R. (1998) Qualitative analysis of gene networks. Pacific Symposium on Biocomputing **3**: 77-88.

Thomas, R. (1991) Regulatory networks seen as asynchronous automata: a logical description. J. Theor. Biol. **153**:1-23.

Troyanskaya, O., Cantor, M., Sherlock, G., Brown, P., Hastie, T., Tibshirani, R., Botstein, D., and Altman, R.B. (2001) Missing values estimation methods for DNA microarrays. Bioinformatics **17**: 520-525.

Vohradsky, J. (2001a) Neural model of the genetic network. J. Biol. Chem. **276**: 36168-36173.

Vohradsky, J. (2001b) Neural network model of gene expression. Faseb J. **15**: 846-854.

Vu, T.T., Vohradsky, J. (2002) Genexp – a genetic network simulation environment. Bioinformatics **18**(10): 1400-1401.

Wang, X., Ghosh, S. and Guo, S.W. (2001) Quantitative Quality Control in Microarray Image Processing and Data Acquisition. Nucl. Acids Res. **29**(15): e75.

White, K.P., Rifkin, S.A., Hurban, P. and Hogness, D.S. (1999) Microarray analysis of Drosophila development during metamorphosis. Science **286**: 2179–2184.

Wolfinger, R.D., Gibson, G., Wolfinger, E.D., Bennett, L., Hamadeh, H., Bushel, P., Afshari, C. and Paules, R.S. (2001) Assessing gene significance from cDNA microarray expression data via mixed models. J. Comp. Biol. **8**: 625-637.

Wu, S., Liew, A.W.C., and Yan H. (2004). Cluster Analysis of Gene Expression Data Based on Self-Splitting and Merging Competitive Learning. IEEE Transactions on Information Technology in Biomedicine **8**(1): 5-15.

Wuensche, A. (1999) Classifying cellular automata automatically: Finding gliders, filtering, and relating space-time patterns, attractor basins, and the Z parameter. Complexity **4**(3): 47-66.

Yeung, K.Y. and Ruzzo, W.L. (2001) Principal component analysis for clustering gene expression data. Bioinformatics **17**(9): 763-774.

Yeung, L.K., Szeto, L.K., Liew, A.W.C. and Yan, H. (2003) Dominant spectral component analysis for transcriptional regulations using microarray time-series data. To appear in Bioinformatics.

Yang, Y.H., Dudoit, S., Luu, P., Lin, D.M., Peng, V., Ngai, J. and Speed, T.P. (2002) Normalization for cDNA microarray data: a robust composite method addressing single and multiple slide systematic variation. Nucl. Acids Res. **30**(4): e15.

Zhang, Y.J. and Liu, Z.Q. (2002) Self-Splittng competitive learning: A new on-line clustering paradigm. IEEE Trans. on neural networks **13**: 369-380.

Index